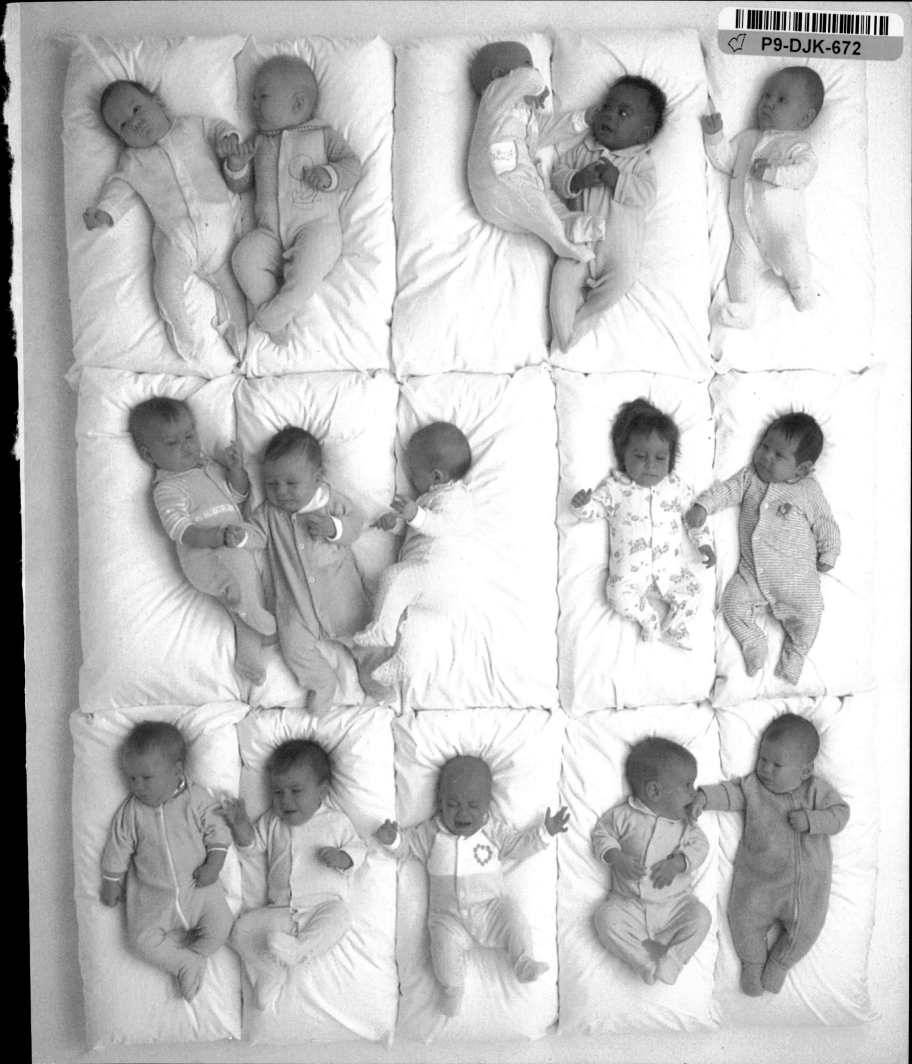

Babies

History, Art, and Folklore

To Alice, Alexandre, and Auguste

To Victor and Espérance

Babies

HISTORY, ART, AND FOLKLORE

Béatrice Fontanel and Claire d'Harcourt

Foreword by Dr. Robert Coles

Translated from the French by Lory Frankel

Harry N. Abrams, Inc., Publishers

Contents

Foreword

When I was a medical student I had the privilege of visiting William Carlos Williams, whose distinguished career as a poet, short-story writer, and novelist did not prevent him from practicing medicine in upper New Jersey for almost half a century. I even had the opportunity to see him at work, talking with his patients, and I'd often hear him remember what it was like to be a turn-of-the-century "general practitioner," a physician who made house calls regularly, who tried with all his might to be of help to sick children and their parents. One day, a tape recorder before us, he carried me back with him to earlier times, reminding me thereby of what I could every day take for granted: "We did our best with the little we had—we fought the fevers with aspirin and cold baths and alcohol rubs. We reported children who had diphtheria—they were quarantined. We waited for the crisis to come for kids who had pneumonia, and along with their mothers and fathers, we wondered if they'd make it—it was win-or-lose time. Now there are antibiotics; then, we tried to be as supportive as we could be—we waited, we hoped and prayed: a big difference between what it was once like to be a doctor and what it's like now, and a big difference between what it was once like to be a patient and what it's like now!"

In his own way, this elderly physician with long pediatric experience was offering a history of a profession, and more: a social and cultural chronicle of how life had been at an earlier time. Nor was the speaker being merely rhetorical or self-serving—his words meant to tell a listener how hard it once had been to treat the young, and so, how heroic were the efforts of those who did so. Rather, Dr. Williams was anxious for someone from a younger generation to understand his own, everyday situation, the assumptions and accomplishments and possibilities he could all too readily take for granted. The past, thereby, would become an important, instructive presence, a means by which what is contemporary gets appreciated for what it is by virtue of what was absent or wanting in earlier times.

In the pages that follow, Dr. Williams' reminders to a young admirer are greatly amplified in the form of a history, actually, of early childhood, rendered by writers, folklorists, and artists. Here a major aspect of mankind's past is chronicled—how babies were believed to originate (even an accurate knowledge of the manner in which conception occurs was not always known) and how they were delivered, fed, attended, assisted in their physical, psychological, and cognitive development. Indeed, upon opening this book, one soon enough enters a world enormously different from ours—a world we can quickly dismiss as benighted or wrongheaded or arbitrary or even wicked or perverse—one that lacked not only the medical competence unavailable to doctors who practiced a few decades ago in the West, but lacked, really, an entire breadth and depth of scientific awareness we simply carry within ourselves and call upon as needed: biology and chemistry and physics and psychology, not to mention medicine, as they constantly inform our sense of things, our notions of the desirable, the unattractive, the utterly required, and the thoroughly wrong.

A while back the French cultural historian Philippe Ariès pointed out that the very idea of childhood, as we define and experience it (and reexperience it as parents, grandparents, teachers) is an expression, a consequence, of our present-day life. Centuries ago life had a different (a faster, a more hazardous) pace to it, so the extended time of dependency and growth that we witness (and foster) in our sons and daughters did not exist. Rather, at seven or eight, say, young people took their place in society as workers, as citizens—rather than as children, never mind schoolchildren. But if that information startles us, we had best prepare ourselves for even more striking surprises as we turn these pages, use our eyes to absorb words and pictures—a narrative exposition of family life as it once happened, with special reference to the baby conceived, carried in the mother's womb, born, nurtured, and brought into a particular social setting, with its various expectations, rules, and customs.

As the reader will soon enough realize, the hopes we now lavish upon the life we conceive, bring into the world, encourage, and sustain were unimaginable to the parents of yore, even as their ways of thinking about babies and being with them, are beyond our own imagining—until we take the stories and illustrations that follow into our thinking lives, and, yes, let such reports, such factuality and anecdotes, become part of our moral sensibility (so that thereby we can put ourselves at least somewhat in the shoes of others and comprehend their outlook, their beliefs).

With this book in our hands we have a chance, then, to follow a bit of advice also spoken by Dr. Williams as he explained in considerable detail a medical past that had only recently yielded to new discoveries: "If you learn what came before you, it'll be easier for you to say goodbye to what you've accepted as the truth—accept the news, the break-throughs of the future." So wise, those words: a reminder to us, who correctly rejoice in what is ours today, in contrast to what others so evidently, tragically, sorely lacked "back then," that some day, generations from now, others will be learning about our lives, about how babies fared in this fast-diminishing twentieth century, this millennium that is almost over, and will scratch their heads, as we do, and wonder about it all—the matter (sometimes, the mystery) of progress as it gets to happen over time and in various ways and places.

Robert Coles is a child psychiatrist, professor of psychiatry and medical humanities at Harvard Medical School, and the James Agee Professor of Social Ethics at Harvard University.

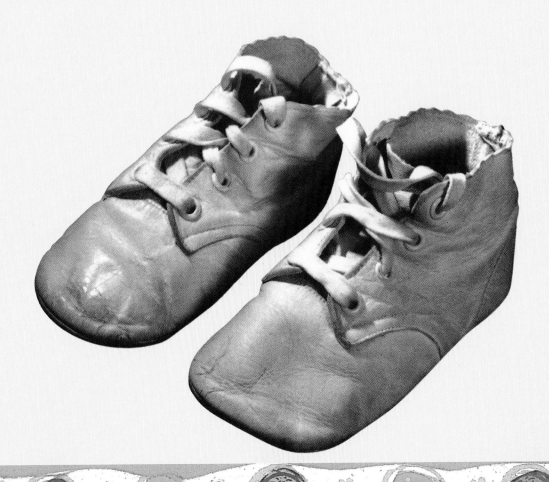

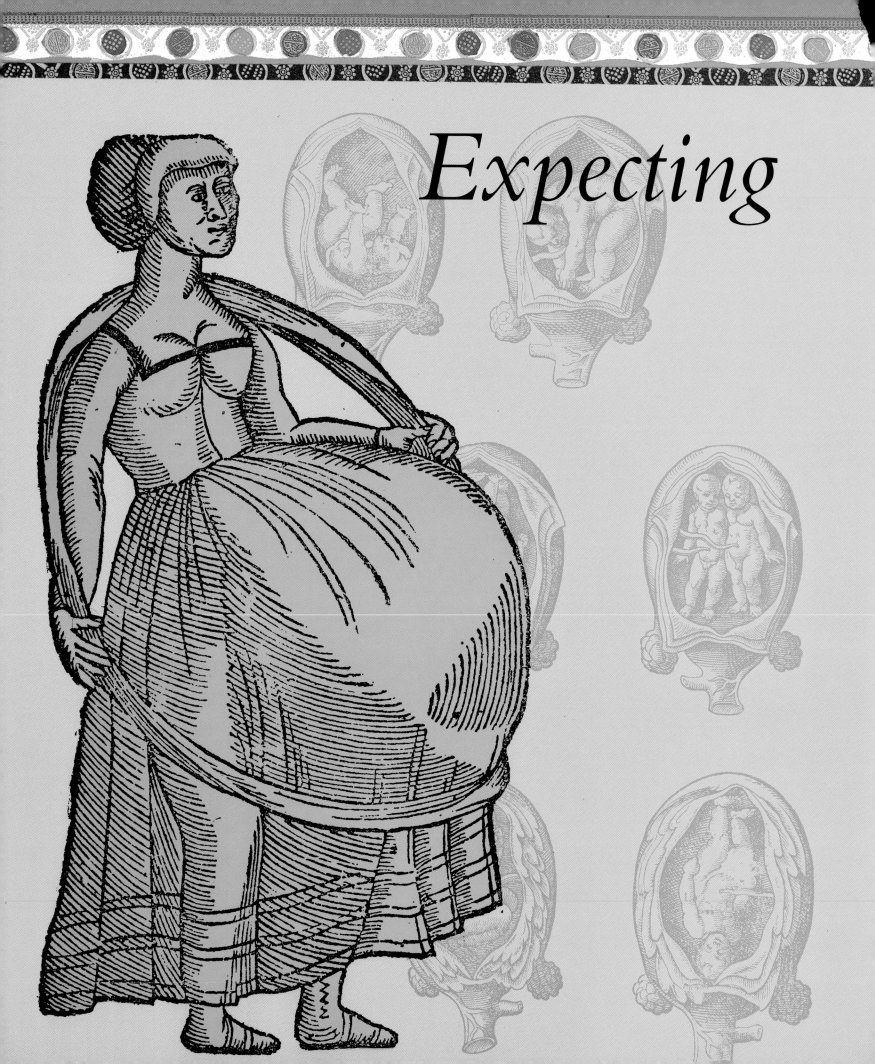

Expecting

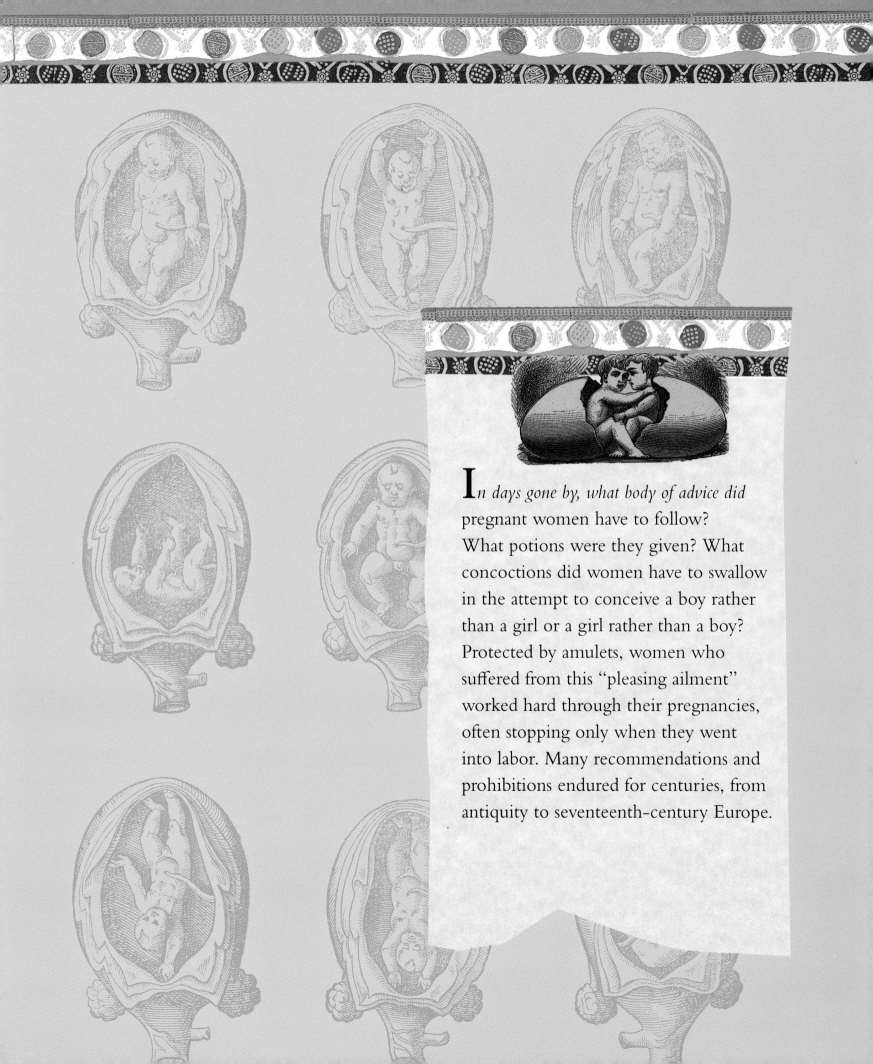

In days gone by, what body of advice did pregnant women have to follow? What potions were they given? What concoctions did women have to swallow in the attempt to conceive a boy rather than a girl or a girl rather than a boy? Protected by amulets, women who suffered from this "pleasing ailment" worked hard through their pregnancies, often stopping only when they went into labor. Many recommendations and prohibitions endured for centuries, from antiquity to seventeenth-century Europe.

"*Pleasing Ailment*" and *Rounded Bellies*

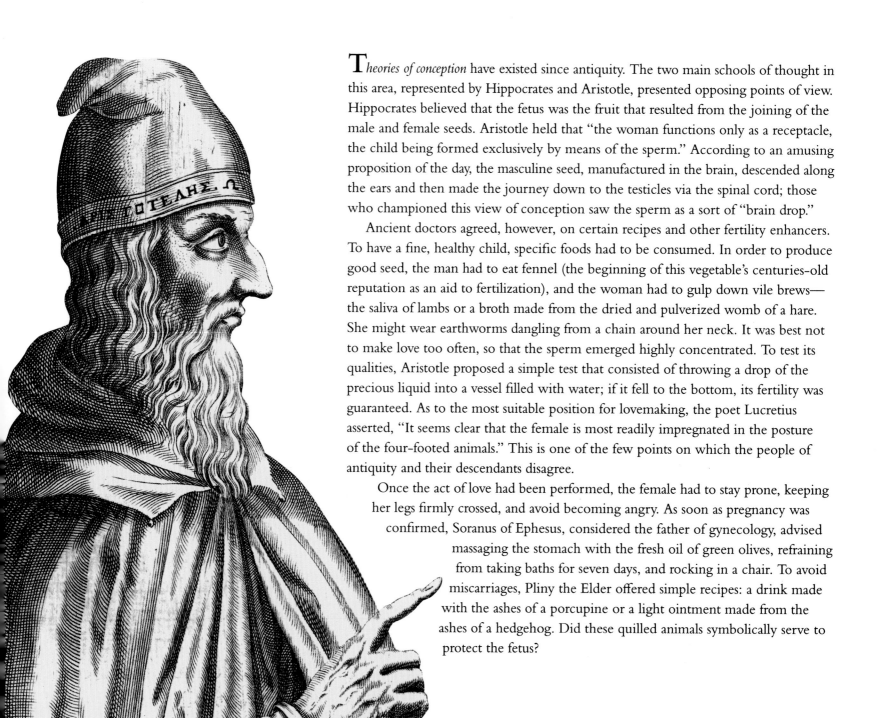

Theories of conception *have existed since antiquity. The two main schools of thought in this area, represented by Hippocrates and Aristotle, presented opposing points of view. Hippocrates believed that the fetus was the fruit that resulted from the joining of the male and female seeds. Aristotle held that "the woman functions only as a receptacle, the child being formed exclusively by means of the sperm." According to an amusing proposition of the day, the masculine seed, manufactured in the brain, descended along the ears and then made the journey down to the testicles via the spinal cord; those who championed this view of conception saw the sperm as a sort of "brain drop."*

Ancient doctors agreed, however, on certain recipes and other fertility enhancers. To have a fine, healthy child, specific foods had to be consumed. In order to produce good seed, the man had to eat fennel (the beginning of this vegetable's centuries-old reputation as an aid to fertilization), and the woman had to gulp down vile brews— the saliva of lambs or a broth made from the dried and pulverized womb of a hare. She might wear earthworms dangling from a chain around her neck. It was best not to make love too often, so that the sperm emerged highly concentrated. To test its qualities, Aristotle proposed a simple test that consisted of throwing a drop of the precious liquid into a vessel filled with water; if it fell to the bottom, its fertility was guaranteed. As to the most suitable position for lovemaking, the poet Lucretius asserted, "It seems clear that the female is most readily impregnated in the posture of the four-footed animals." This is one of the few points on which the people of antiquity and their descendants disagree.

Once the act of love had been performed, the female had to stay prone, keeping her legs firmly crossed, and avoid becoming angry. As soon as pregnancy was confirmed, Soranus of Ephesus, considered the father of gynecology, advised massaging the stomach with the fresh oil of green olives, refraining from taking baths for seven days, and rocking in a chair. To avoid miscarriages, Pliny the Elder offered simple recipes: a drink made with the ashes of a porcupine or a light ointment made from the ashes of a hedgehog. Did these quilled animals symbolically serve to protect the fetus?

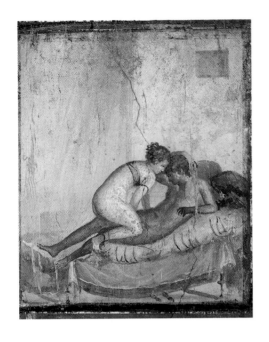

Aristotle believed that semen naturally produced males, and that a female resulted only if its development was disturbed. Saint Augustine specified that the male fetus received a soul on about its fortieth day of life in the womb, while the female's came somewhat later.

OPPOSITE: *Aristotle.* Print. Bibliothèque Nationale, Paris

LEFT: Fresco from the House of the Centenary, Pompeii

BELOW: Marx Reichlich. *The Visitation.* 1511. Alte Pinakothek, Munich

Female Sinners and the Virgin Mary

"Few people, very few people," wrote the historian Georges Duby to indicate Europe's sparse population during the High Middle Ages. Having many children guaranteed continuity of the line for some, additional hands to work in the fields for others. Procreating was both a necessity and a duty for medieval men and women. Woman was a sinner, but she expunged the impurity of her flesh through childbirth. As in previous centuries, certain foods had the reputation of aiding conception: chestnuts, pine nuts, leeks, carrots, asparagus, almonds. Starting on their wedding night, young marrieds were given a soup, sometimes highly spiced, to stimulate sexual union. Infertility, considered a calamity, was often blamed on the female. Recommended treatments included pilgrimages, votive offerings, prayers to the Virgin Mary and all the saints with "specialties" in this area, and a variety of other remedies, such as placing a plaster of nettles over the womb. These might be accompanied by magic rituals forbidden by the Church. The remains of pagan beliefs led some sterile women to bathe in springs and make offerings to the fairies that inhabited them.

Medieval spouses went to bed naked, wearing only caps to protect them from the cold, and they got into bed one after the other. The Church allowed only one position—the man and woman facing each other—unless one of them was too obese; this was a change from ancient times. Opinions on sexual pleasure were divided, however, especially regarding that of the female. In the thirteenth century, Saint Thomas Aquinas condemned it, while other theologians believed it played a role in the beauty of the child. In a wonderful paradox, some were convinced that if the woman repressed her pleasure, it was in an attempt not to conceive, which

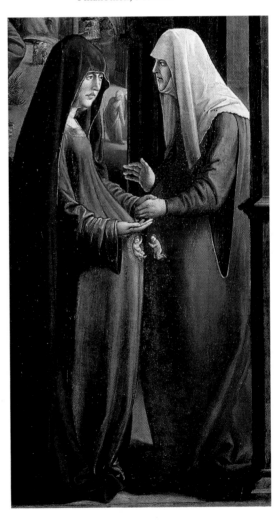

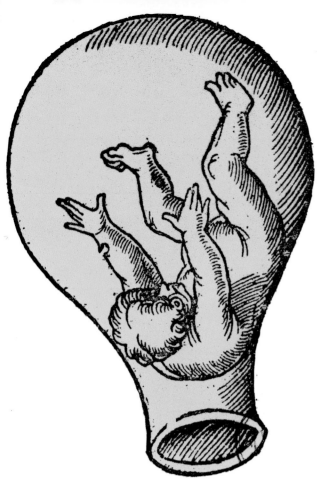

was a sin. To circumvent this problem, they counseled the husband to prolong the lovemaking until the woman came to orgasm. In their book *Histoire des mères* (History of Mothers), Yvonne Knibiehler and Catherine Fouquet state that these religious men even went so far as to invite the wife to fondle herself to achieve it.

In the Middle Ages, the belly of a pregnant woman, considered full of mysteries, was feared. Nevertheless, scientists were fascinated by embryology. Until the eighteenth century, the fetus was depicted in manuscripts and printed treatises as a perfectly finished miniature human being floating weightlessly in a much larger gourd-shaped uterus, amusing itself with all manner of acrobatics. Concerned for the baby's comfort, mothers with very round stomachs deemed themselves fortunate, as they gave the child enough space in which to play. People of the medieval Arab world believed the fetus had an active consciousness, to the extent that pregnant women attended lessons on the Koran in order to give the child a head start on their studies. Christians thought that the baby *in utero* had the ability to pray and appeal to God.

In early-sixteenth-century obstetric texts, authors imagined that the baby amused itself up to the moment of delivery by turning somersaults in a womb shaped like a "gunpowder flask for hunting."

THIS PAGE AND OPPOSITE ABOVE: Prints from a 16th-century treatise on obstetrics

Poetic Diagnoses

Using flowery language and a rich style, sixteenth-century French surgeon Ambroise Paré expressed the theories and prescriptions of the classical authors with a new approach to the relationship between men and women. In his book *De la génération* (On Procreation), he presented all the details necessary to create "a small creature of God," the tender and affectionate term that designated the fetus. To evaluate the quality of sperm— "said sperm must be white, rich, and clear, viscous and globular, and smell like the elder or palm tree"—Paré returned to Aristotle's test. Like the ancients, he advised the man not to set on his wife too often, as the sperm had to be "well ripened and digested, thick and glutinous, full of lively spirits." He held that the seminal fluids—his warm and dry, hers cold and wet—squared off in a battle without mercy. The stronger

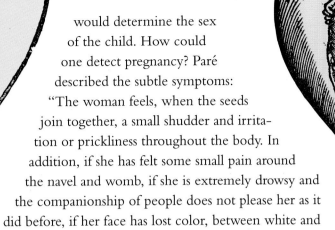

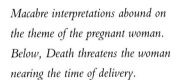

would determine the sex of the child. How could one detect pregnancy? Paré described the subtle symptoms: "The woman feels, when the seeds join together, a small shudder and irritation or prickliness throughout the body. In addition, if she has felt some small pain around the navel and womb, if she is extremely drowsy and the companionship of people does not please her as it did before, if her face has lost color, between white and pale, these are signs of conception. The time for her menses having come round again, instead of having it her breasts become hard and hurt her, due to the blood that distends and enlarges them. Then she is assured of being large with child."

The list of foods capable of assisting procreation grew exceptionally long in the Renaissance and took an extravagant turn. During that period, recommended foods included squab; sparrows; the testicles and combs of cocks; the genitals of bulls; rice cooked in cow's milk and saffron; cinnamon; cloves; pepper; asparagus cooked in a good broth; chestnuts; truffles; mint; arugula; pine nuts; pistachios; and parsley. One recipe gives an idea of external aids: "Take oil of elder in which you have steeped ants and rub this on the kidneys and genital areas." Finally, since the pleasure of the female was necessary for conception, it would not do if sexual relations gave her any pain. Ambroise Paré, delicate and technical, offered advice to certain readers: "The fault arises from the overlength of the shaft; you will need to place a padded bag around it so it will not enter so deeply." What a happy time when the recommendations included eating squab and saffron rice and taking the greatest possible pleasure in making love in order to fabricate "little creatures of God." With the rise of prudishness in the following centuries, the tone would change perceptibly.

As in the past, the parade of absurd concoctions intended to assist procreation or protect the pregnant woman reveals the wealth of imagination of their authors. In the early seventeenth century, Louise Bourgeois, for example, midwife to the queen of France, Marie de Médicis, advised using vaginal irrigations of chamomile, mallow, marjoram, and catmint boiled in three pints of good white wine. To cure the hemorrhoids that tend to afflict pregnant women, she prescribed grinding a good quantity of wood lice, boiling grated apples with rosewater, and applying a mixture of the two to the area. After a fall, a pregnant woman immediately had to take the embryos of seven or eight eggs mixed with finely minced crimson silk.

Starting in the sixteenth century, women began to concern themselves with the appearance of their stomach. To keep it from "being spoiled," "you must cook a pomade of melted lard and rosewater." Unguents and strips of linen gave it support.

Macabre interpretations abound on the theme of the pregnant woman. Below, Death threatens the woman nearing the time of delivery.

BELOW: Miniature from a 15th-century manuscript. Bibliothèque Nationale, Paris

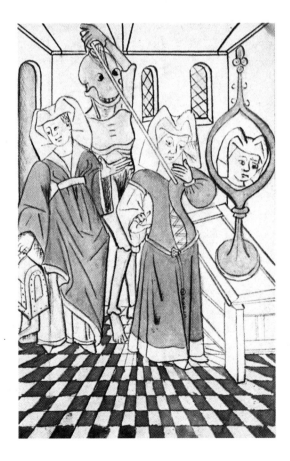

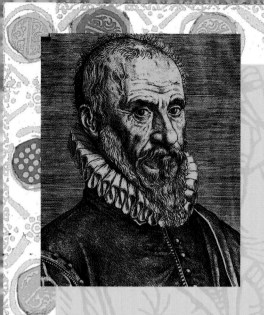

Ambroise Paré, Surgeon and Sexologist

"The man, in bed with his consort and spouse, must fondle her, arouse her, caress her, and stir up her passions, even if he finds her unyielding to the spur: and the cultivator should not rashly enter into the field of human nature without first having made his approaches, which consist of kissing her and speaking to her…: also of fondling her genital parts and nipples until she is stimulated and titillated, to the point that she becomes at one with the male's desire (which is when the uterus quivers) in order that she will grow willing and eager to couple and make a small creature of God, and that the two seeds can meet together: for no female is so ready at this game as any man. And in order to further this business, the wife should apply a fomentation of hot herbs, in good wines and malmsey, to her genital parts and at the same time place in her cervix a bit of musk and civet: and when she begins to feel stimulated and aroused, tell her husband: and they should then join together and slowly consummate their sport, waiting for the one, for the other, giving pleasure to each other. When the two seeds have been discharged, the man should not quickly detach himself, so that air will not find its way to the uterus and modify the seeds, and so that they will mix together better, one with the other: and as soon as the man has gone, the woman should lie very still, and cross and press together her legs and thighs and hold them slightly elevated, so that the seed will not flow out through the movement and the releasing action of the womb: for these same reasons she should neither talk, nor cough, nor sneeze: and she should go to sleep afterward as soon as she can."

Ambroise Paré, 1573

When pregnant, a woman would be bled and purged, and most doctors said she had to abstain from sexual intercourse. In the seventeenth century, the doctor Dionis ridiculed a colleague who counseled abstinence: "Mauriceau could not have made these observations at first-hand, having never had a single child in forty-six years of marriage. For me, who had a wife who became pregnant twenty times and gave me twenty children that she successfully brought to term, I am persuaded that the husband's caresses spoil nothing."

ABOVE: *Portrait of Ambroise Paré.* 1582. Print. Bibliothèque Nationale, Paris

BELOW: *The Bloodletting.* 15th century. Colored print. National Library of the University, Prague

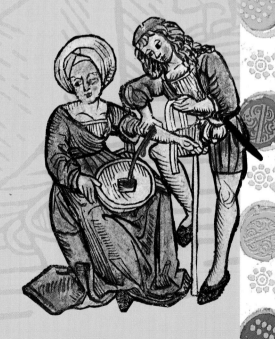

Women also reinforced it with a dog skin, which the obstetrician Jacques Guillemeau, cited by Jacques Gélis in *L'arbre et le fruit* (The Tree and the Fruit), recommended washing several times with rosewater, and then steeping in the oil of Saint-John's-wort, sweet almond, or spermaceti to soften it.

Garlic Cloves and Urine Examiners

The symptoms that supposedly provided clues to the detection of pregnancy were subtle indeed. Shivers, grinding of the teeth, and spasms were considered surefire signs in the seventeenth and eighteenth centuries. One of the most celebrated obstetricians of the time in Europe, François Mauriceau, maintained that conception had taken place "if the man and the woman experienced at the time a greater pleasure than usual, which happens when, during this moment, the vagina has squeezed the penis to advantage, because the uterus, opening up to receive the sperm, sucks the end of the male member in such a way that it is highly excited, and coming itself to receive the two seminal fluids of which it is so fond, mainly that of the man, it causes the woman a sensual and extraordinary thrill in every part of her body. The woman will know that she has retained the seeds if, after coitus, she feels nothing flowing from her uterus, which soon contracts. The penis withdraws from it less moist, drier than usual."

The garlic clove test was another way for a woman to find out if she had conceived. At night, on going to bed, she inserted a clove of garlic in her "reproductive parts." In the morning, if her breath emitted the characteristic odor of garlic, she was not pregnant. If her breath was unchanged, it was thought that the fetus had created an obstacle and was blocking the passage of the odor. "Urine examiners" could also detect pregnancies. A "very ripe" color, observed in a carafe, indicated a positive result.

Aside from the absence of menstruation, which could be due to causes other than pregnancy, and the movements of the fetus, which are often not felt until the fifth month, these diagnoses of pregnancy strike us today as whimsical. However, midwife Louise Bourgeois revealed one of the few methods of knowing "if a woman is with child" that come close to having some merit: "By touching it softly, the midwife can recognize if the uterus is very tightly closed, like the anus of a pullet into which one cannot fit a grain of wheat."

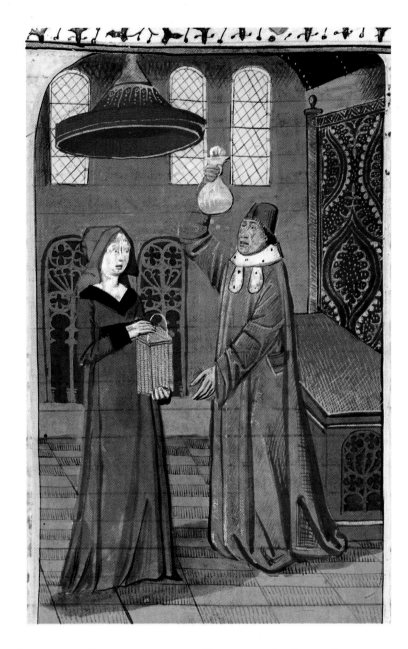

Uromancy served to diagnose illnesses in general and pregnancy in particular, which was considered a kind of illness, especially when the woman was thought to be carrying a girl.

ABOVE: Saint Elizabeth having her urine examined by an apothecary, from the Bible said to have belonged to John XXII. Palais des Papes, Avignon

Aversions and Cravings

The pregnant woman did well to avoid all strong emotions—not only sadness and anger but also joy and delight—for they could trigger spontaneous abortions. The sensitive women of the world especially had to be protected; some suffered miscarriages simply from hearing the sound of artillery. It was also deemed best to avoid disagreeable smells, as even that of a badly extinguished candle was said to bring on early labor. Pregnant women had to refrain from dressing their hair, and it was strongly advised that they abstain from even lifting their arms. The woman was considered to be like a sensitive photographic plate: if she caught sight of a handicapped person, she risked giving birth to an impaired child; if an animal frightened her, she might be delivered of a monster, and so on. In the eighteenth century, such notions led to a controversy between the "imaginationists" and their detractors. The former explained, for example, that a woman who witnessed punishment on the wheel would deliver an infant with broken body. Another European woman, frightened by the sight of a black man, washed herself with hot water, which "enabled" her to bear a white child, but the baby still had black skin between her fingers and toes, for her mother had neglected to wash those areas.

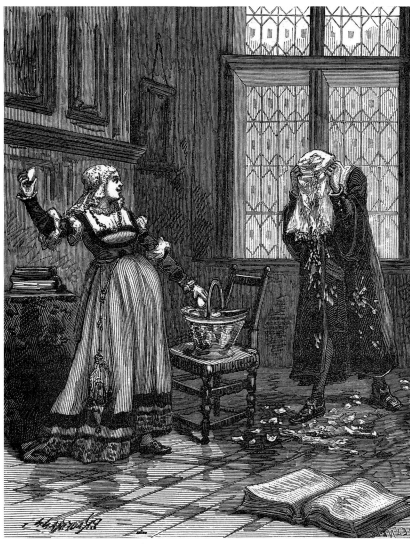

The cravings of pregnant women had to be satisfied at any price, lest their rejection expose the infant to all manner of birth-marks or birth defects. However, Jacques Blondel, who reported this story in his book *Dissertation sur la force de l'imagination des femmes enceintes* (Dissertation on the Power of Imagination of Pregnant Women), published in 1788, found it hard to swallow such nonsense: "How can it be conceded," he remarked, "that tucked into his womb a fetus could pine after a glass of champagne, a piece of Westphalian ham, or a salmon from Newcastle?" Women's cravings, however, might not be simply gustatory. While cravings for coffee and chocolate were known in this period when such things were still luxuries, doctors reported women also had irresistible urges to eat sand, mud, plaster, and spiders. Deeply anchored in traditional ways of thinking, beliefs surrounding cravings served a real purpose, as Pierre Darmon recognized in his work *Le mythe de la procréation à l'âge baroque* (The Myth of Procreation During the Baroque Era): they explained abnormal births that otherwise would be attributed

Certain crafty women took advantage of cravings and uncontrollable urges to explain their babies' resemblance to their lovers or to exact conjugal revenge. Legend has it that a learned German botanist of the sixteenth century elected to let his wife hurl eggs at him to satisfy her desire to do so, rather than risk her having a miscarriage.

ABOVE: Print. 19th century

"*Madame Morin announced that I had a red blemish over my left kidney because my mother had had a craving for cherries. At which old Fournier, who held popular prejudices in deep contempt, replied that he was happy that Madame Nozière had remained content during my gestation with such a modest desire, for if she had really let herself go and dreamed of feathers, jewels, cashmere, a carriage drawn by four horses…I would not have had nearly enough skin to carry the imprint of all these enormous desires. Say what you like, doctor, retorted Madame Caumont, but on Christmas night, my sister Malvina, being in the family way, was gripped by an irresistible urge for a midnight feast and her daughter…—Was born with a sausage hanging from the end of her nose, no? interrupted the doctor.*"

Anatole France, *Le petit Pierre*, 1919

A pregnant woman was seized by a craving to bite the shoulder of a baker. Her husband offered the good man money, and twice the woman was able to give in to her cannibalistic urges. But the baker refused to submit a third time. The unfortunate woman bore triplets, one of them stillborn.

BELOW: Honoré Daumier.
A Pregnant Woman's Craving.
19th century. Print

OVERLEAF: Japanese print. 1881.
Bibliothèque Nationale, Paris

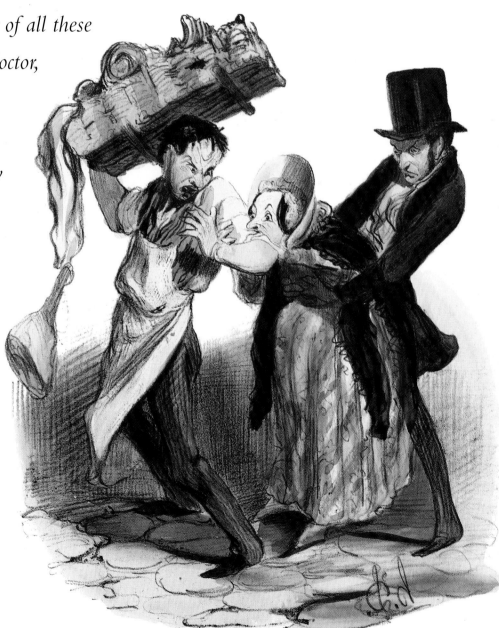

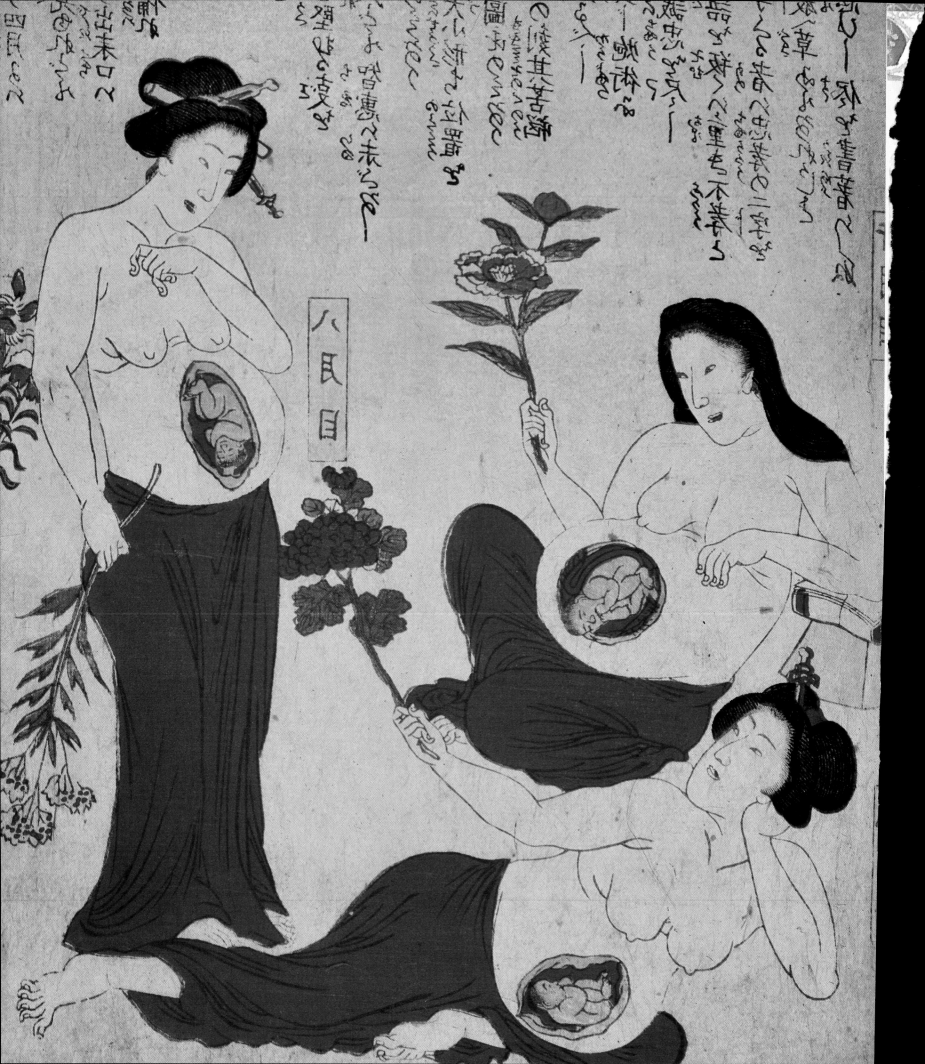

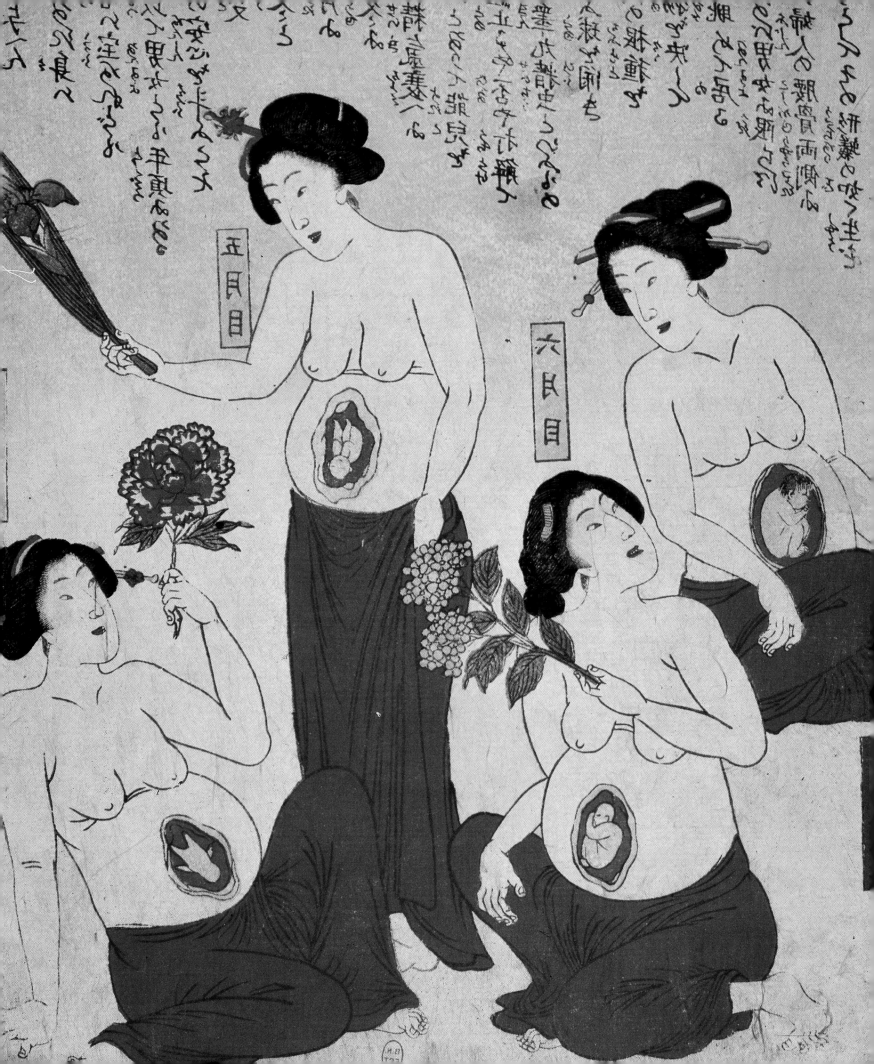

The role played by the female in the process of procreation was judged more or less important depending on the degree of misogyny of the society or the individual. Some deemed her only a receptacle. Doctors unearthed a weighty argument to justify this theory: for them, the fact that the male organs are more "in evidence" than those of the female proved that they contribute far more to the process.

RIGHT: Postcard. 20th century

BELOW AND OPPOSITE: Spermatozoa. Prints from Buffon, *Histoire naturelle*, 1750. Bibliothèque Nationale, Paris

OPPOSITE: Print. 17th century

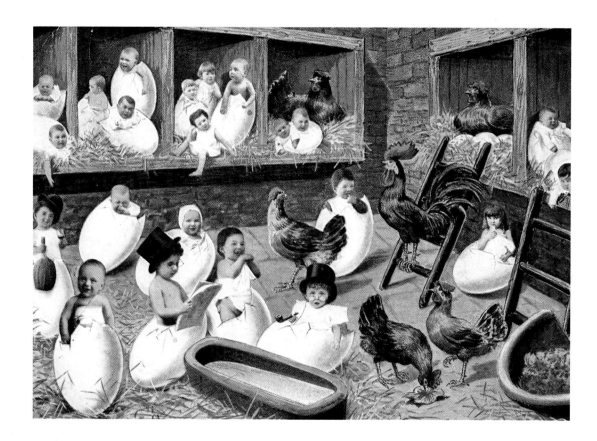

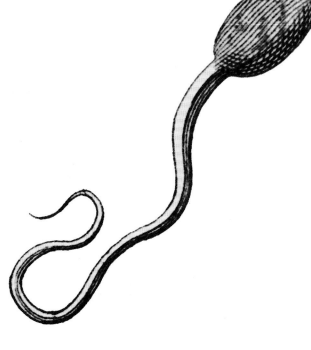

to Satan's intervention. Mothers no longer risked disgrace, imprisonment, or the stake if their newborns were imperfectly formed.

An Ocean of Animalcules

It can be seen that theories and practices evolved little since Hippocrates and Aristotle. In the article entitled "Procreation," the authors of the mid-eighteenth-century French *Encyclopédie* (Encyclopedia) excoriated scientists: "Seventeen or eighteen centuries have passed with nothing new having appeared on the subject, on account of the foolish veneration in which these two masters are held, to the extent that their productions are regarded as the limits of the human mind." However, the invention of the microscope and the research of a handful of scientists led to new discoveries that stimulated the hidebound world of medicine. In 1668, the Danish scientist Stenon first described the ovaries. In 1677, the Dutch Louis De Ham and Antoni Van Leeuwenhoek observed spermatozoa, then called "animalcules," for the first time. A new war began between the "ovists," who believed that the fetus was already formed in the egg produced by the female body, and the "animalculists," who held that the embryo was completely contained in the spermatozoon.

Although the first microscopes had appeared by the early seventeenth century, it was not until the second half of the century that the lenses had sufficient power for meaningful observation. De Ham declared that "a drop of sperm was an ocean in which swam a numberless host of small fish in a thousand different directions." He imparted his discovery to Van Leeuwenhoek, who, thrilled by this ballet, spent whole days with his eye glued to the eyepiece, never tiring of watching "this highly agreeable spectacle." Bristling with life, spermatozoa quickly supplanted the sadly inert egg. Yet the very transports and excesses attributed to the animalcules—it was asserted that the spermatozoa of a ram traveled in herds—led to their demise as the basis for a popular theory. It did not seem very flattering, after all, that humans should issue from this swarming of "worms." And the waste came in for criticism: for one spermatozoon, how many must be sacrificed? This situation even drew an accusation of genocide. The *Encyclopédie* (Encyclopedia) waxed indignant over the fact that the most malicious one left after a "general massacre alone possesses the womb and the egg." By the beginning of the eighteenth century, the ovist theory again came to the fore.

Fertilized by the Wind

In the seventeenth century, science progressed at the expense of women's pleasure: doctors learned that women could conceive without achieving orgasm. Some went even further, concluding that frigid women reproduced more easily— their calmness gave them an edge in retaining the sperm. Husbands no longer needed to exhaust themselves in making love. Nevertheless, another medical misapprehension handed an enormous benefit to certain women: despite the development of the microscope and some real breakthroughs, seventeenth- and eighteenth-century scientists continued to believe that a woman could be impregnated by the wind. In an anecdote recounted by Pierre Darmon in 1637, an aristocratic woman who had given birth to a son claimed that she conceived in a dream during her husband's absence. The doctors came to her rescue, explaining that on a summer night, "her window being open, her blanket in disorder, the zephyr from the southwest, regularly impregnated with the organic molecules of human insects, of floating embryos, had fertilized her."

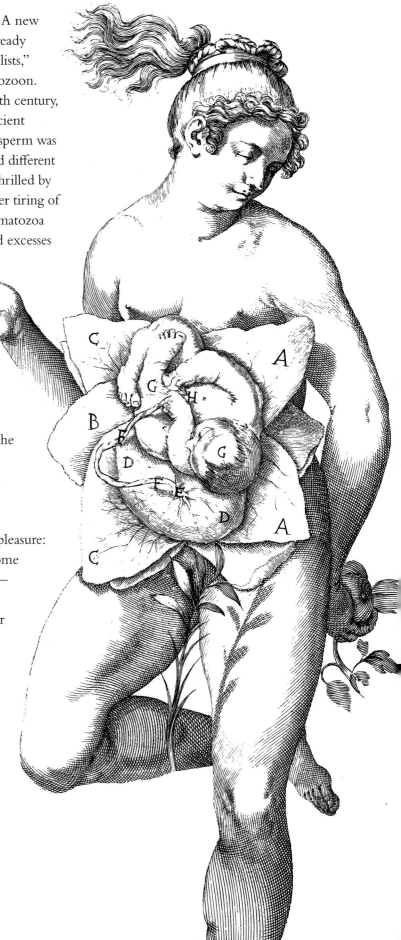

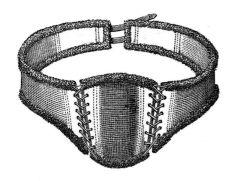

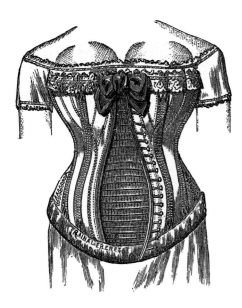

Worn under flowing dresses that hid the stomach, pregnancy girdles were thought to prevent deformity.

ABOVE AND BELOW: Prints. Late 19th century

OPPOSITE: Workers. c. 1900. Photograph from *L'Illustration*

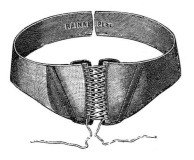

Pregnancy in the Industrial Age

In 1850, the French doctors Pouchet and Négrier explained the laws of ovulation. In 1875, the true way fertilization occurs became known. However, in the nineteenth century, popular traditions still held strong in the European countryside. Depending on the locale, battling infertility involved rubbing the stomach to counter the magic of menhirs, striking bells, or a variety of other procedures. A woman expecting a baby was never supposed to leave her house after sunset and, above all else, she had to avoid urinating outside under a full moon; fertilized by that heavenly body, she would be liable to give birth to a monstrous creature. She must never weigh herself, as this would stop fetal development. Strings and laces were forbidden, so that the fetus would not be strangled by the umbilical cord.

As for Western doctors, they continued to place numerous activities off limits to women in the nineteenth century and even into the twentieth. They forbade using the swing, waltzing, and even singing, for the effects of the voice might harm the child. In 1921, in his *Hygiène de la maman et de bébé* (Hygiene of the Mother and Child), Léon Pouliot warned against strolling through stores, putting the contents of cupboards in order, and going on outings on a streetcar. "Do not go bathing in the sea, unless you are very accustomed to it," Pouliot cautioned, "and even then avoid the shock of a wave hitting the abdomen; with very good reason, swimming is forbidden." On the other hand, he freely authorized certain distractions: "The intimate evening party with friends, ended at an early hour, spent in pleasant conversation or augmented by a round of bridge is perfectly permissible (especially if your husband gives it)." Dr. Lacasse banned bicycling, using the sewing machine, and, above all, going on a honeymoon, which placed the fetus at risk during its first few days. He claimed that "matrimonial tribulations" offered plenty of danger: "It is simply a small assassination à deux, a nice little infanticide," he accused. "Think, Madame, of the day when you do not see your menstruation come, you are no longer an empty casket. Let your lodger enjoy his apartment in peace."

Gaining protection from supernatural powers by using amulets, magic sachets, eagle stones, and so on, most pregnant women made no concessions to their condition in their daily life. Unlike upper-class ladies, who could treat themselves to some rest, the majority of women continued to work up to the last moment.

Prenatal care was developed in the twentieth century. Today, regular visits to the doctor are opportunities for the mother-to-be to have her questions answered and to have her blood pressure, urine, and weight checked. Starting in the 1960s, sonography, discovered in the 1950s, made it possible to watch the formation and development of the fetus directly. Amniocentesis, to check for chromosomal abnormalities, became widespread as well. Although women in rural areas or the inner city may not be able to avail themselves of all such modern techniques, today pregnancy is safer than ever for women in many parts of the world.

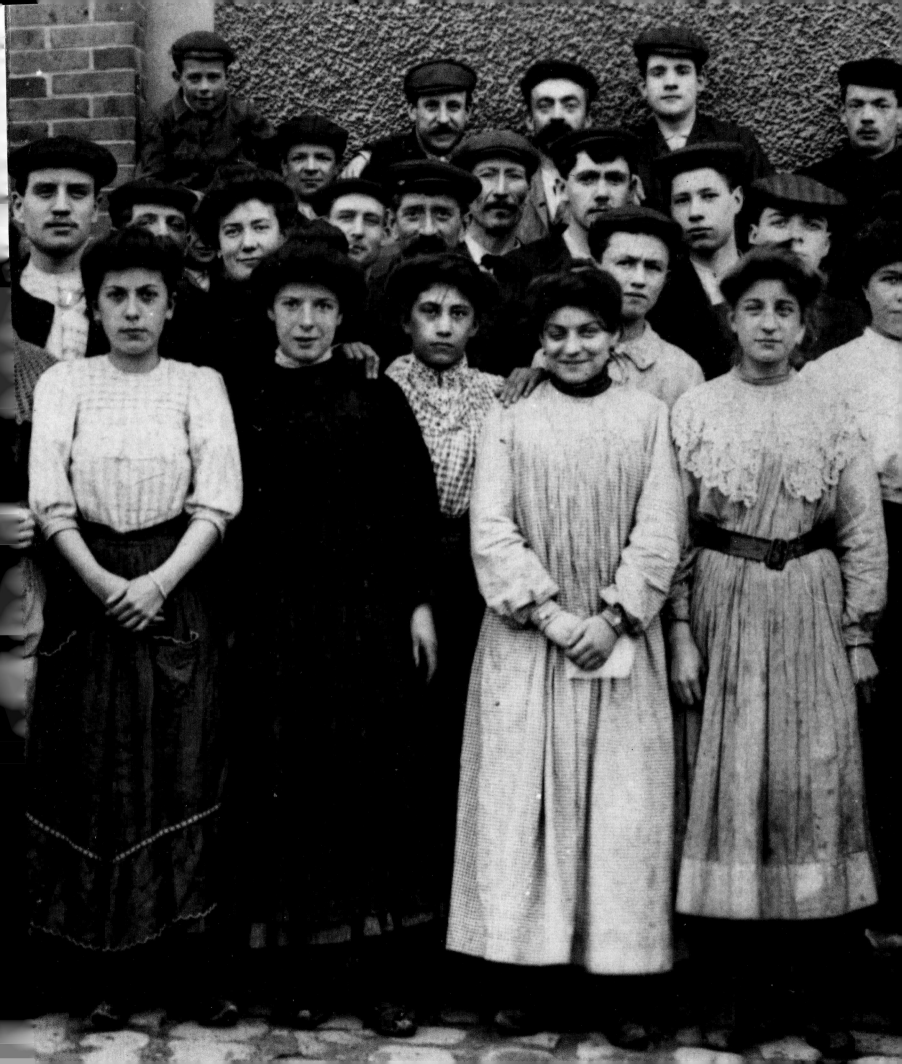

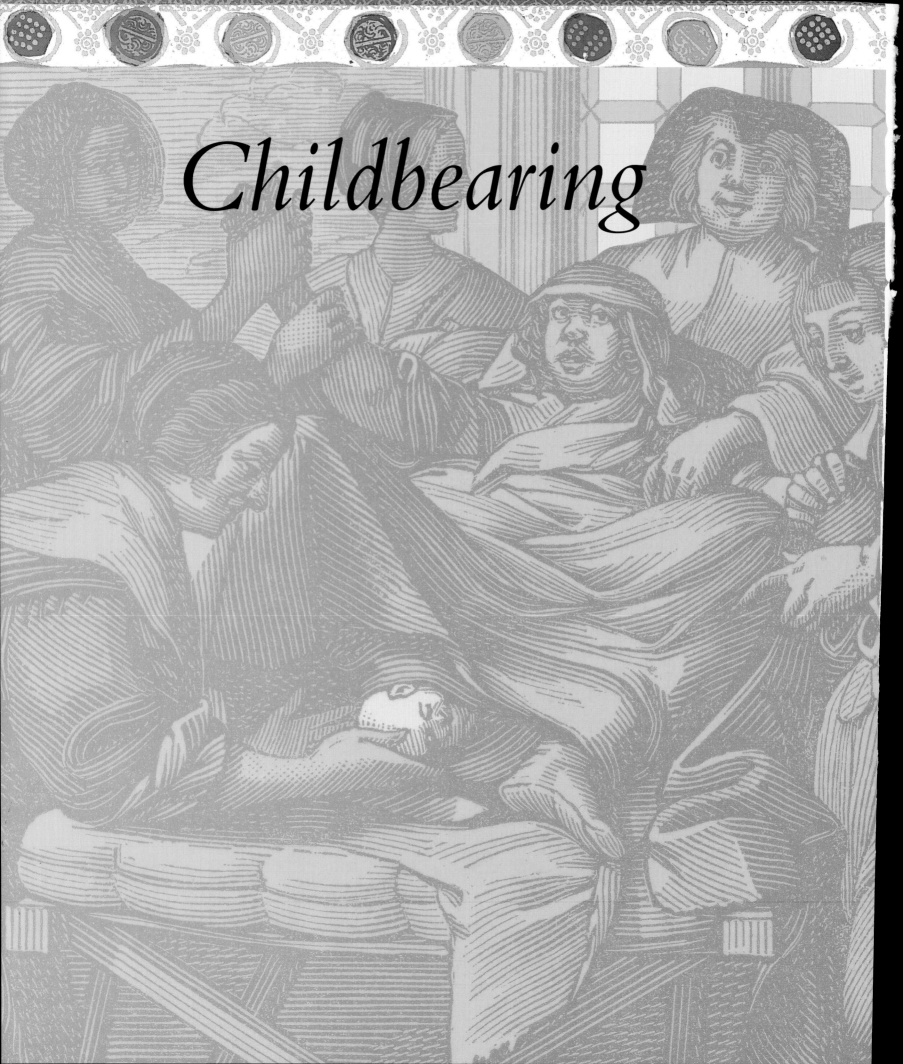

Childbearing

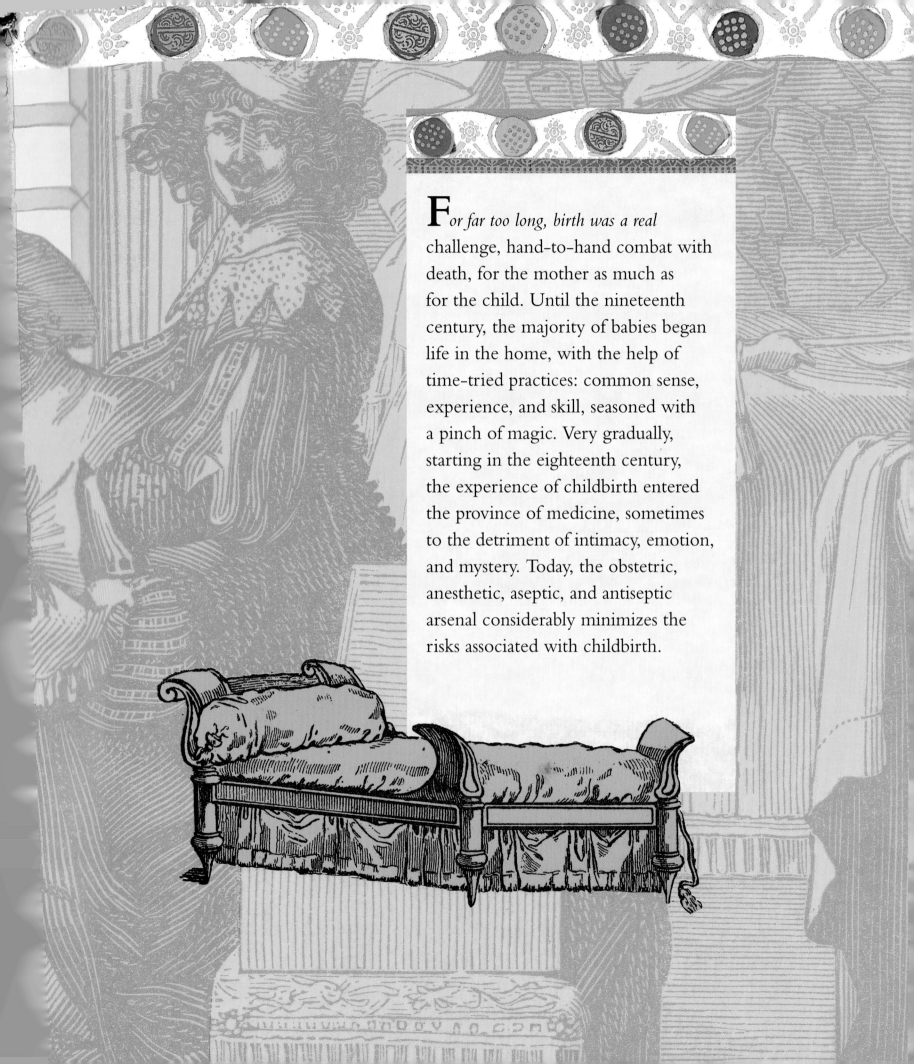

For far too long, birth was a real challenge, hand-to-hand combat with death, for the mother as much as for the child. Until the nineteenth century, the majority of babies began life in the home, with the help of time-tried practices: common sense, experience, and skill, seasoned with a pinch of magic. Very gradually, starting in the eighteenth century, the experience of childbirth entered the province of medicine, sometimes to the detriment of intimacy, emotion, and mystery. Today, the obstetric, anesthetic, aseptic, and antiseptic arsenal considerably minimizes the risks associated with childbirth.

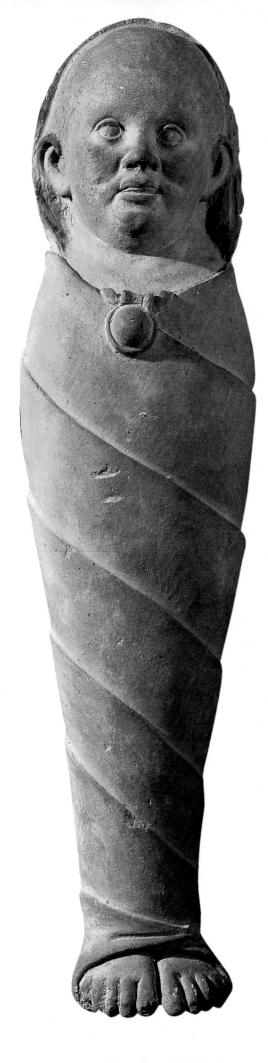

Cries and Whispers

Adorned *with purple* fabrics fringed with gold and strewn with flowers, a room in the villas of wealthy Romans was reserved for childbirth. At the first sign of pain, the patrician mistress of the villa moved to this room and settled herself in a large bed made of rare woods, sitting up, as if for a feast. Women sometimes also made use of special birthing chairs without arms. "With a view to the delivery that proceeds according to nature, it is necessary to keep ready in advance olive oil, hot water, hot compresses, soft sponges, raw wool, bandages, a cushion, fragrant products, a birthing chair or an armchair, two beds, and a conveniently furnished room." How many Romans could afford this wealth of objects and furniture recommended by Soranus of Ephesus in the second century B.C.? A pioneer, this famous doctor already concerned himself with a laboring woman's suffering; he recommended making the women more comfortable by the laying on of warm hands or by the application of cloths soaked in warm oil. Numerous recipes intended to alleviate the pain of or hasten labor also circulated among midwives: fat of viper, gall of eel, or powdered hoof of donkey in a salve on the stomach; tongue of chameleon or skin of snake or hare applied to the abdomen. Pliny the Elder also recommended certain beverages that contained the dissolved droppings of geese, snails, or earthworms. And, Lucinius averred that appealing to the goddess Juno, protectress of pregnant women and childbirths, remained the most certain way of guaranteeing a successful delivery.

Finally, the infant entered the world. The midwife placed the baby on a sheet or shreds of fine papyrus, "this so that it will neither slip nor suffer any bruising, but, on the contrary, it will have a soft but firm hold." Such attentions, however, were not proof of the baby's acceptance by society or its parents. Probably because the Stoics held that the fetus in the womb had no soul, the Roman father could deny life to his child. Soranus entitled one of the chapters in his book "How to Recognize the Baby That Is Worth the Trouble of Raising." After placing the newborn on the ground, the midwife announced its gender and then performed an examination. If the baby was in poor health, it was undesirable to let him live. The standards by which good health was judged, by which this terrible decision was made, were quite precise: the mother had to be in good health during labor, the delivery had to occur between the seventh and ninth month of pregnancy, and the baby had to cry vigorously and have all limbs and organs in good condition. If the midwife declared the baby viable, it fell to the father to accept him as his own by picking him up from the ground. The midwife then cut the umbilical cord with a shard of glass, a sharpened reed, or a crust of bread and cleaned the baby's body with salt. Finally, she washed him in water often augmented with a hefty dose of wine, to help stimulate and fortify him. If the newborn did not win his father's nod, he would be left on a trash heap or simply killed.

The Medieval Midwife

In a small medieval village, news traveled fast among the women: their neighbor, just returned from working in the fields, was in labor. Unlike many country folk in previous centuries, this child would not enter the world amid lovely natural surroundings. Her laboring mother was inside the farmhouse, surrounded by villagers. Among them was an older woman who had already skillfully assisted many others during childbirth; she served as the matron, or midwife. She knew little of medicine or anatomy, but she inspired confidence; the secrets of using plants in a wealth of magico-religious recipes had been handed down to her from her mother, who had gotten them from her own mother. In exchange for her help, the family would offer her eggs or a chicken. A large fire burned in the common room fireplace, heating the space as well as the water in a cauldron hung on the pothook. A deep, wide pan and a large jug would provide the baby's first bath. The husband would not be present for the birth; his job was to go out to gather wood to feed the fire. Childbirth unfolded in a basically female world throughout the Middle Ages and for a long period thereafter. The husband would not be directly involved unless an emergency arose. The doctor

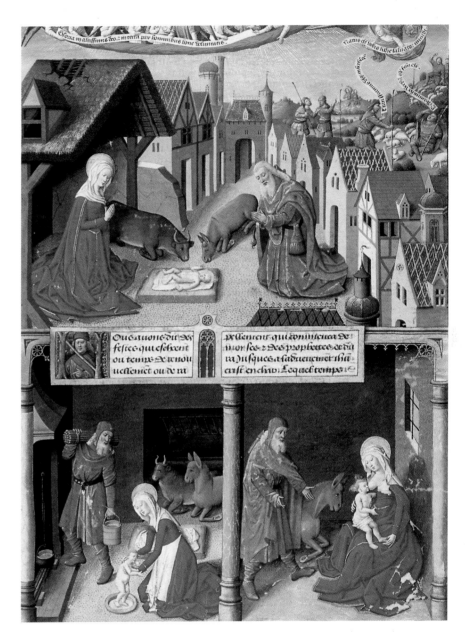

Joseph brings in wood to warm the newborn infant Jesus, taking his first bath in front of the fireplace. During childbirth, the father kept busy with chores.

ABOVE: Illustration from a 15th-century French manuscript. Bibliothèque Nationale, Paris

OPPOSITE: Ex-voto. Etruscan, 4th century B.C. Villa Giulia, Rome

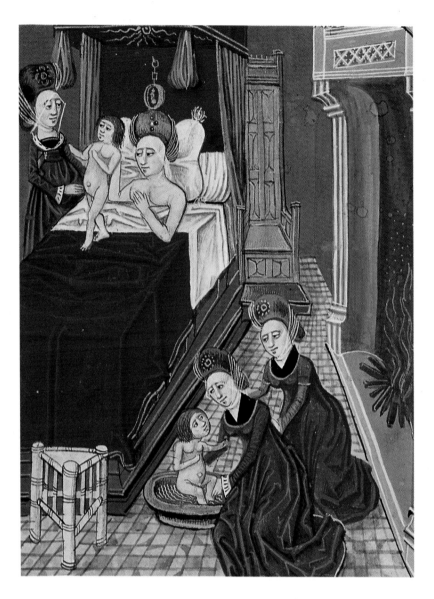

The midwife seems to be testing the walking reflex, the newborn's automatic stepping.

ABOVE: *The Birth of Alexander the Great.* 15th century. Musée Condée, Chantilly

OPPOSITE: *The Birth of Saint John the Baptist.* 15th century. Musée de l'Ain, Bourg-en-Bresse

was also conspicuously absent; it was not until the fifteenth century that he began to take part if complications occurred, and then only for wealthy families.

The mother-to-be sat up in bed, supported by a pile of pillows. Nude beneath the covers, she did not let down her hair. The matron performed by touch only; in fact, until the nineteenth century, a woman gave birth hidden under a sheet or her robe. She could change position as she wished, to stand up or squat. Some medieval treatises even advised her to walk and climb stairs while in labor. She might also sit in a bath infused with soothing aromatic herbs, intended to aid the baby's progress. The midwife and the other women stayed with her throughout the delivery, the midwife offering advice, massages, potions, irrigations, and talismans, and the others giving her both physical and emotional support.

A Bath of Crushed Roses

In the Middle Ages the cries of the mother during labor were considered to be as natural as those of the baby at birth, which signal her vitality. Once the umbilical cord was cut, the matron made a double knot, then covered it with a powder made from dragon's blood (a resinous plant), sarcocolla, cumin, and chervil before making a dressing with a piece of linen soaked in olive oil. Separating the newborn from her mother, the midwife gave the baby a thorough going-over—a comprehensive neonatal exam, which was followed by a gentle cleansing. The midwife tested the limbs for reflexes and the joints for easy movement. If the infant belonged to a sufficiently well-off family, she would be wrapped in crushed roses with salt, in accordance with the advice given by medical treatises. This delicate and refined practice was designed to remove the material coating her skin at birth and to strengthen her limbs. Using her finger, the matron smeared honey on the baby's palate and gums to clean out her mouth and stimulate her appetite. The baby was then dipped several times into a bath of warm water, whose temperature had been carefully gauged with a hand or foot. After being dried, the baby was rubbed with oil, particularly vigorously if it was a male, whose "limbs must be stronger than those of females for hard work." Then the newborn, swaddled in a cloth that a woman had just warmed in front of the fireplace, was put to bed in the shadows, to protect her eyes, still too sensitive to face the light.

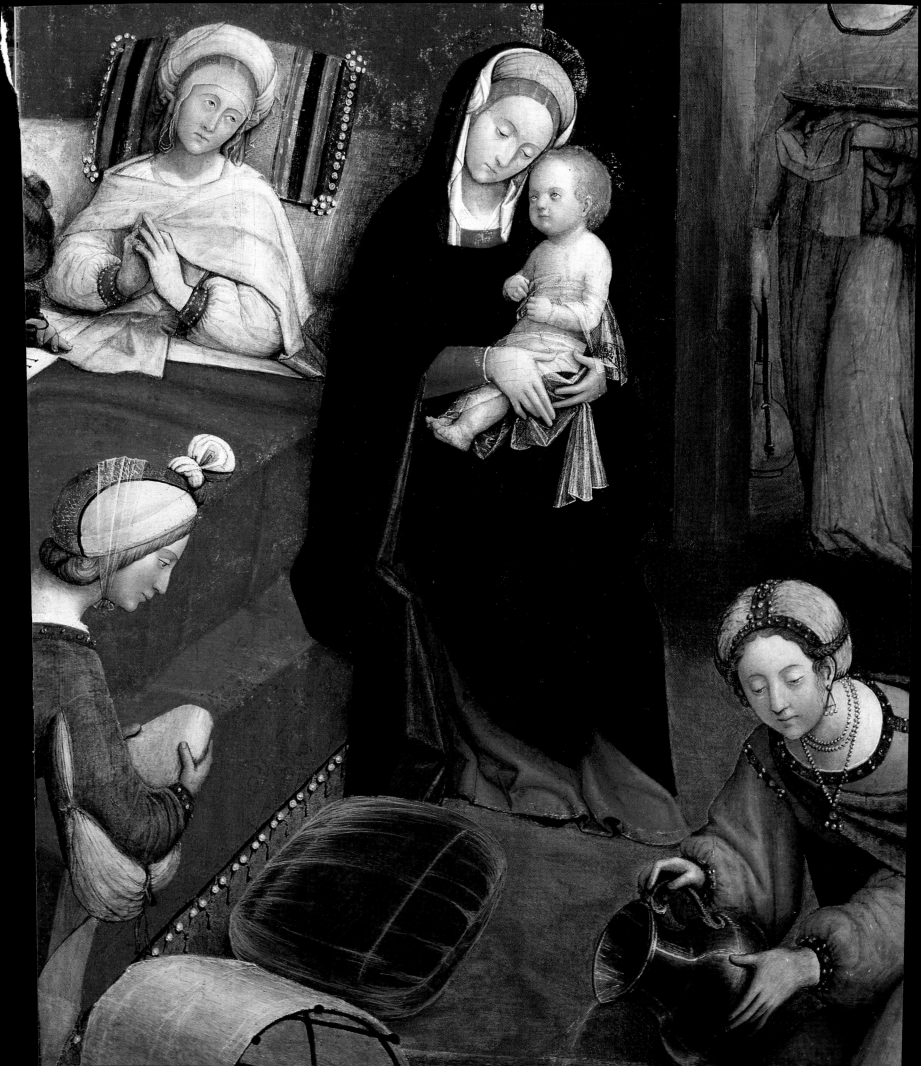

The women who were not fully occupied caring for the baby helped the new mother. They gave her a white smock to wear, remade her bed with clean sheets, brought her water so she could wash her face and hands, and then served her a meal of a glass of wine, broth, and a fowl to help her regain her strength. The new mother then received visits from her women friends and relations. It was for them that the mothers-to-be of medieval high society transformed their bedrooms into luxurious nests called "lying-in rooms."

In fifteenth-century Italy, rich families began to imitate the extravagant luxury of lying-in rooms of the court. The walls of their rooms were hung with rare fabrics, and the floors were strewn with flowers in summer and thick rugs in winter. A large bed, surrounded by curtains and heaped with fur blankets, formed the centerpiece. A huge armchair upholstered in velvet, small footstools and silk cushions for the visitors, and a richly sculpted wooden chest containing the layette often completed the furnishings of the places that welcomed princes and princesses to the world. The new mother, "more bedecked than a bride," settled herself in bed. A dresser with a number of different sets of shelves, according to the expectant mother's rank, was

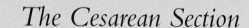

The Cesarean Section

In the canton of Thurgovie in Switzerland in the year 1500, the wife of Jacob Nufer, who gelded pigs in his area, was expecting a baby. Her labor began, and it proved to be long and difficult, and still the baby did not emerge. Thirteen midwives bustled about the poor woman, but they could do nothing for her. "As her pains increased more and more and the baby still did not come, the husband conveyed to his wife that if she had confidence in him, he would try an operation that, by the grace of God, might succeed.... The husband opened her belly in a single thrust of the knife, as if he were operating on a piglet. On his first try, he pulled out the baby." He sewed up his wife's wound, and the following year she gave birth to twins; the first child lived to the age of seventy-seven.

This account of what was claimed to be the first cesarean on a living woman was given by François Rousset in his book Traité nouvel de l'hystérotomie

placed in the room. Relatives, friends, and acquaintances filed in, bearing the most exquisite gifts, and were offered wine, quince pastries, and pies from gold and silver plates laid on the dresser. This indulgent show of sumptuousness continued until the ceremony of churching replaced it.

The Churching Ceremony

Poor peasant women did not have a choice: a few days, perhaps only a few hours after delivery, they went back to work in the fields. In better-off households, the new mother was directed to rest for about a month (according to the Bible, forty days), and during this period she was considered impure. Tarnished by the sin of the flesh that led to conception and by the blood that continued to flow since delivery, she risked contaminating everything she touched. Rich or poor, the new mother did not recover her purity until she had undergone the churching ceremony. When this important day arrived, she arrayed herself in a new dress and went to church to offer a candle to the Virgin Mary. The priest welcomed her and sprinkled her with holy

The many, and highly realistic, depictions of cesareans carried out on dead women in the Middle Ages lead one to think that this operation was relatively common at the time.

BELOW: *The Birth of Caesar.* 15th century. Miniature. Musée Condé, Chantilly

OVERLEAF: Domenico Ghirlandaio. *The Birth of Saint John the Baptist.* 15th century. Church of Santa Maria Novella, Florence

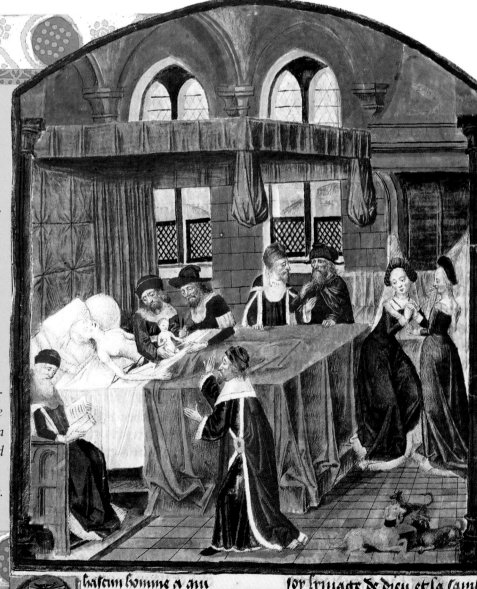

ou enfantement césarien (New Treatise on Hysterotomy or Cesarean Birth), published in 1581. Cesareans had been performed on dead women since antiquity to save the infant when possible. Romans carried out the operation in the desire to populate the empire; in the Middle Ages, the operation was required by the Church to ensure that there would be a sufficient number of baptized people on Judgment Day. (The number of such cesareans, intended to guarantee eternal life to the baby, grew throughout the seventeenth and eighteenth centuries.) In the eighteenth century, progressive surgeons, called on to save the lives of both mother and child, became increasingly interested in this operation on the living woman. In practice, however, its use remained the exception, not the rule, and controversy concerning its worth raged. Until the mid-nineteenth century, the cesarean took more lives than it saved: more than one woman and one child in three died. Only when anesthesia became available and, even more important, when surgeons adopted the principles of asepsis and antisepsis—in the second half of the nineteenth century—did the operation finally become less dangerous.

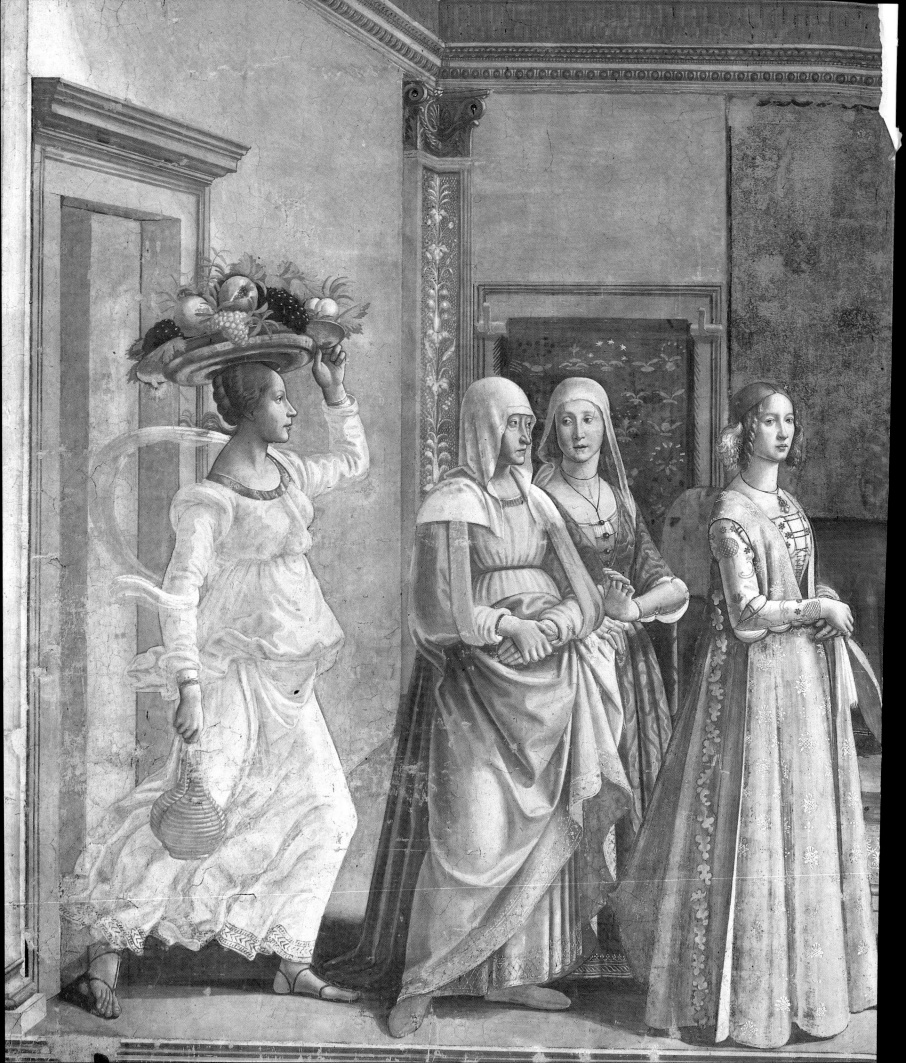

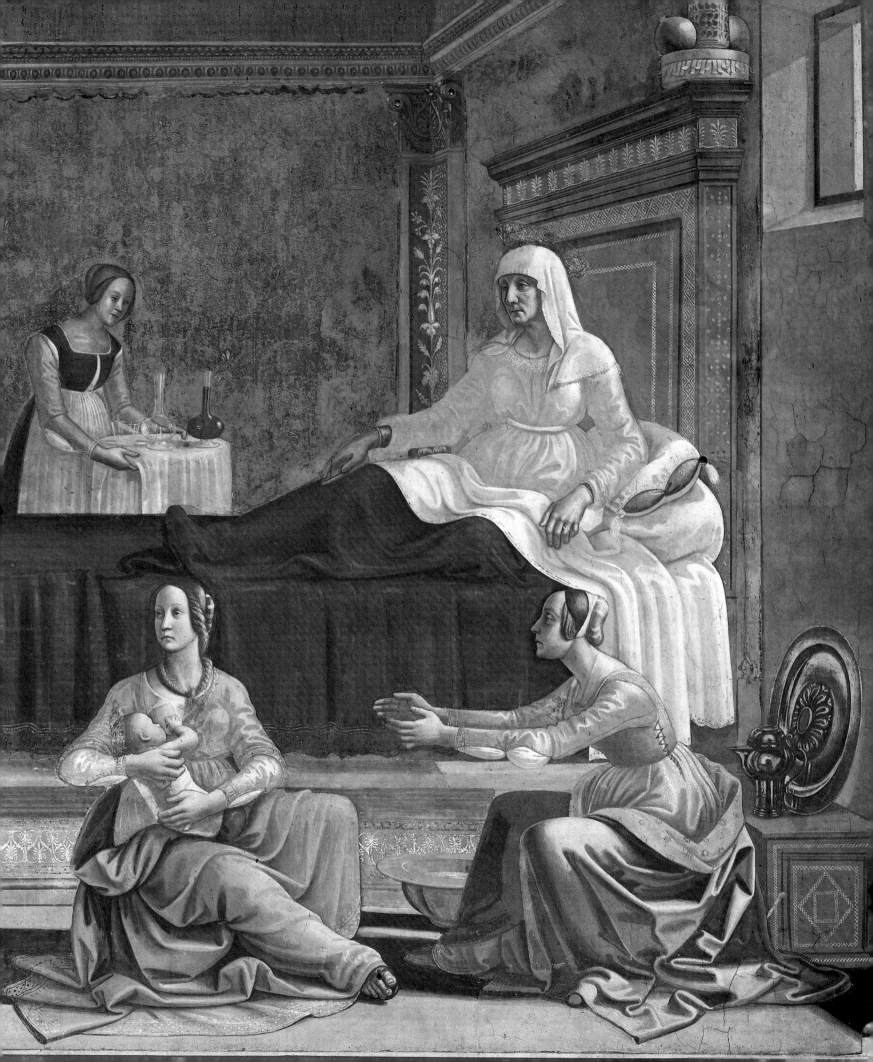

The childbirth sachet was composed of several cloth envelopes that contained a variety of objects: medallions, rosary beads, statuettes and miniature reliquaries, and wads of tiny parchments covered with religious writings and magic formulas.

BELOW: Childbirth sachet.
Musée des Arts et Traditions
Populaires, Paris

OPPOSITE: Pfullen-Dorfer retable.
c. 1500. Municipal Museum,
Stuttgart

water. This purification reintegrated her into the Christian community, and she was then free to resume her customary tasks. The postpartum period of retreat was enforced so strictly that women who had to attend to their affairs before it had elapsed resorted to such stratagems as going out with a roof tile on their heads to indicate symbolically that they had not left their houses. Wealthy women often took full advantage of this period of rest by lounging about, surrounded by gossiping friends, indulging themselves in good food and wine.

Pilgrimage and Relics

Until obstetrics made some progress in the nineteenth century, childbirth remained a struggle with death. How was the delivery carried out in seventeenth- and eighteenth-century Europe? To ensure a successful delivery, women turned to religious rites as well as magical practices and objects. Far from being restricted to peasants isolated in the countryside, these beliefs were shared by queens and middle-class women alike. The childbirth sachet, handed down from generation to generation, was said to guarantee a favorable outcome. Its contents had to be kept secret, perfectly sealed, or it might lose its power. How many generations of expectant mothers have also appealed to the saints, especially the Virgin Mary and Saint Margaret, during their pregnancy and labor? The pregnant woman might go on pilgrimage to one of many sanctuaries dedicated to these all-powerful saints, or she might content herself with wearing the sash of one or the other. A sash of Saint Margaret that belonged to the Benedictines of the church of Saint-Germain-des-Prés in Paris was "rented" to women about to give birth. The Virgin Mary's sash turned up in various places in France. Rumors of the miracles and favors granted to women who had simply touched it came to the ears of King Louis XIII, who procured it for his wife, pregnant after more than twenty years of marriage. Several hours before labor began, she tied on this relic and then later successfully brought into the world a healthy son, the future Louis XIV.

Not everyone had the means to borrow the sash of the Virgin, nor even to touch it. Most women made do with a large glass of water containing the fragments of a tiny image of Mary or of a paper scrawled with several verses from the Bible—a pious drink that could substitute for pilgrimages and relics.

Amulets and Talismans

Worn on the upper part of the body during pregnancy to keep the baby in the belly, protective objects were placed lower down during labor—on the

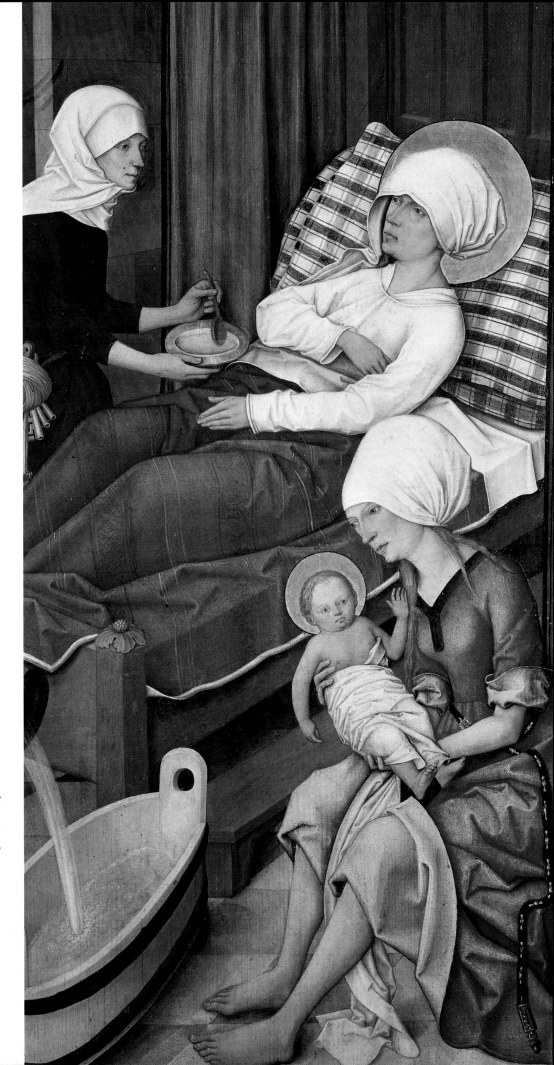

"During my labor, strengthen my heart to bear the pangs that accompany it, so that I will accept them as the consequences of your punishment of our gender for the sin of the first woman. In the light of that curse, and of my own offenses in marriage, I suffer with joy the sharpest pains. Although the sanctity of marriage has made this conception legitimate, I confess that it is tainted with the poison of lust. If it is your will that I die during childbirth, I worship you, I bless you, and I bend to your will."

Antoine Godeau,
Instructions et prières chrétiennes
(Christian Instructions and Prayers),
1646

The Deception of the Rabbits

"The doctrine of spontaneous generation had gained so much credit since the beginning of the century that many people were persuaded that a sole could give rise to a frog.... A well-known London surgeon named Saint André wrote about this doctrine in 1726.... One of his women neighbors, poor but bold, resolved to take advantage of the surgeon's theory.... After eight days, this woman called on him to attend her in her hovel; she told him she was feeling sharp pains as if she were in labor.... She gave birth to a small rabbit, which survived. Saint André showed everyone his neighbor's son.... The woman found this calling so profitable that she gave birth every eight days. Finally justice intervened; she was taken in; a small young rabbit that she had obtained and had buried in an orifice not meant for it was flushed out. She was punished; Saint André went into hiding. The newspapers found this rabbit warren a source of great merriment."

Voltaire (cited by G. J. Witkowski)

belly or around the thigh. The best known of these amulets was a hollow stone with small fragments inside, which tinkled when it was shaken. Said to come from a nest of raptors, this "eagle stone," which symbolized the fetus moving in the uterus, was a rare and precious object, handed down from generation to generation in wealthy families. Tying this "pregnant stone" to the left thigh, encircling the belly with a snakeskin, wearing a necklace of red coral, laying a magnet on the lower abdomen to attract a child, lighting a long candle that will be consumed by the end of labor—such magical practices came down through the ages. Rural matrons still had a long list of routines that they applied throughout labor: untie all knots and undo all bolts—even set loose the cows in the barn—to facilitate the baby's passage; put pepper in the woman's nostrils to promote expulsion through sneezing; shake her as if she were a plum tree; frighten her to start her contractions; sit the expectant mother "on the bottom of a warm cauldron" to soften her genital area, or lubricate it with melted butter or lard; place the husband's nightcap on the wife's belly, or have her pull on his pants.

Crying Up a Storm

First of all, relatives, neighbors, and matrons hastened to stuff all the cracks very carefully in the doors and windows of the room where the birth would take place. The least chill could be fatal to

These protective medallions guaranteed the woman in labor a successful delivery.

BELOW: Corsican medallions. Musée des Arts et Traditions Populaires, Paris

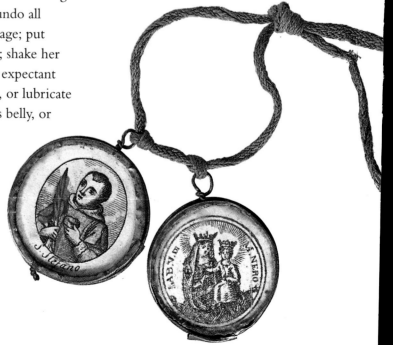

mother as well as child, but more important, evil spirits could take advantage of the smallest crack to enter the room and cast a terrible spell. To heat the room, the large fire in the fireplace was carefully tended. If the delivery took place in the stable, which was not uncommon until the nineteenth century, the animals would also heat up the air. The presence of numerous women called "flies," who moved about, cried, or whispered, also surely raised the temperature of the room. If the heat of the closed space was considered insufficient, the expectant mother was given highly spiced drinks to "enflame the womb." The air could quickly become dangerously suffocating in the common room of the peasant family, with the additional presence of five or six friends, just as in the royal bedroom.

To prevent any possibility of substituting the royal baby, a harrowing formality—from the queen's point of view— arose in the seventeenth century. At the first sign of labor, the king, princes, and princesses, along with the ministers and ambassadors, gathered around the mother-to-be. The chancellor, an unimpeachable witness, got on his knees at the end of the bed. Representatives of the public were also admitted to the royal bedchamber, though they had to stay behind partitions. This ceremony continued through the following century.

In 1778, at the time of the birth of Marie-Thérèse of France, Madame de Campan recounted in her memoirs that Queen Marie Antoinette came close to death. "When the doctor Vermond loudly proclaimed, 'The queen is going into labor!' the floods of the curious that rushed into the room were so numerous and so tumultuous that this movement nearly killed the queen. The previous night, the king had taken the precaution of having the immense tapestries surrounding the bed of Her Majesty attached with ropes; if not for this precaution, they would surely have fallen on her. It was no longer possible to move in the room, which had so filled up with such a mixed crowd that one might have thought oneself on a public square. Two Savoyards climbed on the furniture to more readily see the queen, situated opposite the fireplace on a bed arranged for the delivery. Was it this noise, or the sex of the child—which the queen had the opportunity to learn, it is said, by a prearranged sign from the princess of Lamballe—or was it the fault of the doctor, who inhibited the natural progress of childbirth? The blood rushed to her head, her mouth worked, the doctor cried out, 'Air, warm water, I must bleed the foot!' The windows had been sealed; the king opened them with a force that could only have come from his tender

"The king did me the honor of asking if I would like to be the remueuse [the woman in charge of changing the swaddling clothes] of Monsieur the Dauphin, and that I would receive the same wages as the wet nurse. I begged His Majesty to be so kind as to agree that I should in no way abandon the ordinary practice of the midwife, so that I could always be able to serve the queen," wrote midwife Louise Bourgeois.

ABOVE: Arthur Rackham. Illustration for the fairy tale *The Sleeping Beauty in the Wood.*

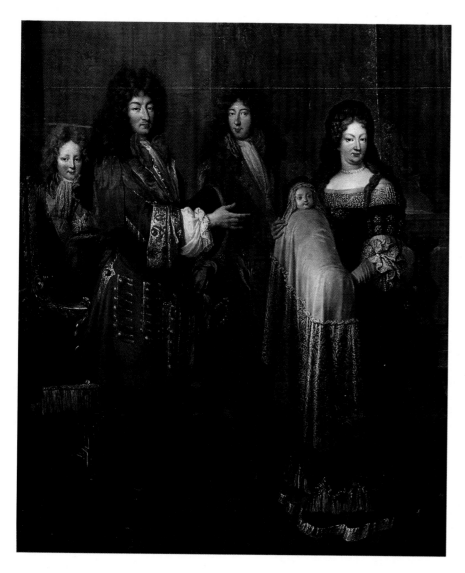

Once the chancellor had announced the dauphin's gender, the royal baby was swaddled and carried to his suite in a silver basin. A watch was mounted around his cradle.

ABOVE: Antoine Dieu. *The Birth of Louis de France.* 1715. Château de Versailles

RIGHT: Print. 1808. Bibliothèque Nationale, Paris

OPPOSITE: A. Gilli. *The Newborn.* 19th century. Musée du Petit-Palais, Paris

feelings for the queen, these windows being very high and glued with bands of paper over their entire length. The servants of the bedchamber, the ushers dragged by the collar the indiscreet curious who did not stir themselves to clear the room. This cruel tradition was abolished for all time. The princes of the family, the blood princes, the chancellor, and the ministers certainly sufficed to witness the legitimacy of a hereditary prince. The queen returned from the gates of death."

Up until the nineteenth century, childbirth was a public act, for the most exalted as for the most humble. Once the child was born, the matron's work was far from over. She had to usher the newborn into the world following rituals that were practiced in some areas into the beginning of the twentieth century. First of all, she had to separate newborn from mother by cutting the umbilical cord, in a spot that depended on whether the child was a boy or a girl. "The good women wanted to calculate the best length of the cord to leave, since they thought that the male member would use it as a template, and that it would become longer if what hung from the navel was left longer." The cut cord and the placenta, which until the nineteenth century was considered to be the infant's double, could not be thrown away. Instead, depending on the place, they were buried, burned, or hidden in the foundations of the house; sometimes the mother might carefully preserve the umbilical cord to bring happiness to the child after he had grown up. Then the midwife bathed the newborn thoroughly in front of the fire with melted butter or water mixed with wine. She often cleaned the baby's insides by making him drink several spoonfuls of sugared wine, which gave him strength. Finally, she sometimes took it upon herself to shape the baby, this still unformed small being. She energetically kneaded his head "to make it round or long," following the propensities of the time and place. With a fingernail she let grow for this purpose, she also cut the string beneath the newborn's tongue to release it and make sucking on the breast easier.

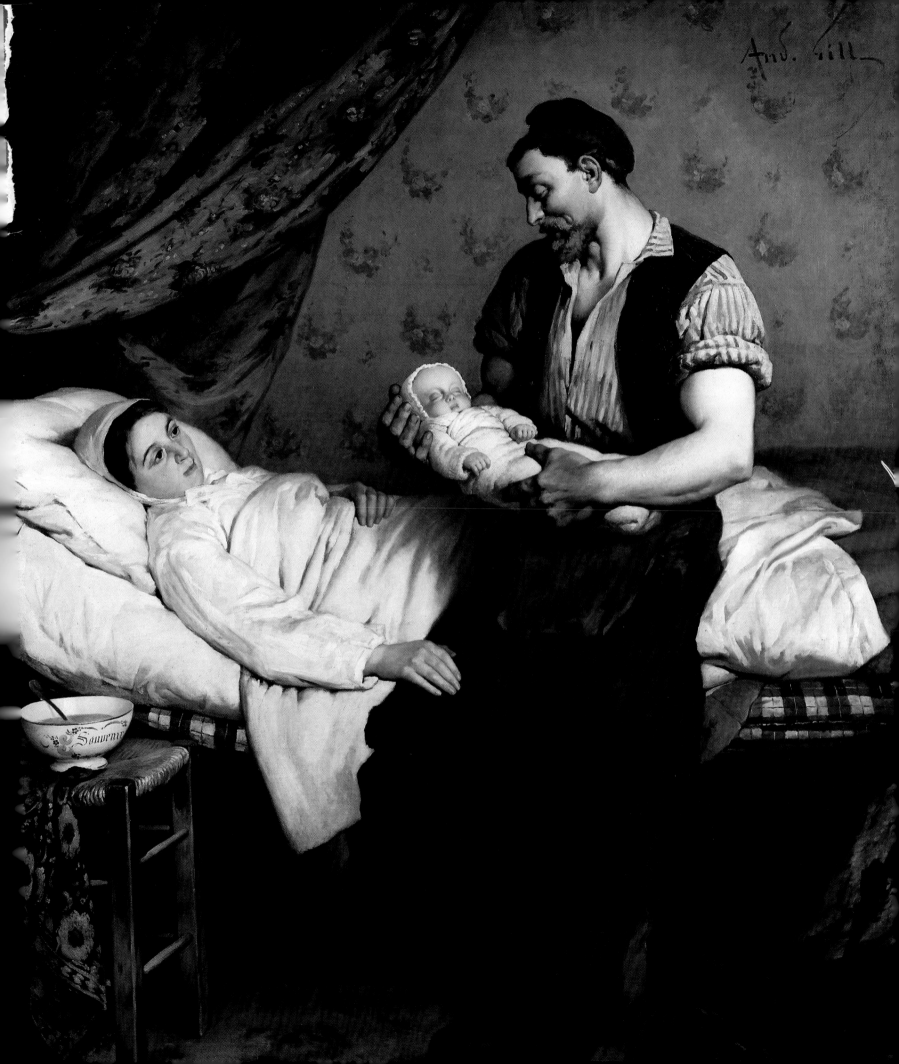

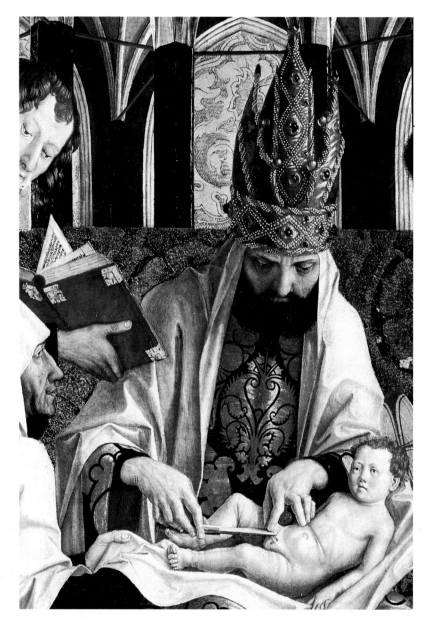

Circumcision, a religious ceremony celebrated by Jews, Muslims, and various other peoples, is a ritual that welcomes the baby into the community, like baptism for Christians.

ABOVE: Michael Pacher. *The Circumcision.* 15th century. Church of Saint Wolfgang, Austria

Processions and Ceremonies

Several hours or days after birth, the midwife or one of the women who assisted at childbirth led a procession conveying the infant to church to be baptized. The midwife was not only responsible for the smooth progress of the delivery, but she was also in charge of the salvation of the infant's soul, even more so than that of his body. Thus, she had to be versed in the baptismal formulas to be able to perform the ceremony herself if an infant's life was in jeopardy. The souls of infants who died unbaptized were condemned to wander endlessly, and their bodies could not be buried in cemeteries. To guard against that great danger, even baptism *in utero*, whose validity was long the object of controversy, was practiced. If, after all, the infant survived, these "spiritual rescues" had to be followed by the sacrament duly performed in the proper fashion, administered at the church by the parish priest.

The procession that accompanied the candidate for baptism tended to be impressive. At the beginning of the ceremony, the priest asked the godfathers and godmothers what name they had chosen for the infant. This name was often the same as that of the father or mother, a grandparent, or godfather or godmother—a sign that the infant from then on belonged to the familial community. It was also the name of a saint, under whose protection the baby was placed. Until the end of the fifteenth century, infants were then unswaddled near the baptismal font so that they could be completely immersed in the water. As this proved dangerous to the babies' health, making them vulnerable to blasts of cold air, immersion was soon thereafter forbidden, and the priest made do with sprinkling water on their heads. The ceremony concluded, the procession that accompanied the baby to church set off again and, among the middle and lower classes, found its way to the inn or tavern to celebrate the event.

The mother, meanwhile, was bid not to set her feet on the ground. In rural areas, she might stay in bed with soiled sheets wearing a dirty nightgown for up to a week—a far cry from the attentions of the Middle Ages. A popular belief that white linen brought on hemmorhages took root during the seventeenth and eighteenth centuries and lasted until the beginning of the twentieth. (The churching ceremony was considered to be of such importance during this period that it was carried out even if the mother had died in labor.)

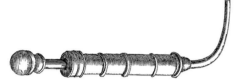

This syringe was used by seventeenth-century doctors to administer intrauterine baptism.

Naked and held by his godfather above the baptismal font of his parish, this newborn has been in the world for little over a day. The priest applies the holy chrism, a mixture of olive oil and balsam, on his head. The priest will baptize and then dry the baby before covering his head with a small white bonnet called the chrisom, which is impregnated with holy oils. After the ceremony, the celebration begins, and the baby receives gifts from his godparents and guests.

RIGHT: Rogier van der Weyden. *The Seven Sacraments.* 15th century. Musée des Beaux-Arts, Anvers

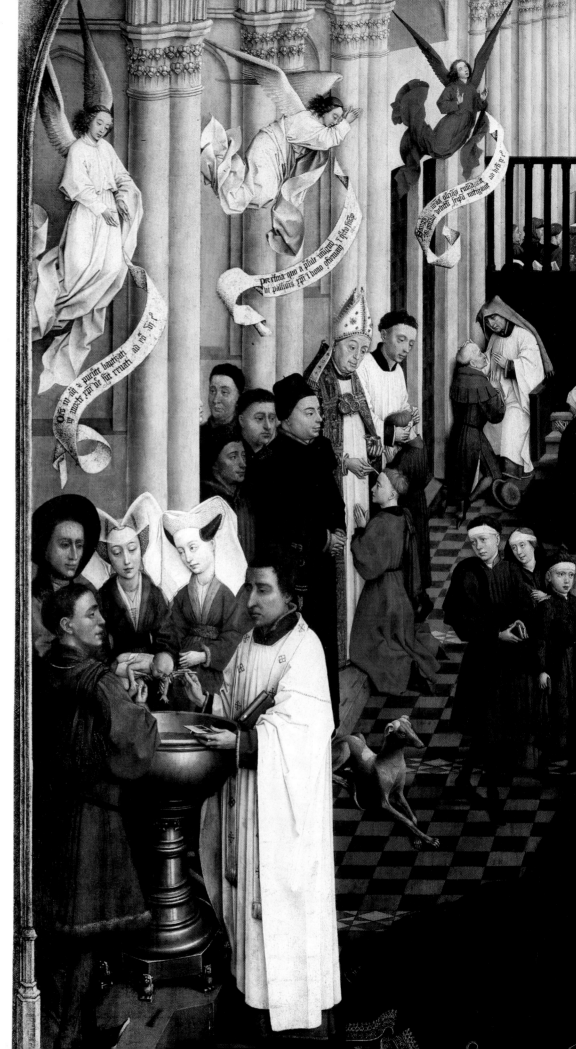

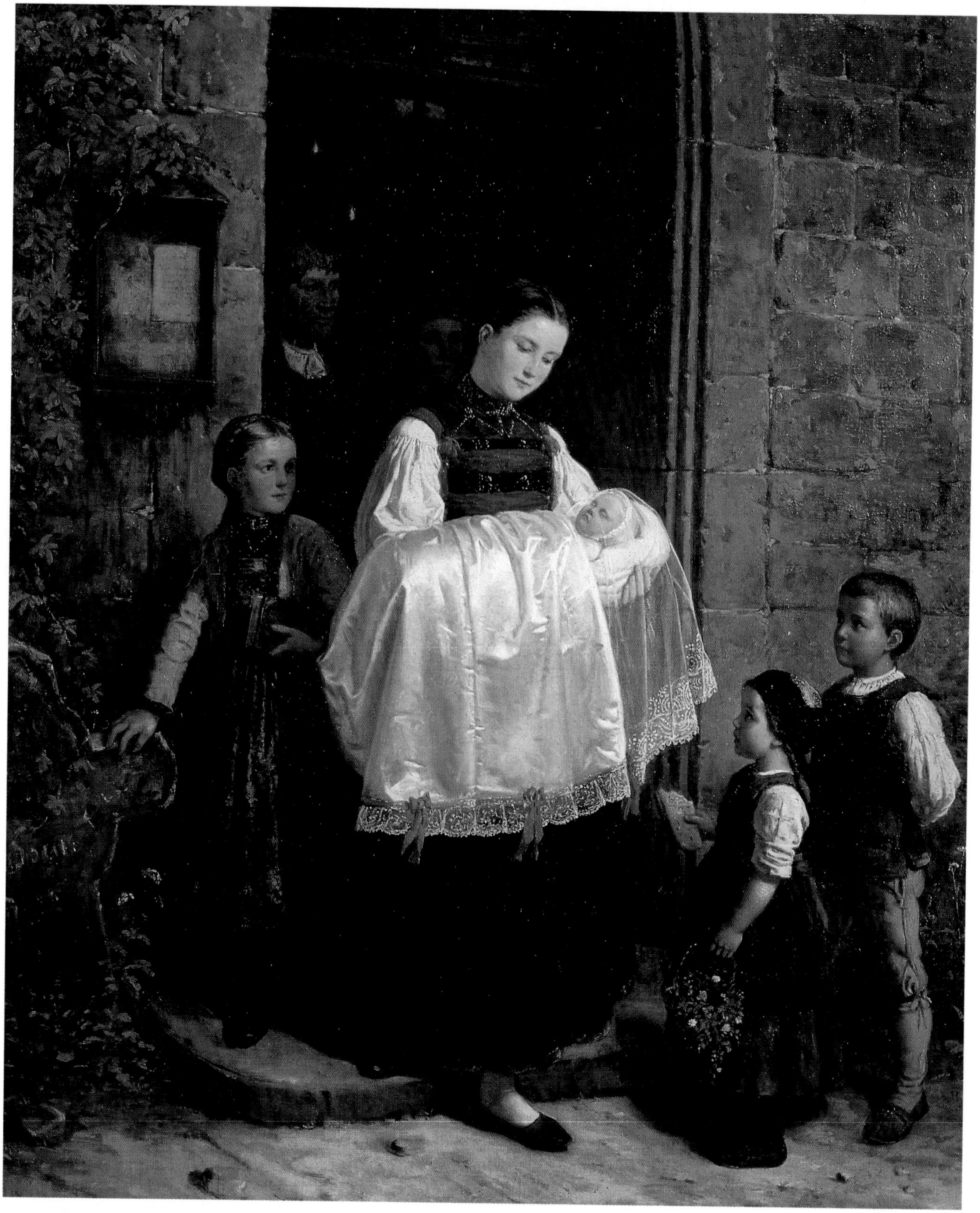

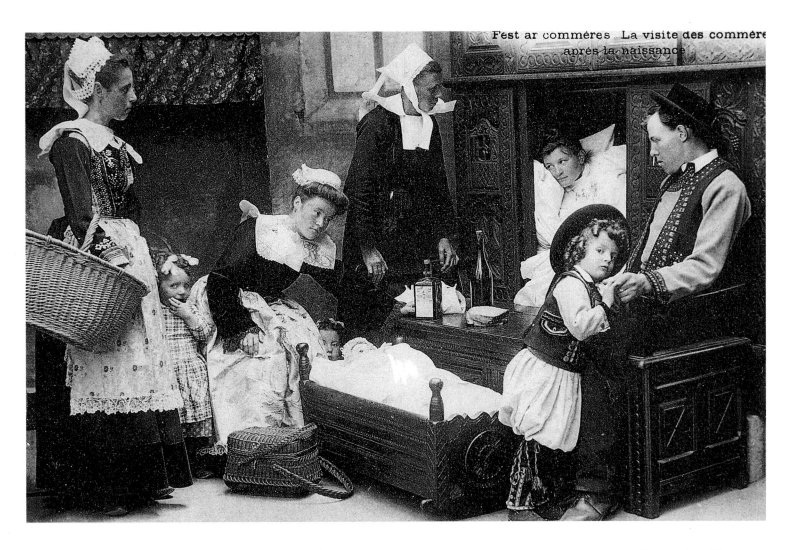

Fest ar comméres La visite des comméres
après la naissance

*Settled in her enclosed bed, this
Breton woman who has just given
birth receives the neighbors who
have come to visit her.*

ABOVE: Postcard. 1905

OPPOSITE: Hubert Salentin. *The
Return from the Baptism.* 1859.
Victoria and Albert Museum,
London

OVERLEAF: Peasant family from
la Sarthe. Late 19th century.
Photograph

After the baptism took place, close neighbors came to visit the mother. The
father sometimes slipped into bed in her place; he would pretend to be suffering
the effects of a painful childbirth and then take the baby in his arms. This custom,
called *couvade*, allowed the man to be symbolically recognized as the father. Alerted
by word of mouth, other neighbors came to visit, their hands filled with foods that
they offered as they pronounced the customary wishes for the infant: "May God
bless you and make you straight as a match, healthy as salt, full as an egg, sweet as
sugar, and good as bread." Until the baptism, infants were kept away from outside
influences, protected by amulets or, later, wreaths and rosaries.

The welcome given to newborns in poor families—in the nineteenth century
as in every age—greatly differed from that accorded the infant of the wealthy. In
middle-class Paris, for example, anyone who was anyone received a small announce-
ment, informing them of the birth of the child and inviting them to offer their
congratulations on a given day and at a given time. During these visits, a nurse,
wearing a splendid silk dress that was customarily given to her for this moment, held

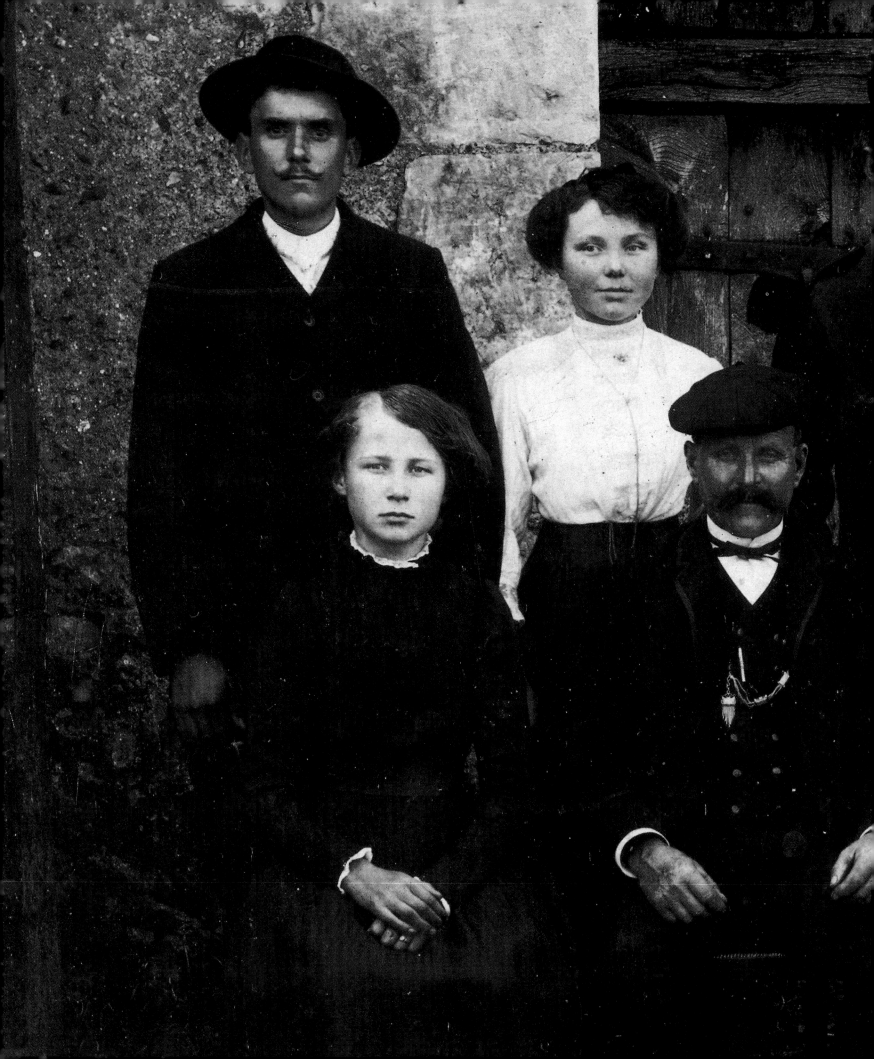

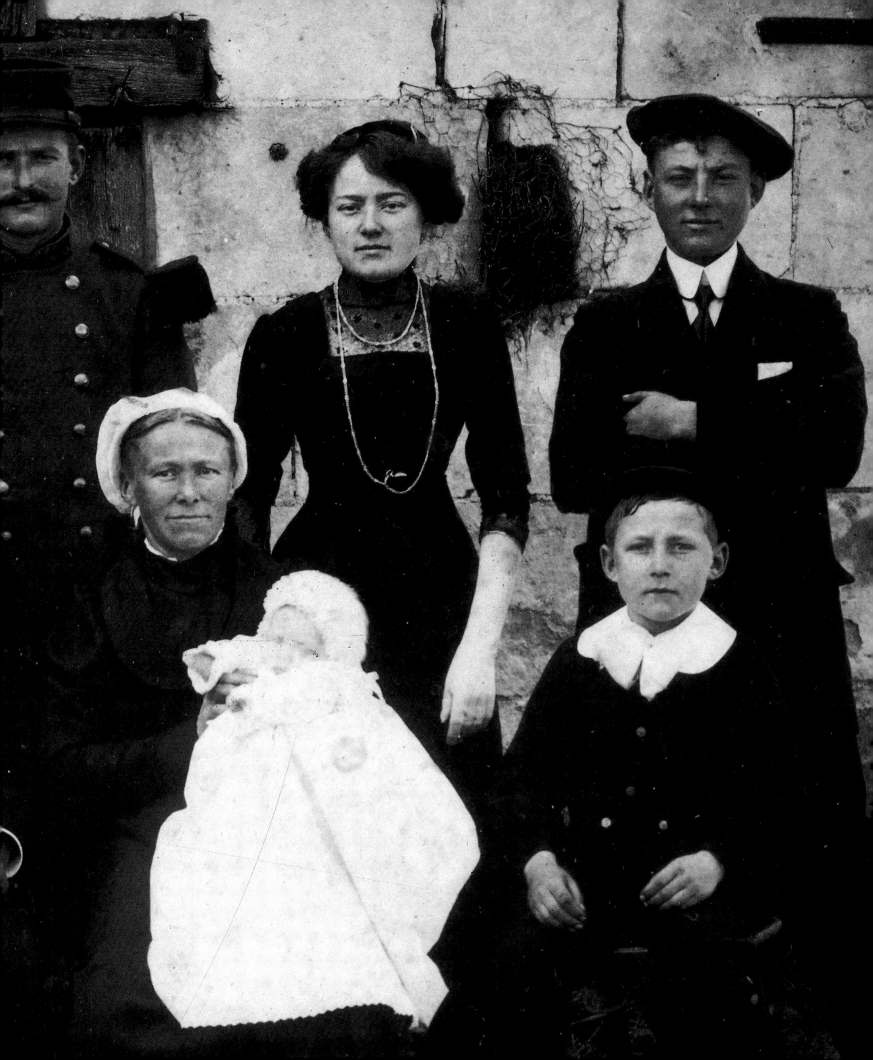

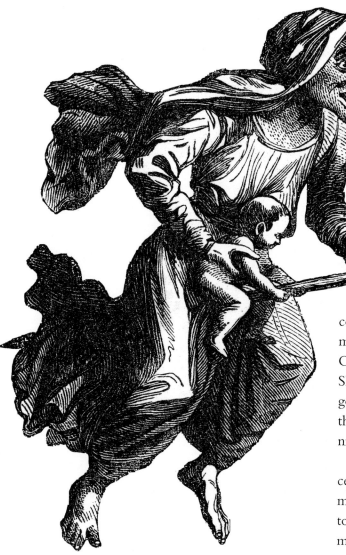

This witch, a caricature of the midwife, goes to a Black Mass carrying a stolen baby.

OPPOSITE LEFT: Anatomic model. 17th century. Ivory

OPPOSITE RIGHT: After J. Rueff. Childbirth scene using the birthing chair. 16th century. Print

the baby. The wet nurse also dressed for the occasion. If the baby was a boy, everything—the mother's outfit, the baby's cradle, the wet nurse's ribbons—was in blue, the color of the protecting heavens. If it was a girl, everything was in pink; this flattering color was chosen simply to differentiate her from a boy.

The "Good Mother" or the Witch

In Europe in the seventeenth and eighteenth centuries, and often later, a midwife almost always presided at childbirth. She rushed over, bringing a pair of scissors to cut the umbilical cord, a piece of thread, and a small pot filled with an unguent made according to her secret recipe. As in the Middle Ages, the matron of the village was an older woman, one who herself had many children.

To learn her profession, she had assisted another matron in the community at many childbirths. Few eyewitness accounts of the life of the country midwife of this era have come down to us, with the exception of a diary kept by Catherine Shrader, a Dutch midwife of exceptional temperament and sensitivity. She recounted her career as a traveling midwife—the long distances she covered going from hamlet to hamlet through snowstorms, the exhausting hours, the four thousand babies she helped bring into the world until she reached the age of ninety-one.

In France, it was not until the sixteenth century in the cities and the seventeenth century in the countryside that formal training began to be established for the midwife. In 1587, the first statute regulating the profession appeared: whether called to work for "queens, princesses, ladies, damsels, middle-class, or poor women, midwives will behave honestly and virtuously and will not use either unseemly words nor gestures and before arriving will have removed their rings from their fingers, if they have any, and washed their hands."

The "good mother" possessed a body of knowledge based on tradition and experience. The mystery and superstition that surrounded her work often led to accusations of sorcery: midwives unscrupulously performed abortions, were given to using babies for all manner of demonic practices, were in league with the devil. Was it to counteract this "matron-witch" or to ensure the baptism of all newborns that the institution of a matron chosen by the community was encouraged by the Church starting in the seventeenth century?

Elected by all the women of the parish, she took an oath in their presence and in front of the parish priest. This solemn pledge was cited in the book *Entrer dans la vie* (Coming into the World) by J. Gélis, M. Laget, and M.-F. Morel: "I swear and promise to God in your presence to live and die in the Catholic faith, apostolic and Roman, to acquit myself with the greatest possible correctness and faithfulness

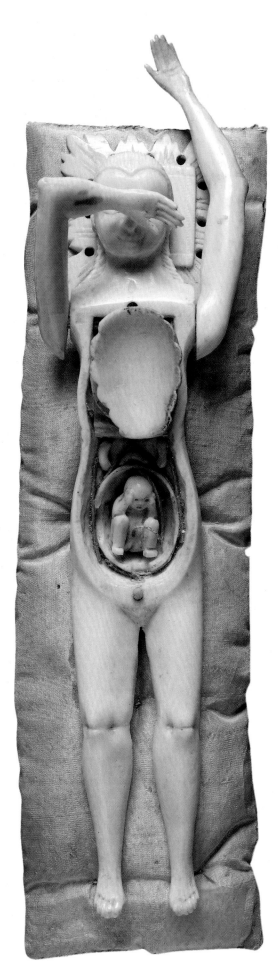

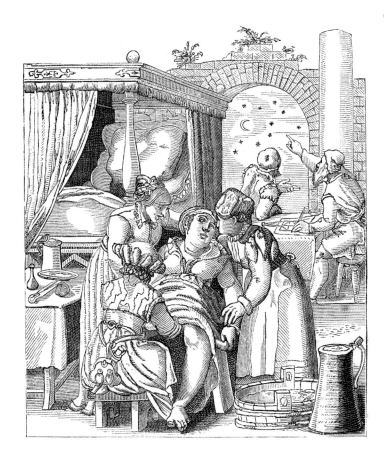

of the post that I am undertaking, to help women in childbirth and never to allow either the mother or the child to run any risk through my error. And when I notice an urgent peril to make use of the advice and the rules of the surgeon and other women who I know to be experienced in this role. I promise also never to reveal the secrets of families nor of any persons that I assist." She then obtained from the priest a certificate of good morality.

The Beginnings of Obstetrics

A speculum pierced with holes to facilitate fumigations with fragrant herbs, invented by Ambroise Paré; a sexual embrace just before childbirth to "shake up the infant and make it come out more easily" or the application of a sheared sheepskin on the mother's belly, methods recommended by the doctor Jacques Guillemeau; gentle murmurs of comfort, prescribed by the surgeon Mauriceau—until the eighteenth century, the obstetrical tools and techniques of European doctors were hardly more scientific than the midwives'. In the sixteenth and seventeenth centuries, scientific writings on the subject began to increase but, in practice, childbirth remained the exclusive province of the "good mothers." Even city dwellers and rich families called on doctors only as a last resort, so one's arrival was usually an ominous portent.

Even queens called on midwives. In fact, Louise Bourgeois became famous: "Having qualified as a midwife, I served a great number of women, poor as well as those just getting by, ladies as well as damsels, and those up to the rank of princess."

Seated, Squatting, Kneeling, Lying Down...

"I have often noted that one of the things most essential for a woman in labor is to be well placed, for the relief of the mother as well as the child: if the woman wishes to and is able to walk until she is ready to give birth, I find that very beneficial... if she has a low seat on which there is a pillow in front of a table, for when she feels her labor pains coming, she can get on her knees.... Others want to get into bed from the first sign of labor." Early-seventeenth-century midwife Louise Bourgeois let her patient adopt the position that best suited her. This attitude reflects reality; for many centuries, women went through childbirth in a variety of positions, including standing or crouched. Neighbors who came to assist the woman in labor gave her significant physical support: the woman leaned on them, or sometimes she sat on a companion's or her husband's knees. Holland even made a profession of it, the schooster; veritable live birthing chairs, these people had the job of holding the woman on their knees throughout the delivery. In one village, a carpenter had acquired such a reputation that all the women in labor wanted to give birth on his knees. Exhausted and tired of the many interruptions to his work, he built a chair that could replace him.

In the sixteenth century, the ancient custom of birthing chairs was revived: midwives had their chairs, or one that belonged to the community, brought to the house of the expectant mother some time before childbirth. Wealthy families sometimes had their own birthing chair, a precious family piece.

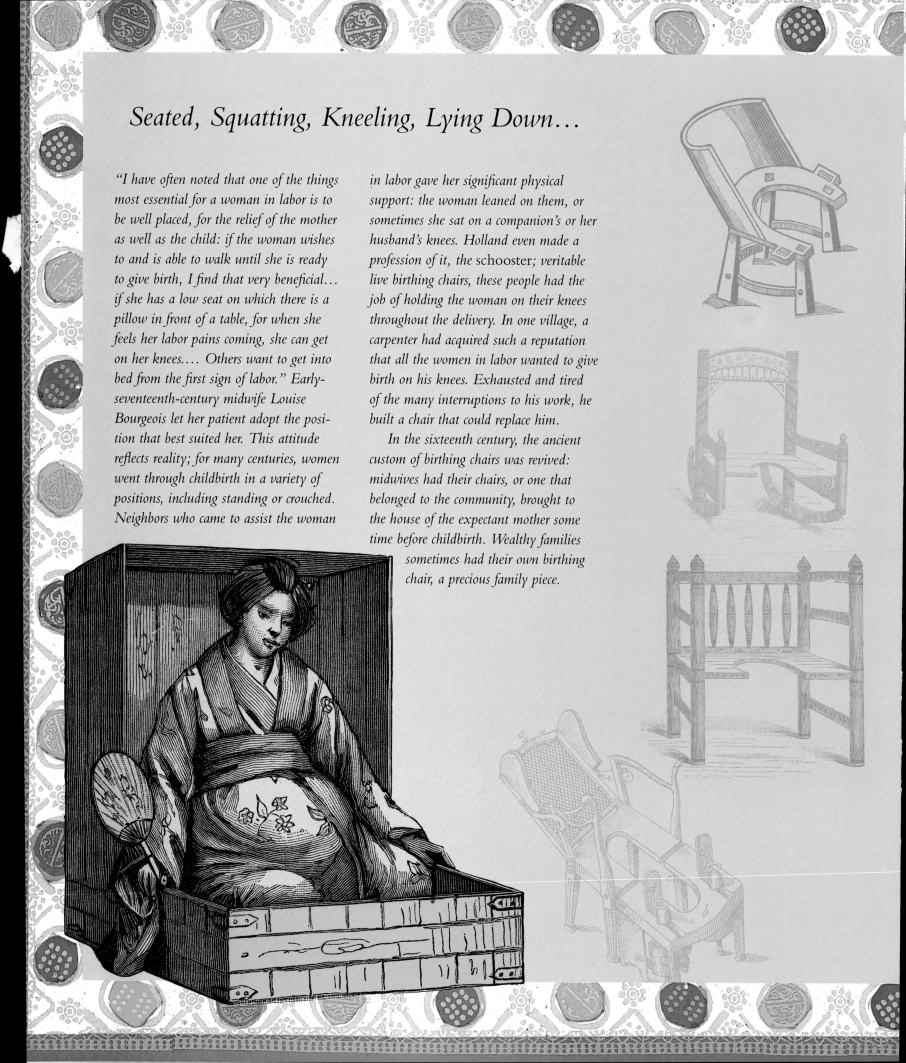

In Holland, every married woman who was fairly well-off brought her own in her trousseau. Easily taken apart and reassembled, and easily transported, these "childbirth devices" were developed to permit various positions—seated, sitting up with legs straight out, or even reclining. They represent a first step toward the medicalization of childbirth, in which the woman, kept immobile, must let herself be "nursed." The second stage in this process was the gradual transformation of the chair-bed into labor bed. Starting in the eighteenth century, obstetricians championed the prone or semiprone position to make it easier for them to work, and these positions were mandated by hospitals, where they are still in use today.

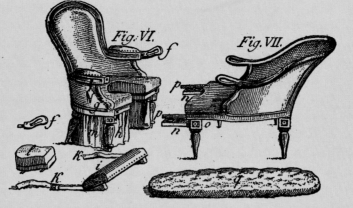

Seated in front of the woman in labor, the midwife waits for the arrival of the baby, assisted by a woman who holds the mother-to-be firmly against the back of the birthing chair.

BELOW: Childbirth scene. 16th century. Print

OPPOSITE LEFT: A Japanese woman in labor on her knees in a special wooden box comparable to the birthing chair

OPPOSITE RIGHT: Various birthing chairs. 19th century. Prints

ABOVE RIGHT AND BELOW: "Bed of misery" and birthing chairs used in the 18th century. 19th century. Prints

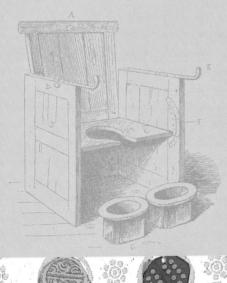

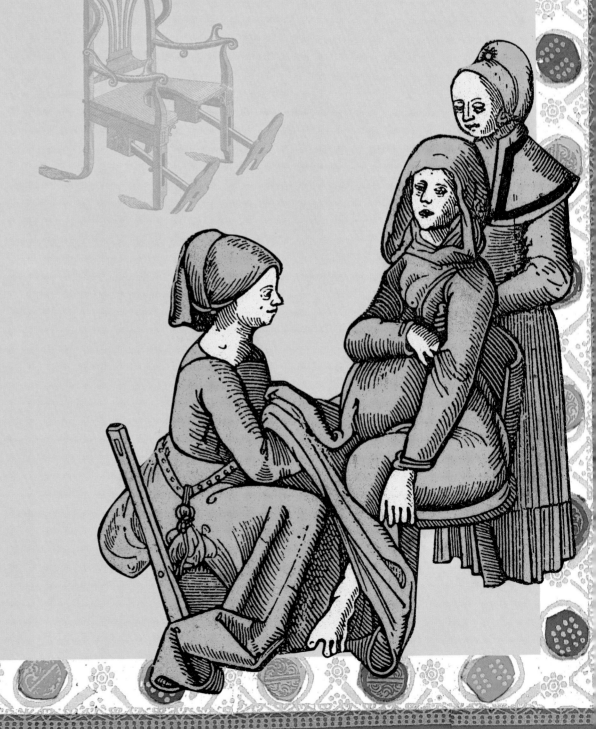

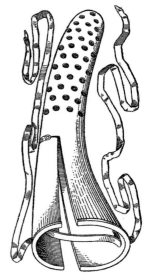

Even higher than that—when she attended Queen Marie de Médicis herself, Bourgeois wrote: "The relics of Madame Saint Margaret were on a table in the room, and two monks from Saint-Germain-des-Prés prayed to God without a break. The Queen's labor lasted twenty-two and a quarter hours.... While she remained in labor for such a long time, the king rarely quit her side.... The Queen wanted to give birth on her chair; where, once she was seated, the princes ranged themselves below the grand pavilion, opposite her. I was on a small seat in front of the Queen. Once she had given birth, I placed Monsieur the Dauphin in the linens and swaddling clothes in my bosom, without letting on to anyone else what the child was.... After the delivery, the King had his own adjoining bed made up, where he went to sleep as soon as she was well." The royal family was imitated by all the ladies of the court and the city; they all relied on midwives. Most male doctors did not enter the domain of obstetrics until the eighteenth century. Partly for reasons of discretion and partly to challenge the midwives, King Louis XIV called on the services of a doctor when his mistress Mademoiselle de La Vallière went into labor.

ABOVE: An irrigation speculum invented by Ambroise Paré

BELOW: A delivery in Holland during the seventeenth century. Everything happened under a sheet.

An Attack on Modesty

Scandal! In 1573, Ambroise Paré published a work entitled *De la génération de l'homme et manière d'extraire les enfants du ventre de leur mère* (On the Procreation of Man and the Method of Extracting Infants from the Abdomen of Their Mother). The medical school decried this immorality: the world of childbirth did not belong to men. Several years earlier, in Hamburg, Dr. Wert, who had disguised himself as a midwife in order to attend a delivery, was denounced, condemned to death for Satanism, and burned alive. Up until the end of the seventeenth century, the prejudice that would not allow men, in the name of decency, to intervene in childbirth tolerated few exceptions. In the early eighteenth century, the doctor Philippe Hecquet heaped disapproval on his colleagues who dared to breach this taboo in his book *De l'indécence aux hommes d'accoucher les femmes* (On the Indecency of Men Attending Women in Childbirth). At the end of the same century, the great doctor Baudelocque added: "The touch is the most dangerous of all the senses and leads to lubricity.... To what dangers do

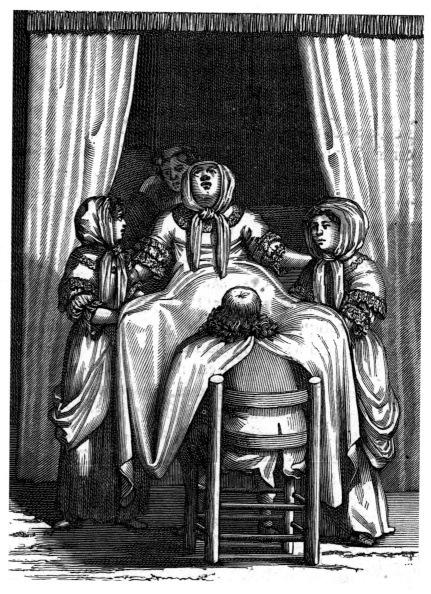

Christians who put themselves in the hands of a doctor expose themselves?" The doctor was not immediately accepted. And though he was allowed to touch, he was not allowed to look. A sheet tied around his neck helped him to resist temptation.

In a day when men's fashions called for them to be shaved and powdered, French doctors were advised to cultivate a repulsive appearance. The famous doctor François Mauriceau challenged this practice: "There are men who say that a surgeon who wants to practice delivering babies must be slovenly or, at the very least, untidy, letting grow a long, dirty beard, in order not to arouse the slightest whiff of jealousy on the part of husbands of women who send for them to give them help. Such a manner of dressing resembles that of a butcher rather than of a surgeon, whom women already fear sufficiently without adding such a disguise." In other countries, where effectiveness and pragmatism were valued over false modesty, the doctor had long since been accepted at childbirth. The modesty of the English decreed only that the woman lie on her left side, so that she and the practitioner could not look at each other.

The Trial of the Matrons

Women and infants died by the thousands. Until the end of the eighteenth century, stillborn babies, often pulled out of their mother's bellies in pieces, were numerous. For every 1,000 live births, 250 would die during their first year, 150 of them in the first month. Seventeenth- and eighteenth-century women, who averaged four or five children, had a one in ten chance of dying during or after childbirth. In the eighteenth century, this dramatically high death rate began to attract attention, and the French government took alarm at the prospect of depopulation. The medical profession, which had made tentative moves to become involved in obstetrics in the seventeenth century, took advantage of this new awareness to gain full acceptance. It ferociously attacked midwives; superstition, sorcery, ignorance, and incompetence, doctors claimed, characterized the methods of these "good women." In 1782, one doctor went so far as to lend his voice, in a satirical pamphlet, to the unhappy fetuses: "We do not have safe passage into the world. It is with the greatest appre- hension that we dare show ourselves, being continually ill treated by certain women

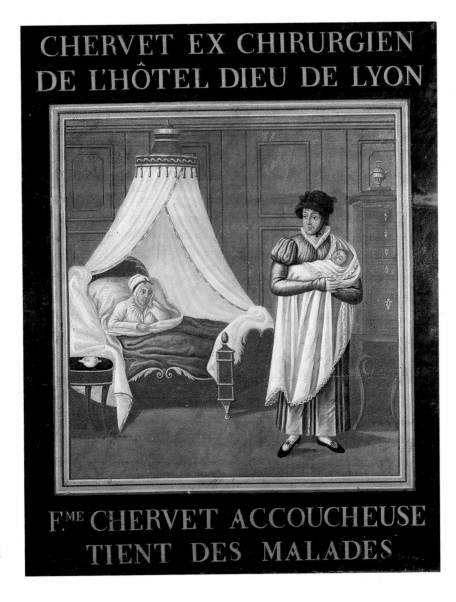

CHERVET EX CHIRURGIEN DE L'HÔTEL DIEU DE LYON

F.^{ME} CHERVET ACCOUCHEUSE TIENT DES MALADES

In wood, in canvas, in japanned tole, midwives have hung out their signs since the sixteenth century. In the nineteenth century, they lit painted lanterns at night, beacons for young women in distress.

ABOVE: Midwife's sign. 19th century. Musée Dauphinois, Grenoble

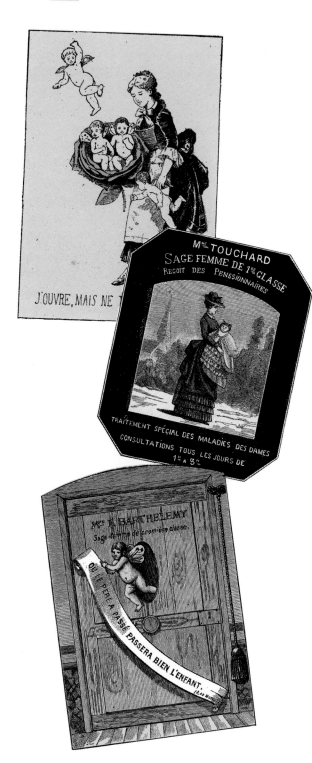

Midwives' signs—decorated with pictures and personalized with mottoes—existed in great variety.

ABOVE: Prints. 19th century

that are called matrons. They murder us, they flay us, they lacerate us pitilessly; often, they treat us even worse: they decapitate us, they give us black eyes, they bruise our limbs, they pull us to pieces; finally, innocent victims, we expire amid all these outrages." Throughout the eighteenth century, the surgeon-obstetricians worked to persuade the public that the midwives were responsible for the high rate of mortality among women and infants during labor. The male doctors came out the big winners of this trial, as evidenced by the decree issued by the parliament of Paris in 1775, which forbade women to practice surgery. Even the moves toward the professional training of midwives served to reinforce the power of the obstetricians.

School for Midwives

In the eighteenth century, the French royal administration, uneasy about the high infant mortality rate, decided to give midwives formal training. Manuals appeared throughout the countryside. The best known, which became a veritable catechism for generations of midwives, was written by the doctor Baudelocque. Parish priests read these manuals to illiterate matrons. An extensive program of classes for midwives was undertaken throughout the kingdom of France. A woman named Madame Angélique Boursier du Coudray was sent by the king to travel the roads of various provinces, where she attempted to inculcate the rudiments of the art of the delivery. To make the principles of obstetrical science understood "even to women of little intelligence," she gave public demonstrations using a mannequin she had fashioned out of wood and cloth. In this way, she trained more than five thousand midwives.

This great enterprise, however, had only a limited effect, for the many illiterate rural women could not benefit from it. Also, as it turned out, almost all the midwives who earned the official certificate issued by Madame du Coudray moved to the cities to serve a wealthy clientele that could afford to pay them. In rural areas, the "good mothers" continued to deliver babies, sometimes into the early part of the twentieth century.

As opposed to the midwife, who exemplified the old ways, the obstetrician symbolized progress; he represented the benefits of an enlightened eighteenth century. Hundreds of obstetrics manuals were published. The guild of surgeons officially separated from that of the barbers; obstetrics became an independent science, distinct from surgery. Maternity hospitals and schools of obstetrics, where anatomy, physiology, and embryology were taught, gradually took root all over Europe. Scientific publications were widely disseminated. At Strasbourg, an obstetrics institution that would become the mother of all those in Europe was founded. In Paris, the first chair in obstetrics, taken by Baudelocque, was established in 1806 and became famous throughout Europe. The century of the Enlightenment was also that of the great obstetricians: Baudelocque in Paris, Deventer in Amsterdam, Fried in

In the fifteenth century, Leonardo da Vinci was fascinated by anatomy and the study of the fetus in utero.

RIGHT: Leonardo da Vinci. *Atlas of Anatomical Studies.* Royal Library, Windsor Castle, Great Britain

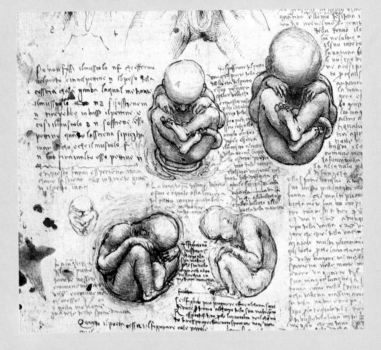

"The number of useless tools has always increased, until we now have dozens of deformities brought on by forceps, retroceps, hooked forceps, etc. Never have women and fetuses been so mechanized as in this century of the mechanical," wrote the outraged Professor Pajot in the nineteenth century.

BELOW: Early forceps

Hooks, Forceps, and Levers: The Obstetric Arsenal

Why did difficult deliveries used to be more common? Many women who had suffered from nutritional deficiencies in their youth had a pelvis deformed by rickets, too narrow or misshapen; it was an opening through which the infant could not pass.

Such deliveries often involved the use of various primitive tools. It should be mentioned that these instruments of torture—the pincers and head-hooks of the doctors, the cruel hooks of the village matron—were reserved for desperate cases, where the life of the mother was at stake. The matron might even grab a tool found in the house—the end of an oil lamp, a ladle, or a fireplace shovel—making use of the hooked end to accomplish a bad piece of work as quickly as possible.

In early-seventeenth-century England, Peter Chamberlen and his sons, all obstet-ric doctors, developed an instrument made of two jointed elements that could be introduced separately into the woman's body to pull out the infant during a diffi-cult childbirth. Working under a sheet, like all their colleagues during this period, they successfully—and jealously—guarded the secret of their invention. One of them, however, finally sold it to Dutch obstetricians, who kept its use to them-selves until the middle of the eighteenth century.

The development of these "iron hands" had a revolutionary effect on obstetrics. It saved the lives of many women in labor as well as their babies, and thus gave obstetricians a clear edge over midwives, who were forbidden to use this tool. In practice, the doctor often hid the forceps from women in labor, who were terrified by the "irons."

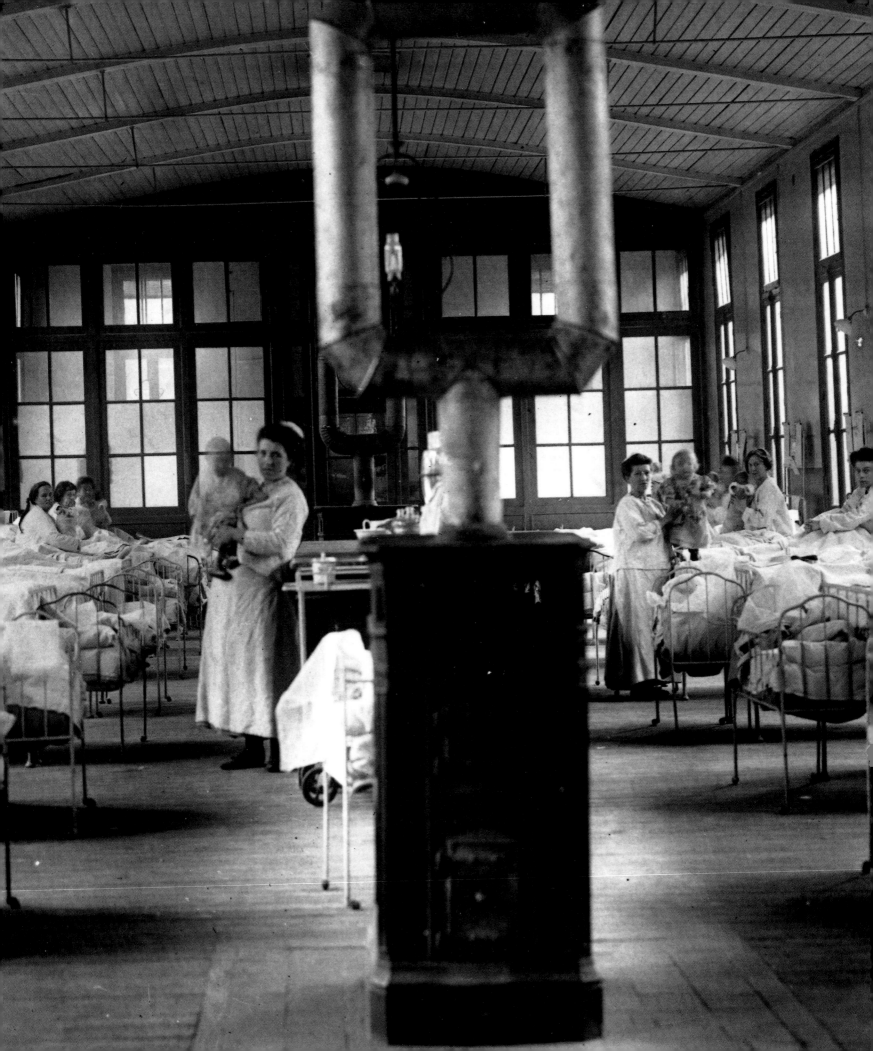

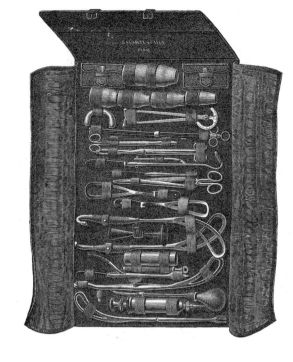

This is what the maternity ward of Port-Royal, in Paris, looked like at the beginning of the century.

LEFT: Photograph. 1910

ABOVE: Obstetric surgical kit. 19th century. Print

Strasbourg, Vespa in Florence, Hunter in England. The European medical student got his training by making a grand tour of the continent's universities. Still, until the nineteenth century, the clientele of these men of science was generally limited to the upper classes of European urban society and remained more numerous in the northern countries than in the southern ones.

"The general arrangement of the Hôtel-Dieu [a Paris hospital] is to put many beds in the wards. The dead are mixed in with the living; in the wards, the air grows stagnant with no means to freshen it, and the light scarcely penetrates, and is heavily laden with moist vapors. The Saint-Joseph ward is devoted to pregnant females. Married or immoral, healthy or sick, they are all brought together here. Three or four in this condition sleep in the same bed, exposed to insomnia and contagion from their diseased neighbors, and in danger of hurting their infants. Women in various stages of labor are crowded four or more to a bed. The heart sinks at the very thought of this situation, in which they infect one another. The majority perish or leave languishing," reported an analysis on the state of the Hôtel-Dieu hospital in 1789.

Since the thirteenth century, the maternity wards of this famous hospital accepted the most disadvantaged women in society. These women became "guinea pigs," on whom all the doctors of the seventeenth and eighteenth centuries cut their teeth, making it possible for this place with deplorable conditions of hygiene to become a great obstetrical teaching center, renowned beyond the borders of

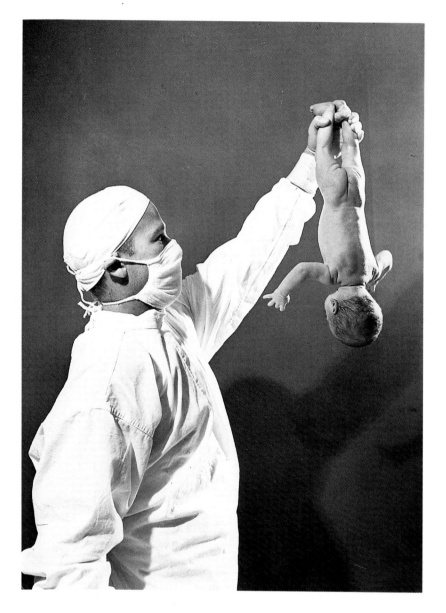

In the 1950s, the newborn baby was held by her ankles.

ABOVE: Photograph

OPPOSITE: Robert Mayne. Photograph

OVERLEAF: Child-care classes for future parents in San Francisco, 1926

France. Following the French Revolution, an attempt was made to improve the fate of the mothers and to create a maternity hospital in the former abbey of Port-Royal. During the nineteenth century, many hospitals established special wards for childbirth.

Puerperal, or childbed, fever was rampant at this time. "The maternity hospital was suffering from one of these terrible epidemics of puerperal fever that blew the breath of mortality over human fertility, a poisoning of the air that emptied itself out as it ran along the rows of beds of women in labor…. One would think it was the plague going by and blackening the faces in a few hours…the black plague of the mothers!" wrote the Goncourt brothers in 1865. Until the end of the nineteenth century, women in maternity wards and hospitals died like flies, exterminated by what was long believed to be a fatal epidemic. Due to this infection alone, one mother in ten did not emerge alive from the hospital.

In 1850, a pioneer obstetrician in Vienna, Phillipp Semmelweis, attempted to demonstrate for the first time that puerperal fever was actually spread by doctors themselves—some would come directly to a childbirth from an autopsy without even disinfecting their hands. Many established doctors denied the microbial origins of puerperal fever and refused to wash their hands before operating. Until Pasteur's work on bacteria, which led to the germ theory of infection, these men could not be convinced of the necessity for aseptic and antiseptic practices, which would eventually put an end to this scourge.

The Medical Delivery

Up to the end of the nineteenth century, and often during the first half of the twentieth, women who had a choice preferred to deliver their babies at home or, eventually, at the residence of approved midwives. Hospital maternity wards contained only very poor or very young expectant mothers and, later, serious cases or those with complications. It has only been in the last fifty years that childbirth at the hospital has become the norm. The progress in obstetrics has allowed childbirth to become more comfortable; in many cases, the focus can now be the pain involved and ways to alleviate it.

For a very long time, all that women could count on to soothe their suffering

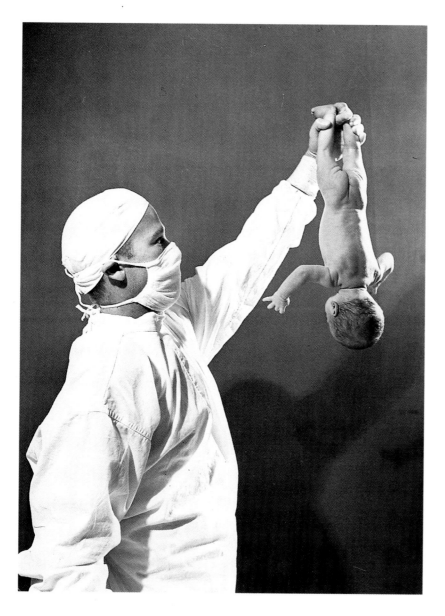

In the 1950s, the newborn baby was held by her ankles.

ABOVE: Photograph

OPPOSITE: Robert Mayne. Photograph

OVERLEAF: Child-care classes for future parents in San Francisco, 1926

France. Following the French Revolution, an attempt was made to improve the fate of the mothers and to create a maternity hospital in the former abbey of Port-Royal. During the nineteenth century, many hospitals established special wards for childbirth.

Puerperal, or childbed, fever was rampant at this time. "The maternity hospital was suffering from one of these terrible epidemics of puerperal fever that blew the breath of mortality over human fertility, a poisoning of the air that emptied itself out as it ran along the rows of beds of women in labor.... One would think it was the plague going by and blackening the faces in a few hours...the black plague of the mothers!" wrote the Goncourt brothers in 1865. Until the end of the nineteenth century, women in maternity wards and hospitals died like flies, exterminated by what was long believed to be a fatal epidemic. Due to this infection alone, one mother in ten did not emerge alive from the hospital.

In 1850, a pioneer obstetrician in Vienna, Phillipp Semmelweis, attempted to demonstrate for the first time that puerperal fever was actually spread by doctors themselves—some would come directly to a childbirth from an autopsy without even disinfecting their hands. Many established doctors denied the microbial origins of puerperal fever and refused to wash their hands before operating. Until Pasteur's work on bacteria, which led to the germ theory of infection, these men could not be convinced of the necessity for aseptic and antiseptic practices, which would eventually put an end to this scourge.

The Medical Delivery

Up to the end of the nineteenth century, and often during the first half of the twentieth, women who had a choice preferred to deliver their babies at home or, eventually, at the residence of approved midwives. Hospital maternity wards contained only very poor or very young expectant mothers and, later, serious cases or those with complications. It has only been in the last fifty years that childbirth at the hospital has become the norm. The progress in obstetrics has allowed childbirth to become more comfortable; in many cases, the focus can now be the pain involved and ways to alleviate it.

For a very long time, all that women could count on to soothe their suffering

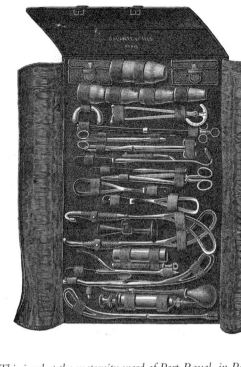

This is what the maternity ward of Port-Royal, in Paris, looked like at the beginning of the century.

LEFT: Photograph. 1910

ABOVE: Obstetric surgical kit. 19th century. Print

Strasbourg, Vespa in Florence, Hunter in England. The European medical student got his training by making a grand tour of the continent's universities. Still, until the nineteenth century, the clientele of these men of science was generally limited to the upper classes of European urban society and remained more numerous in the northern countries than in the southern ones.

"The general arrangement of the Hôtel-Dieu [a Paris hospital] is to put many beds in the wards. The dead are mixed in with the living; in the wards, the air grows stagnant with no means to freshen it, and the light scarcely penetrates, and is heavily laden with moist vapors. The Saint-Joseph ward is devoted to pregnant females. Married or immoral, healthy or sick, they are all brought together here. Three or four in this condition sleep in the same bed, exposed to insomnia and contagion from their diseased neighbors, and in danger of hurting their infants. Women in various stages of labor are crowded four or more to a bed. The heart sinks at the very thought of this situation, in which they infect one another. The majority perish or leave languishing," reported an analysis on the state of the Hôtel-Dieu hospital in 1789.

Since the thirteenth century, the maternity wards of this famous hospital accepted the most disadvantaged women in society. These women became "guinea pigs," on whom all the doctors of the seventeenth and eighteenth centuries cut their teeth, making it possible for this place with deplorable conditions of hygiene to become a great obstetrical teaching center, renowned beyond the borders of

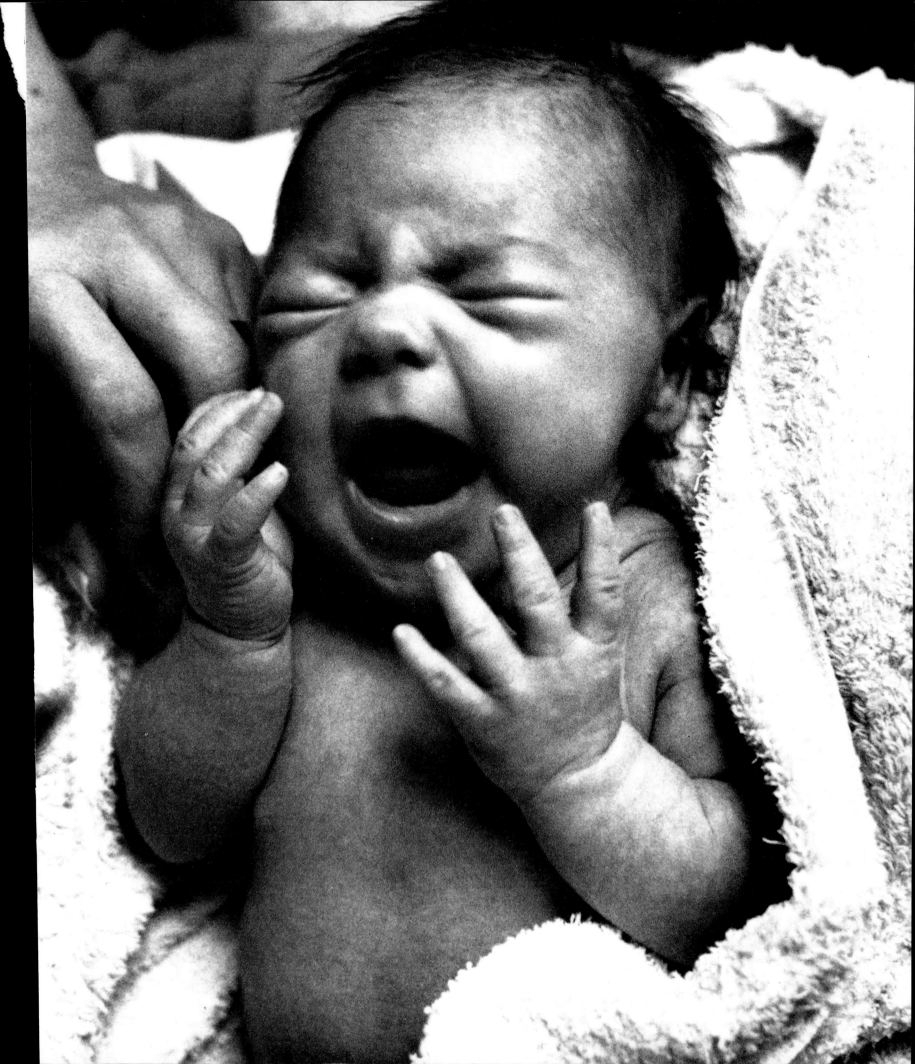

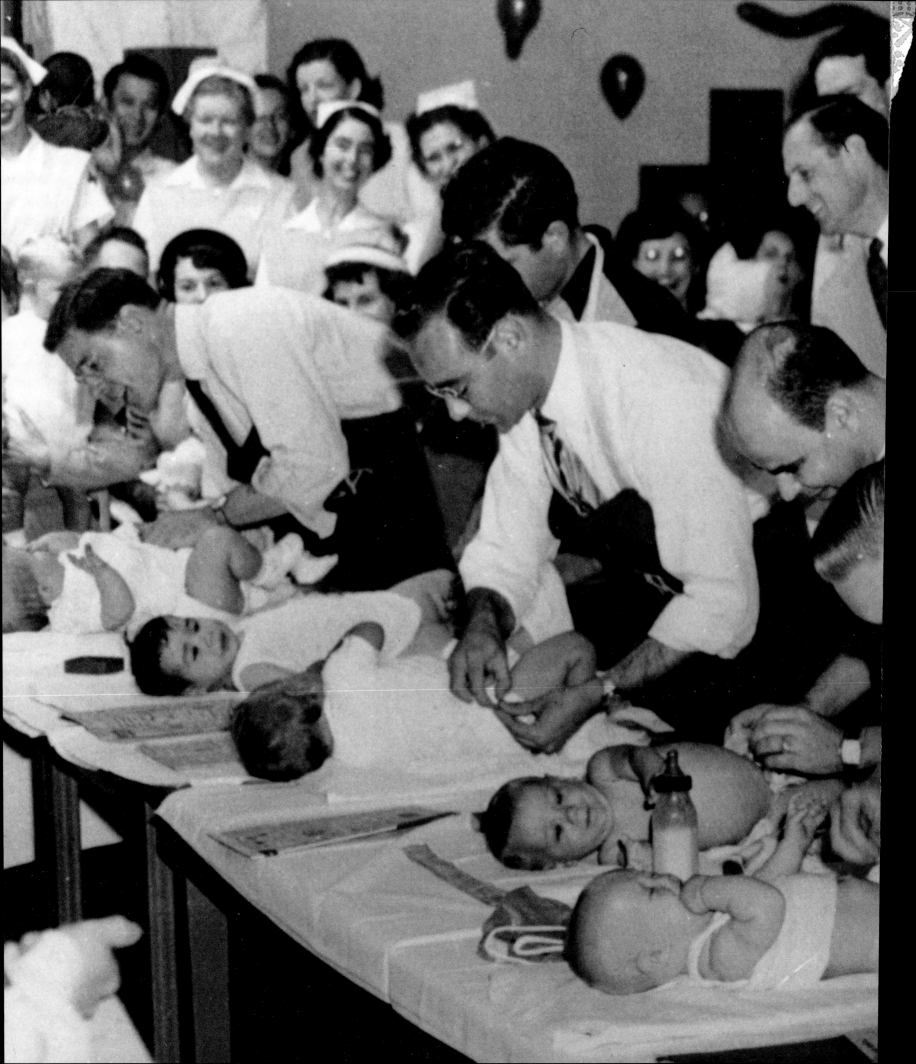

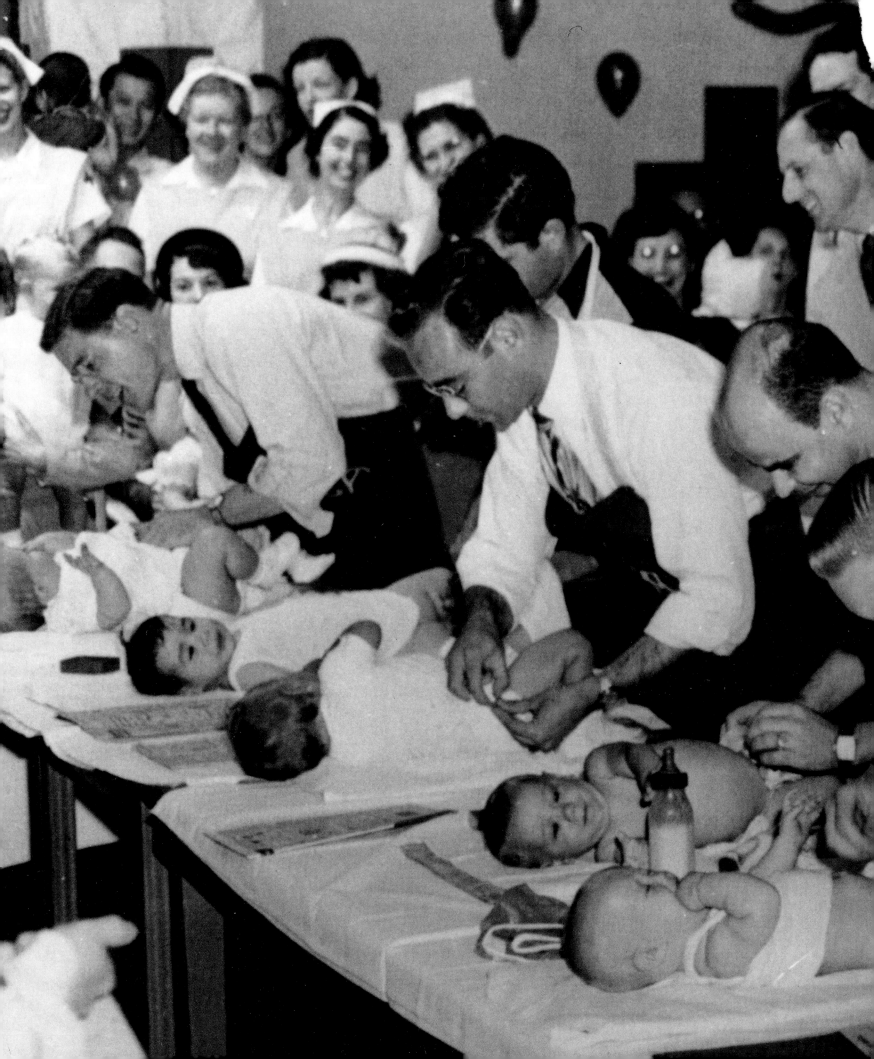

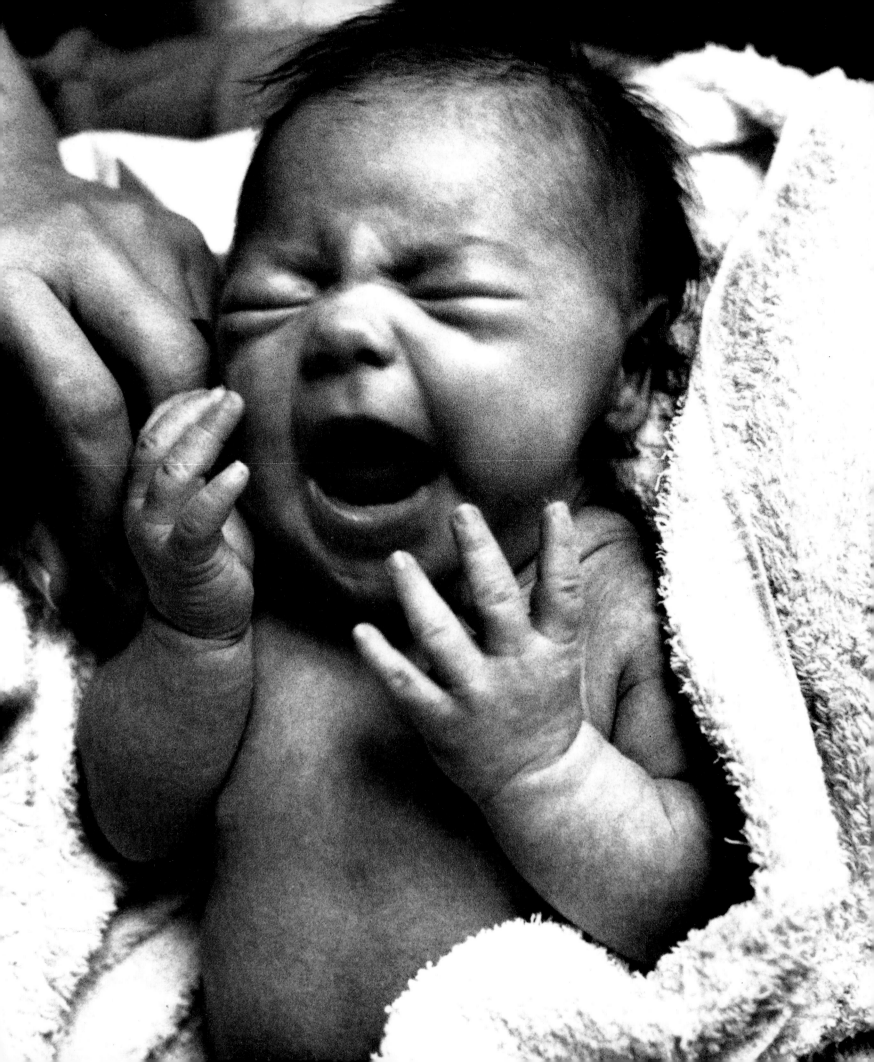

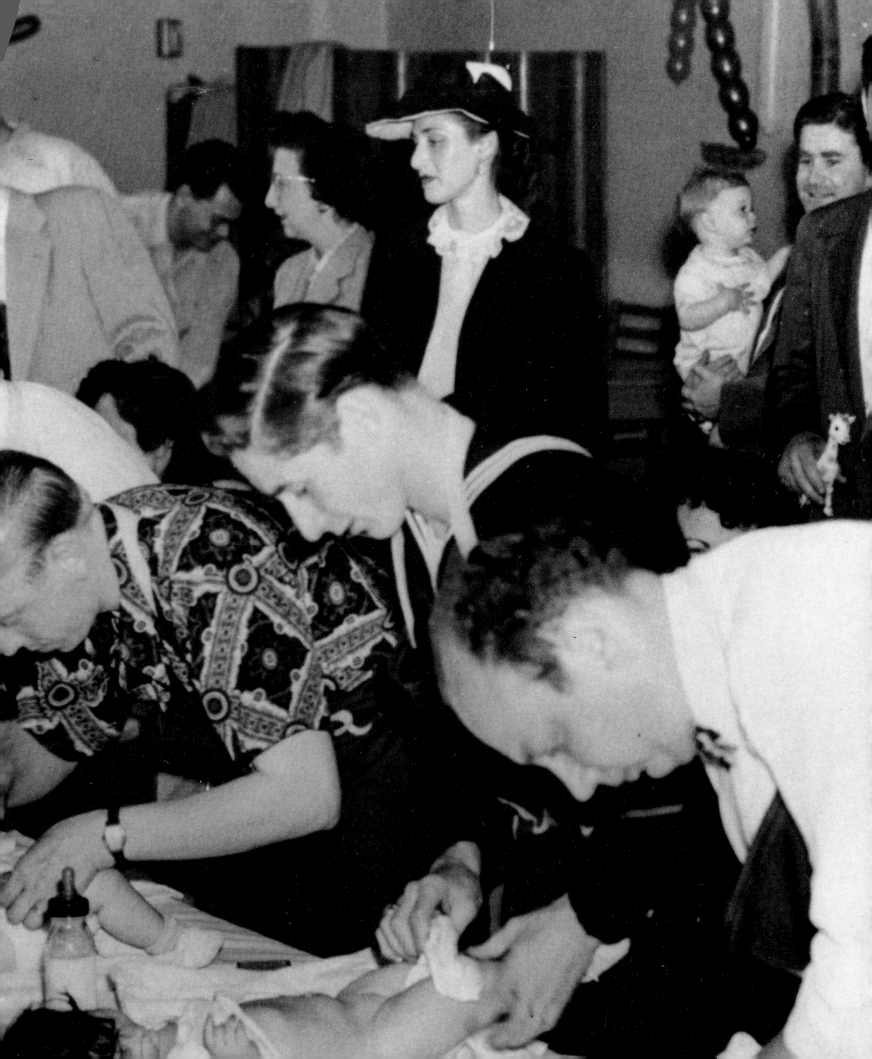

were soft, reassuring words, chunks of salt to crush in their clenched hands, or intoxication, from the wine that matrons often proffered to help make contractions endurable. In mid-nineteenth-century England, deliveries typically began to be carried out under anesthesia, with the help of two substances, ether and chloroform, used for the first time in obstetrics. Queen Victoria was the first woman to be put to sleep with chloroform during labor, for the birth of her eighth child.

In the twentieth century, other analgesics and anesthetics were discovered, including today's epidural. After World War II, obstetrics and pediatrics suddenly made great strides. Gains in hygiene and comfort in hospitals have encouraged expectant mothers to go there. In the 1960s, open wards were divided into rooms holding three or four women. Childbirth education programs such as Lamaze, as well as various relaxation techniques, have been developed to help a laboring woman feel more in control of the event.

Today, many women criticize the sometimes excessive medicalization of childbirth. To many, a hospital birth has become a surgical act in which the woman is hooked up to a monitor and stretched out on a table under glaring lights and the stares of two or three strangers, her feet in stirrups. The typical labor and delivery—and everything surrounding them—have indeed changed, and not all the changes have been for the good. For this reason, a tendency toward the humanization of hospital deliveries has been emerging over the last two decades. In creating a softened, quieter atmosphere, in placing the newborn infant on the mother's stomach, in generally demedicalizing the experience, some hospitals and birthing centers are seeking to establish—or reestablish—around childbirth an environment in which tenderness, security, and emotion carry as much weight as medical techniques.

The epidural anesthetic was described for the first time by the American Dr. Corning in 1885. After being rediscovered in 1901 in the Tenon hospital by two French doctors, it once again fell into oblivion. It came into use in obstetrics after 1970.

BELOW: Maternity cards for French Social Security

OPPOSITE: Newborn. Photograph

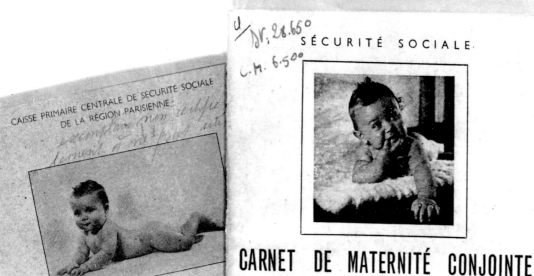

SÉCURITÉ SOCIALE

CARNET DE MATERNITÉ CONJOINTE

CAISSE PRIMAIRE CENTRALE DE SECURITÉ SOCIALE DE LA RÉGION PARISIENNE

CARNET DE MATERNITÉ ASSURÉE

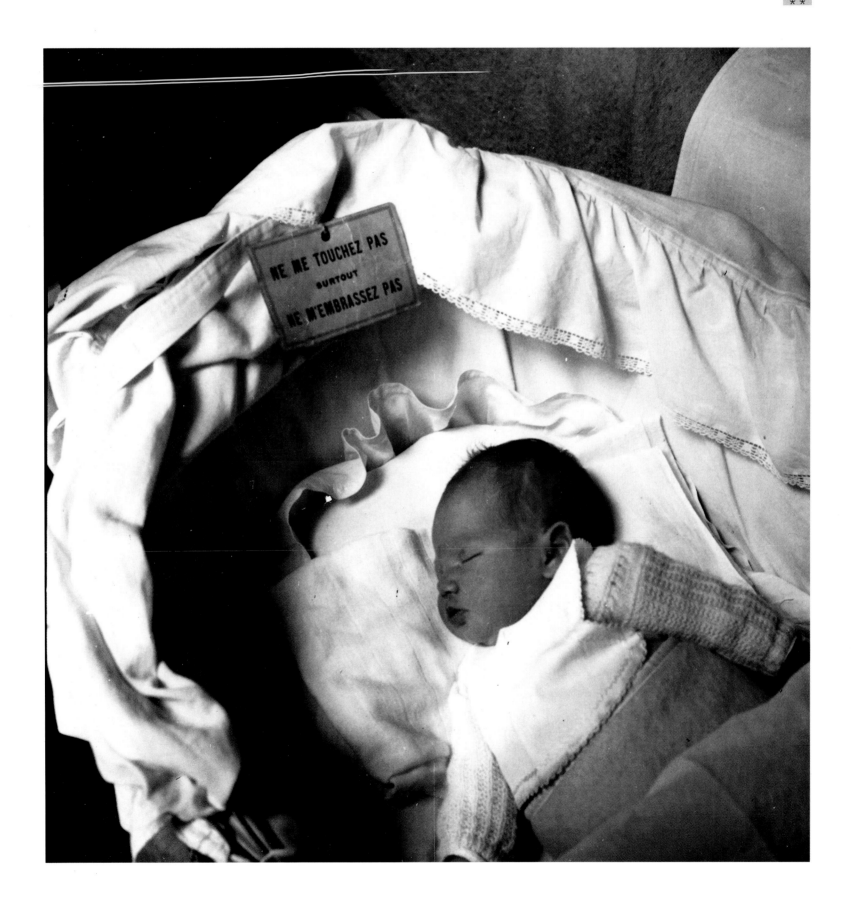

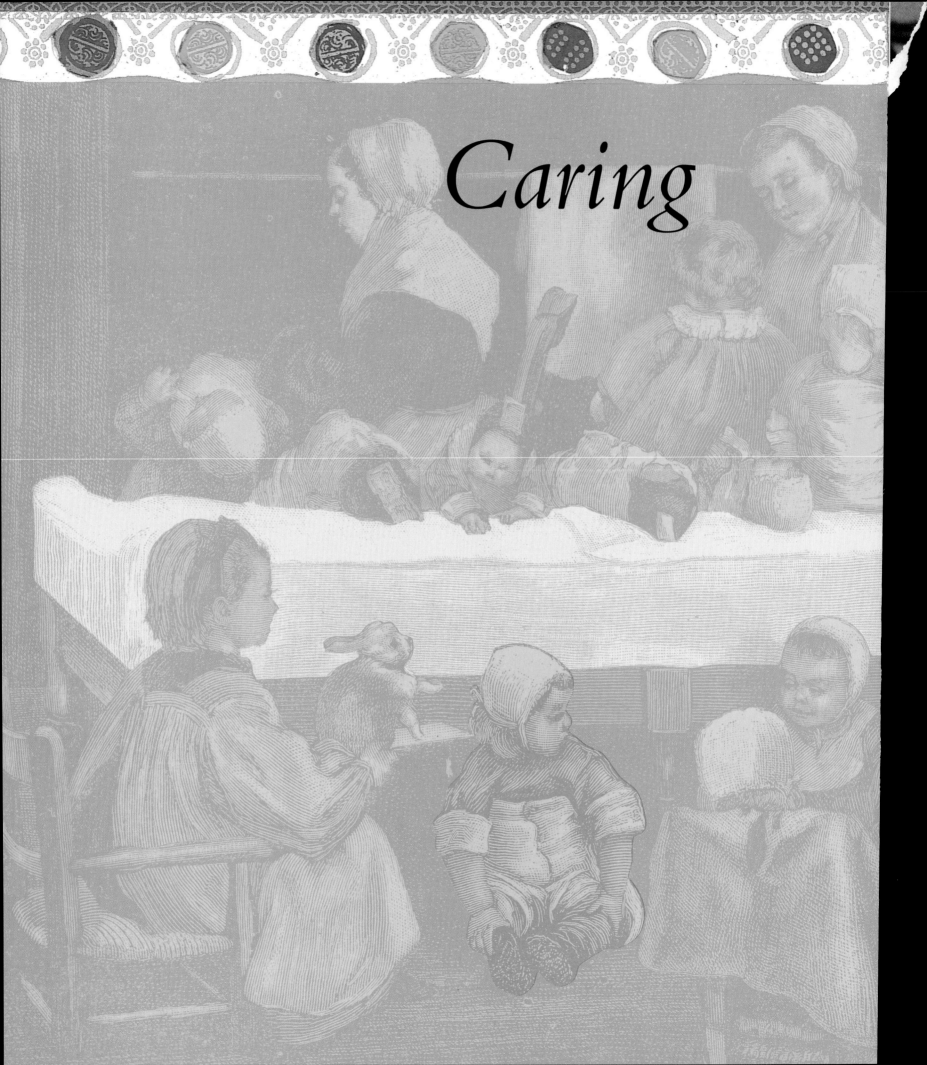

Caring

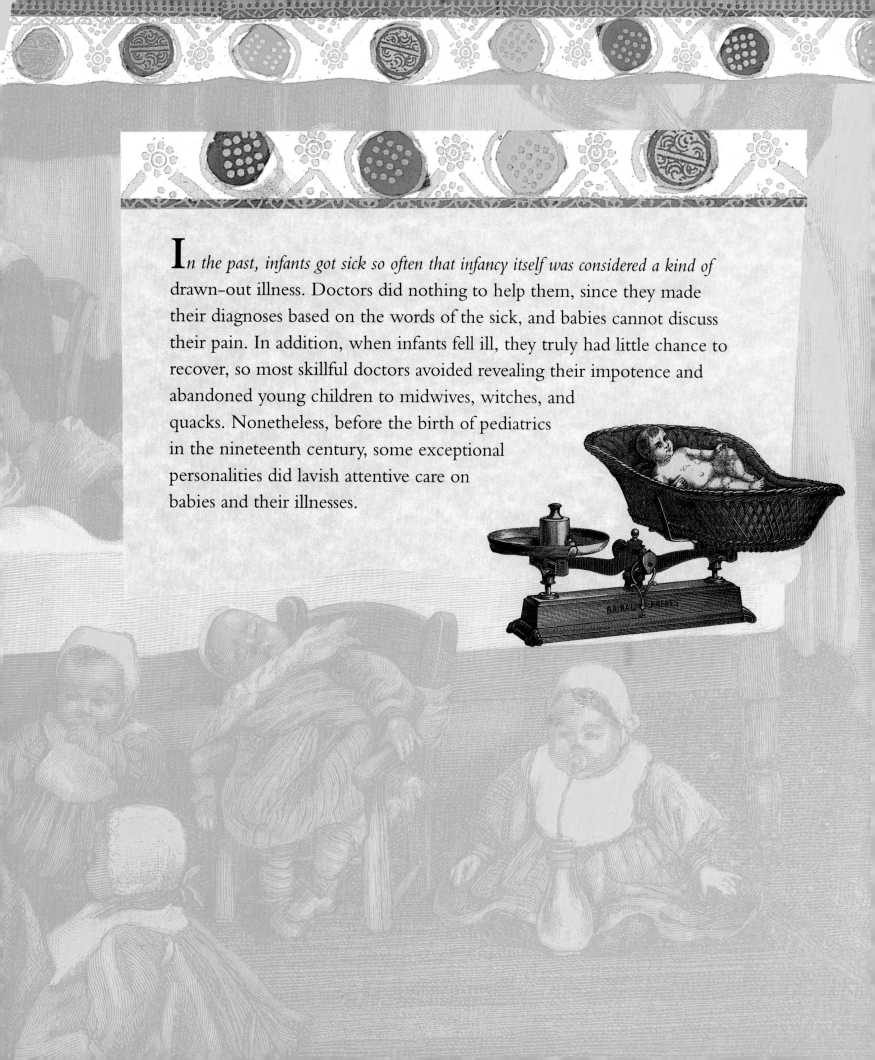

In the past, infants got sick so often that infancy itself was considered a kind of drawn-out illness. Doctors did nothing to help them, since they made their diagnoses based on the words of the sick, and babies cannot discuss their pain. In addition, when infants fell ill, they truly had little chance to recover, so most skillful doctors avoided revealing their impotence and abandoned young children to midwives, witches, and quacks. Nonetheless, before the birth of pediatrics in the nineteenth century, some exceptional personalities did lavish attentive care on babies and their illnesses.

From Cooked Mouse to Antibiotics

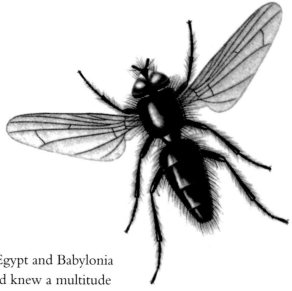

The matriarchal civilizations of ancient Egypt and Babylonia handled babies with great gentleness and knew a multitude of remedies to treat them. Those revealed in Egyptian papyruses add a large dose of magic to many standard ingredients. To treat urinary infections, an old roll of papyrus cooked in oil was smeared on the baby's belly. In desperate cases, the baby had to ingest a cooked mouse. The bones of the animal, preserved in a cloth, were hung from the sick one's little neck. Poppy mixed with wasp droppings calmed a crying infant. Newborns wore stones with curative powers—lapis lazuli, jasper, malachite—around their necks. According to Herodotus, Egyptian doctors were highly specialized; there seemed to be a doctor for every illness. In Babylonia, a demon was attributed to every pain: Utukku was responsible for sore throats, and Labartu victimized mainly women and newborns. An incantatory magic formula on a papyrus dated about 1450 B.C. orders the demon of the illness and of death to leave the body of the threatened infant: "Disappear, ghost who emerges from the shadows, who enters on the sly. Have you come to kiss this child? I will not allow you to kiss him. Have you come to calm him? I will not allow you to calm him. Have you come to harm him? I will not allow you to harm him. Have you come to take him? I will not allow you to take him." In their preventive medicine, Babylonians and Egyptians paid particular attention to insects. Crushing flies, those vectors of fevers so fatal to babies, was a veritable institution for these peoples. Mothers and servants chased after them relentlessly with their flyswatters.

Medications from Antiquity

While newborn babies of Greek or Roman antiquity might legally be killed or abandoned, once they were accepted by their parents, they were cared for attentively. Barley, honey, dates, figs, and olive oil or oil of roses—these were the ingredients of the Mediterranean civilizations' perfumed medications. Soranus of Ephesus detailed the ills specific to babies and prescribed mild remedies. For thrush, he advised painting the mouth with a balm of lentils or a pomade of poppies, and he criticized the custom of Syrian nurses, who twined hair around a finger and then dipped it in milk and honey, which they used to clean the ulcers. He praised the use of poultices of chicory or barley powder to treat rashes and itching. Inflammation of the tonsils was treated with toasted cumin, applied under the chin. For babies cutting their first teeth, a long massage with chicken fat soothed irritated gums. If the pain was too strong for this remedy, Soranus gave instructions to surround the baby's head and jaw with soft, clean woolens and to pass olive oil and warm sponges over the gums. A baby with a bad cough would be given lozenges made with pine nuts, licorice juice, and toasted almonds to suck on.

Some ancient doctors evidently concerned themselves with care specifically for babies; the Roman Celsus already recognized that infants should not be given the same care as adults. Others expressed doubts about certain treatments, inspired more by superstition than by common sense. Pliny the Elder seemed dubious on the subject of a treatment intended for hernias in infants: "Take a male lizard, set it to chew the affected part through a gold, silver, or purple fabric, then with a reed hang it in a fireplace above the smoke. When it dies, the infant is cured."

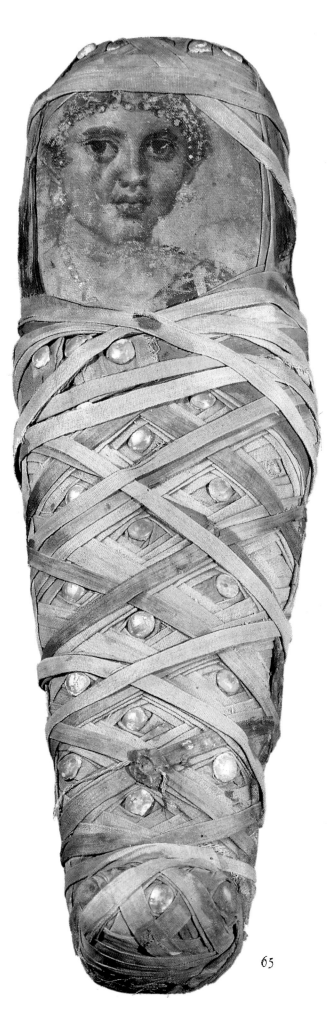

A Roman epitaph reads: "Here lies lamented a very young girl, extremely sweet. She lived six months and eight days; a rose, she flowered and faded in the same moment."

RIGHT: Mummy with funerary portrait of a child. 1st–4th centuries A.D. Egyptian Museum, Berlin. Photograph: Erich Lessing/Magnum

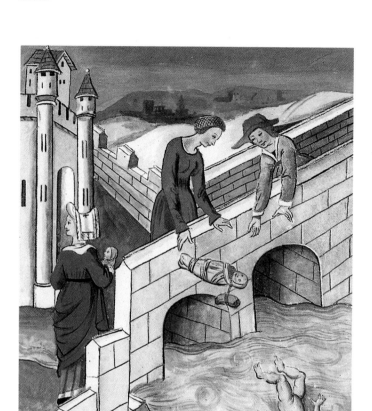

In Rome, women threw unwanted children into the Tiber. The pope's servants were charged with saving them and putting them in a foundling hospital.

ABOVE AND BELOW: Miniatures copied from a 15th-century manuscript. Bibliothèque Nationale, Paris

The devil replaces an infant with a demonic creature in an Italian-style cradle that rocks from front to back.

OPPOSITE: Martino Di Bartolomeo (1389–1434). *The Life of Saint Stephen.* Städel Museum, Frankfurt

The Healing Saints

The Madonna and Child was one of the most popular subjects in medieval art. The many painters who depicted these tender scenes, very grounded in reality, displayed a real solicitude for the small child. In fact, people of the time tried to protect children with a variety of magic charms; "preventive medicine" in the Middle Ages made use of all sorts of amulets. The baby was embellished with crosses, animal teeth, pieces of coral, sachets containing plant seeds or mole paws, garlic necklaces…all intended to stave off the two great woes of infancy: toothache and the worms that were thought to weaken babies' fragile bodies, bringing on fevers and convulsions. In reality, infantile cholera and respiratory diseases were the principal causes of death among very young children—and wolves' teeth did little to fight them. Skin ailments were both more common and less fatal. Babies suffering from diaper rash had their derrieres left exposed to the air, dried by the heat of the fire, or wrapped in a dirty cleaning cloth said to have therapeutic qualities.

When a child fell seriously ill, however, parents found themselves with no recourse. A third of all European children died before the age of five. Only the urban wealthy could afford to call in doctors. People who lived in the country placed their faith less in remedies made from plants and more in saints, the first pediatricians of Christianity. Thus, as soon as a child became ill, parents closed up shop, abandoned their worldly goods, and went off on a pilgrimage. Saint Apotheme, Saint Gibrian, Saint Blaise, Saint Nicholas, Saint Louis—on whose tombs sick children were laid down—were some of the saints specializing in protecting children. The most unusual, undoubtedly, was Saint Guinefort, a healing saint who was none other than a dog. His powers were linked with the disturbing concept of the changeling: when French peasants saw their child burning up with a fever, growing weak, and crying, they wanted to believe that it was no longer their child but a creature put in its place by forest sprites. So they prayed to Saint Guinefort, a greyhound killed while defending its young, to compel the devil to give back their real baby. If the child survived, the sprite was defeated. If the child died, the mother had the odd consolation of believing that the child who had perished was not her own. In the thirteenth century, the Church started to

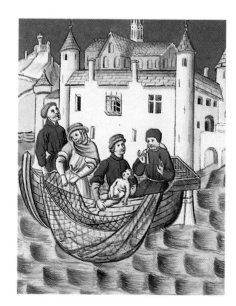

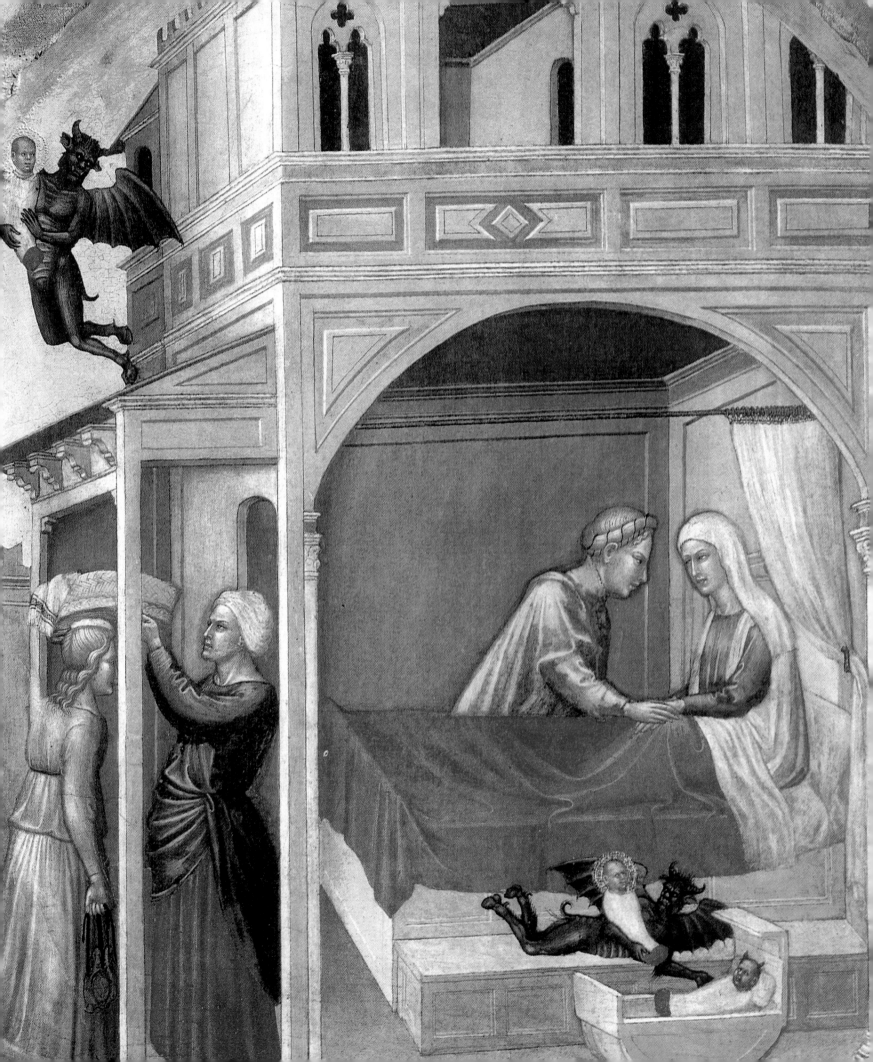

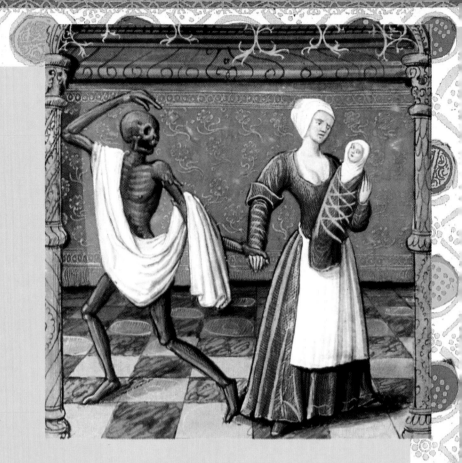

Worms, Enemy of the Infant

"What a great number of illnesses I noticed right away! As on the sandy dunes of Libya that intersect the eddying Nagrada stream, the Numidian hunter who strays onto these desert banks or enters an extremely thick wood notices a multitude of ferocious beasts. On one side, a lion with a terrifying face, there a cruel tiger, here a leopard, and on the other side, a dragon with glistening skin and monsters bred by a mixture of snakes of different species: hesitating, he looks all about him and not knowing of all these monsters which he ought to attack and which to avoid, he remains motionless; in the same way, a great number of illnesses presented themselves to my mind, which, not knowing which to start with nor which to end with, I remain in doubt.... I must speak to you of worms, known for a similar peril in which they also place infants, of these dangerous worms, strange

kinds of poisons, which by cruel bites pick away at the guts when the child is filled with milk, which grows tainted in his stomach, and which from there passes into the abdomen, where it fastens itself to the intestines like moss that cannot be removed. Wise nature then takes recourse in art. Working hard to overwhelm that which it cannot drive away, from these same impurities it produces worms, which spread throughout the intestines. But before these insects have devoured everything in their path, they apply their voracity to the entrails by means of dangerous bites.... This is why it is essential to kill such enemies. With worm powder that you mix with sweet apples in the pap. Mix as well some cumin with gall of beef and make a poultice that you place on the infant's belly."

Scévole de Sainte-Marthe,
Paedotrophia, 1680

To cure the infant, doctors often treated the nurse or the mother. During deadly epidemics, however, both adult and child were often struck down, and death then led away this fragile and indissoluble couple.

ABOVE: The dance of death. 15th century. Miniature. Bibliothèque Nationale, Paris

fight this belief. It could take the idea of the changeling in stride, but it balked at the notion of a saint with four paws. It had the animal dug up, burned the woods where the rituals were practiced, and forbade the cult. However, six centuries later, Saint Guinefort became popular once more.

While the Church played a repressive role in fighting such superstitious practices, there is an area in which its intervention had a positive and lasting effect on the history of children's medicine: the establishment of the foundling hospital. In 787, Datheus, archbishop of Milan, founded the first asylum for abandoned infants. Others were later opened in Montpellier (1010), Marseilles (1190), Venice (1380), and Florence (1421). In 1198, Pope Innocent III, moved by the number of corpses of babies found in the Tiber river, devoted a section of the Santa Maria hospital to the care of foundlings. All of these refuges open to orphans served as the fore-runners of the first children's hospitals.

The First Pediatric Texts

In the Middle Ages, not a single book was devoted to pediatrics. The care of children, however, made up key chapters in treatises on medicine. This was due not to a misunderstanding of the nature of childhood, but instead to the encyclopedic spirit of the time, which linked together the realms of knowledge rather than dividing them up. With the development of printing and the growth of knowledge, doctors throughout Europe published a new type of work. A far cry from the books of the medieval compilers, these tomes judged the medical writings of antiquity with a somewhat more critical eye. Nonetheless, working parallel to popular medicine, steeped in symbolic and magical treatments, the "scientific" medicine of the early Renaissance prescribed for children enemas, bloodletting, purges, emetics, diets, and potions. Some authors gave evidence of more sensitivity and observation. Simon de Vallambert, in his book *Manière de nourrir et de gouverner les enfants dès leur naissance* (How to Nurture and Regulate Children from Their Birth), published in 1565, accurately described the sick child: "He cannot hold up his head straight, leaning it on his shoulders or on the person holding him; and if he always wants to be carried and does not want to stay in his cradle, and if, while being carried, he tosses about, wants, does not want, to be put down, wants to be held and walked all the time, does not want that at all, and if he is sung to or caressed he grows annoyed, taking no pleasure in the songs or the caresses, one could reasonably guess that the child is sick." When caring for breast-fed

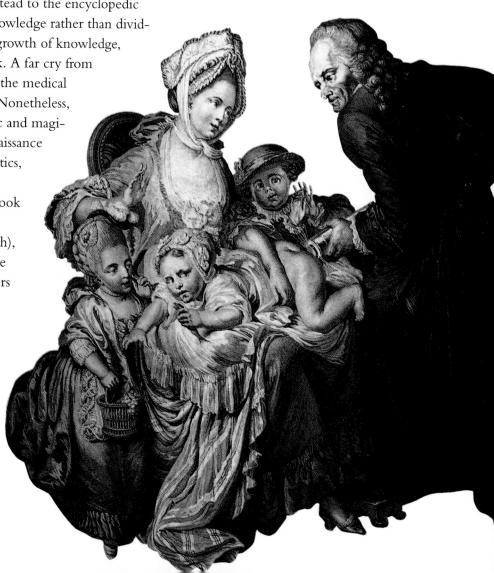

In 1565, Vallambert, who in many other ways seemed to be far ahead of his time, said it was necessary to give children enemas and suppositories, following the policy of the authors of antiquity.

BELOW: Print. 18th century. Bibliothèque Nationale, Paris

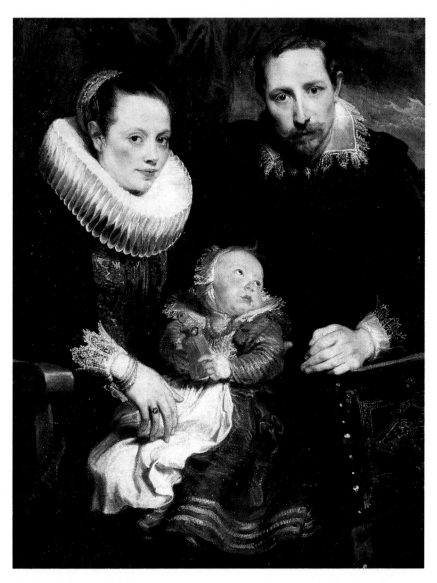

infants, Vallambert preferred to treat the wet nurse, who served as a sort of filter for medications. For those who had been weaned, he stated that "one should be sure that medicines given to children not taste unpleasant or horrible, because if they flatly refuse to take them or conceive a dislike for them, they do more harm than good." For fevers, he directed parents to make sure not to give their children too little to eat, to see that they were not overheated, to make them drink water or infusions often, to give them baths, and to induce sweating. He approved of bloodletting—for the wet nurse! For smallpox and measles, he prescribed orange or lemon juice and pomegranate wine in a fruit salad. The child with measles would be wrapped in a red blanket or a scarlet sheet, or perhaps in a winding-sheet dampened with decoctions of fig and fennel. Bowls of hot water were put in the bed "while the face and the nose of the patient had to be gently fanned, lest he falls into a faint from the heat." In order to protect the eyes from smallpox pustules, the doctor rubbed the eyebrows with acacia and aloes with a bit of saffron and put an eyewash of coriander in the eyes. He recommended treating the pustules with fresh butter or the fat from boiled lard, for "when the pustules of smallpox are very ripe, they can be lanced with a gold or silver needle." It was right to fight against smallpox, for it caused many fatalities and left survivors horribly disfigured.

In Some Thoughts Concerning Education *(1693), John Locke warned that parents should not be too quick to call a doctor when their children were sick. He felt that children should be given the least amount of medicine possible.*

ABOVE: Anthony Van Dyck. *Portrait of a Family.* 17th century. Hermitage, St. Petersburg

OPPOSITE: Print. 18th century. Bibliothèque Nationale, Paris

The "Republic of Children"

In the seventeenth century, science made some impressive breakthroughs: the circulation of blood was described; microscopy was introduced; and the physiology of digestion as well as respiration was unraveled. However, the chapter on children's medicine contained nothing new. This time, a period of religious strife, major epidemics, and serious famine in Europe, imposed extremely difficult living conditions on children, many of whom were abandoned wholesale or mutilated, so that they would be more effective beggars. Holland, the "Republic of Children" (according to historian Simon Schama), offered a notable exception. The first popular books on child-rearing in the modern mode appeared there, in relatively inexpensive editions. Attacks of cholera, emergency treatments, and toilet training—not to mention the first games—were all discussed. Even before Western medicine had the least idea of the role played by vitamins, some Dutch doctors knew that the best way to cure rickets was to increase the consumption of fresh fruits and vegetables.

In Colonial America, the death rate was enormous. Children were often expected to die in infancy and early childhood, and many families lost more than half of their children. In eighteenth-century France, philosophers exalted new values: nature, freedom, and maternal love. Chardin and Greuze painted scenes of family intimacy. Doctors concerned themselves more practically with the "preservation of children," for even in the seventeenth century, one child in four did not live past its first year. Starting in the 1750s, infant pathology aroused a real and sustained interest. The contribution of English doctors— Cadogan, Armstrong, Underwood—marked the history of pediatrics, culminating at the end of the century with Edward Jenner and his development of a vaccine, the first effective protection against smallpox, which was ravaging Europe. Nonetheless, Jean-Jacques Rousseau gave an overwhelmingly grim description of the state of children's health in *L'Emile*: "[Nature] continually trains children. It toughens their constitution with all manner of tests, it teaches them early on what pain and suffering are like: their emergent teeth bring them fever; acute colics bring them convulsions; fits of coughing leave them choking; worms cause them distress; plethora infects their blood; various germs ferment in them and bring them dangerous rashes. Almost the entire early life is taken up with illness and danger." Thus, the London physician William Cadogan, an army surgeon, evinced pleasure in his book *An Essay upon Nursing, and the Management of Children* that "the Preservation of Children [has] become the Care of Men of Sense." He considered it a mistake to leave children in the care of women who did not have the education and knowledge to carry out their task properly. He

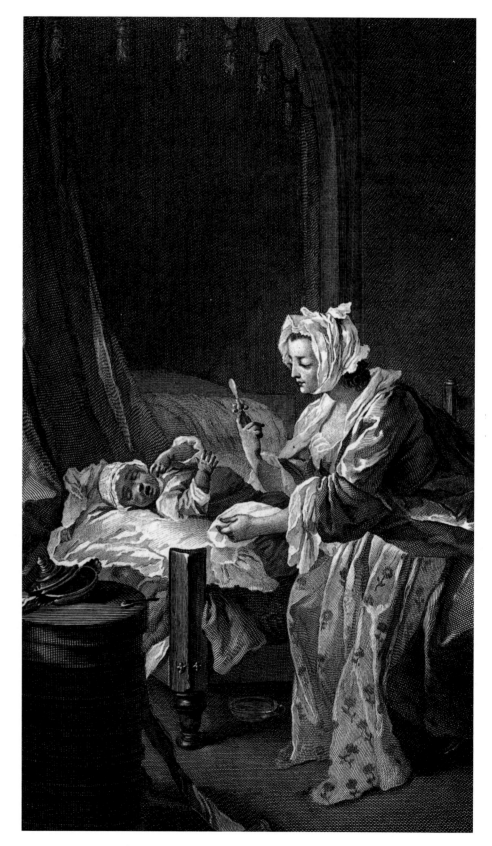

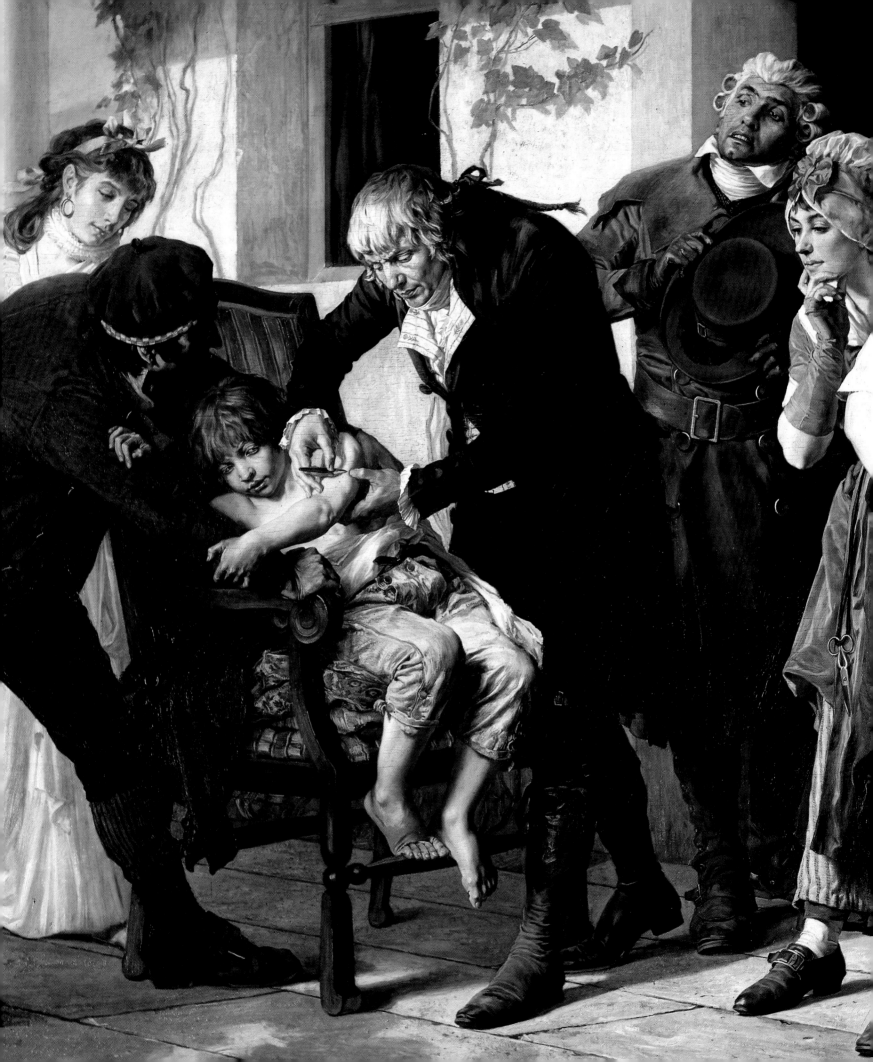

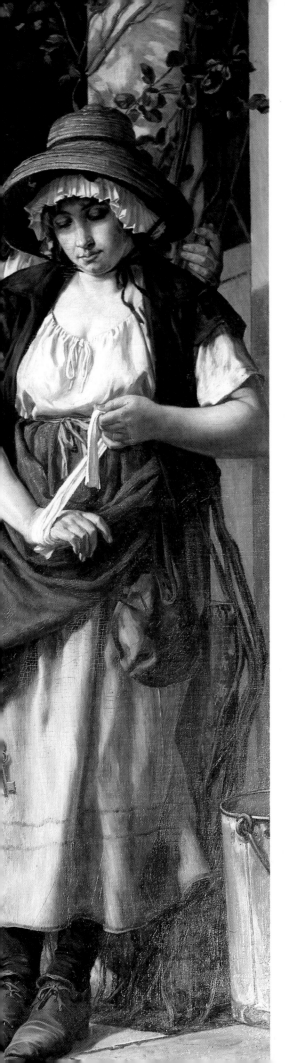

noted the large gap between the way children were raised among the common people and among the wealthy: "The Mother who has only a few Rags to cover her Child loosely, and little more than her own Breast to feed it, sees it healthy and strong, and very soon able to shift for itself; while the puny Insect, the Heir and Hope of a rich Family lies languishing under a Load of Finery, that overpowers his Limbs, abhorring and rejecting the Dainties he is crammed with, till he dies a Victim to the mistaken Care and Tenderness of his fond Mother."

Smoke and Drink

Until the middle of the seventeenth century, resuscitating a newborn was not the province of doctors. When they did intervene, they used midwives' techniques, which sometimes worked. The midwife took wine or brandy into her mouth and blew it in the baby's mouth or sprayed the baby's face. Louis XIII was very weak at birth, and the midwife Louise Bourgeois turned to Henri IV and said, "Sire, if this was another baby, I would put wine in my mouth and give it to him for fear that his weakness would last too long." The king answered, "Act as you would toward another." She did, and the infant came to. To warm the baby, the midwife might lay the placenta, sometimes fried in a pan with wine, on his stomach. She might rub the newborn with cider, vinegar, or brandy. She might blow tobacco smoke into his lungs. She might tickle the soles of his feet with the feather of a quill.

A new willingness to save the lives of newborns appeared more clearly at the beginning of the eighteenth century. Mauriceau was among the first French authors to devote a chapter specifically to resuscitation, especially to condemning certain methods, such as placing a clove of garlic or a piece of onion in the newborn's mouth, as well as placing the placenta on the baby's stomach, as its weight worked against the establishment of good breathing. Nicolas Saucerotte noted in one of his books, "I had the great happiness to recall to life a great number of infants who seemed to be dead on coming into the world, by blowing air into their lungs, rubbing them, tickling them, and exciting their organs of smell and taste." Before the eighteenth century, all efforts had been focused on saving the mother. With the progress in obstetrics, including the development of forceps, mothers finally had a better chance to survive. This encouraged doctors to turn their attention to the newborn.

In the eighteenth century, smallpox terrorized parents, carrying off one in ten babies each year. In 1796, Jenner discovered that the vaccine protected the recipient from the full-fledged form of the disease.

LEFT: Mélingue. *Jenner's First Vaccination.* 1879. Académie de Médecine, Paris

A sick child would be immersed in the water of a spring said to have miraculous powers. If the baby balked, his mother would wet his blouse in the spring and put it on him later. Clothing could also help to make a prediction. In Brittany, for example, parents placed the blouse on the surface of the water. If it floated, the child's illness would turn out to be benign; if it sank to the bottom, her days were numbered. However, the parents could always choose to interpret the outcome in a way that left some hope of their child's recovery.

RIGHT: Eugène Fines. *Spring of Miracles.* 19th century. Musée des Jacobins, Morlaix

OPPOSITE: Saint Nicholas. 18th-19th century. Print

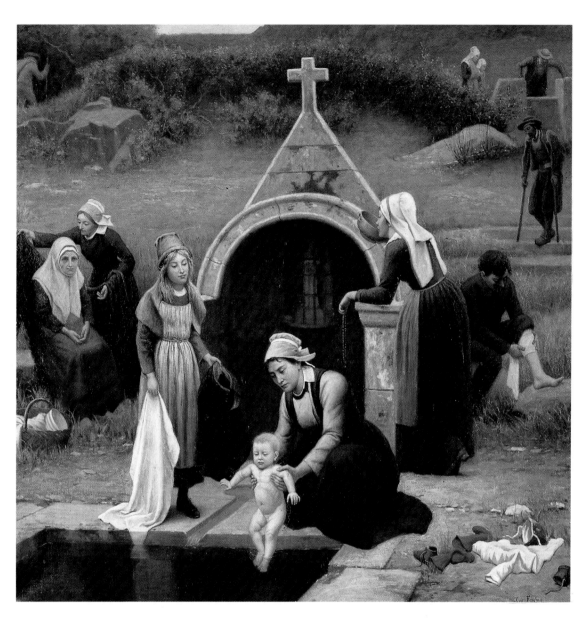

Magic Springs and Dust of Saints

Until the end of the nineteenth century, popular medicine—obviously much denounced by the medical establishment, which produced its share of both progress and errors—continued to wrap the baby in a bundle of magic protections. The role such remedies played was far from minor, for they enabled the parents of sick children to have hope, a critical element in the process of healing. As in the Middle Ages, pilgrimages and prayers to saints remained a major focus. When a seriously ill child revived, parents dedicated her to the Virgin Mary or the saint who saved her. Saint Quintin specialized in coughs and whooping cough, a terrible disease among infants; Saint Blaise in sore throats; Saint Apollonia in toothaches; and Saint Nicholas in stomach upsets (infantile diarrhea often proved fatal). A baby suffering from colic had her stomach measured with a skein of thread, which was next passed around the neck of a statue of Saint Nicholas in the church. Or a bit of dust from the stomach of the statue was mixed with broth. To guard against worms, thought to eat at, prick, enfeeble, and even "piss on the heart" of the baby, parents gave their babies garlic to eat (they also wore a collar of garlic), wine to drink, and a poultice of worms on their stomach; and, most important, parents prayed to Saint Medard. Ailing babies—or, in their place, others wearing their clothes—were also plunged into the water of springs said to have miraculous powers.

Crystal Teething Rings or Moles' Paws

In all periods, teething, a crucial phase in the baby's development, has been a time parents dread. Exhausted, babies became vulnerable to the many ailments that could besiege them, such as diarrhea and bronchitis. To guard against these ailments, parents hung a sachet from the baby's neck that contained the paw of a mole killed in a particularly cruel way: first a wire was run through it, and then it was decapitated. The mole's suffering was intended to replace that of the baby. The symbolic value of this animal doubtlessly derived from the fact that it possesses sharp teeth and that it digs its path underground, like the tooth that pierces the gum. Babies also wore teething necklaces, originally made from stalks of ivy or peony roots, long enough to be chewed. The wealthy used nobler materials—coral or amber—which possessed prophylactic qualities. Infants also chewed on teething rings, sometimes set with a wolf's tooth, sometimes made of crystal. Ambroise Paré observed that wet nurses added small bells to these rings, so the baby could "play" with them. Bells, sometimes hung over the cradle, had the additional role of keeping evil spirits away. Amber necklaces were thought to give protection from croup and prevent irritations in the folds of the neck. A piece of toasted rye put into the mouth and changed every day absorbed all the evil spells cast against the newborn. A coin given to the infant to touch was wrapped and hidden under a stone; a passerby who picked it up would become saddled with the ailment. In fact, in many cases, a remedy consisted of transferring the ailment to a symbolic object.

Children Lost and Found

At the end of the eighteenth century, more than five thousand children arrived every year at Paris foundling hospitals. Louis Sébastien Mercier gave a dismal

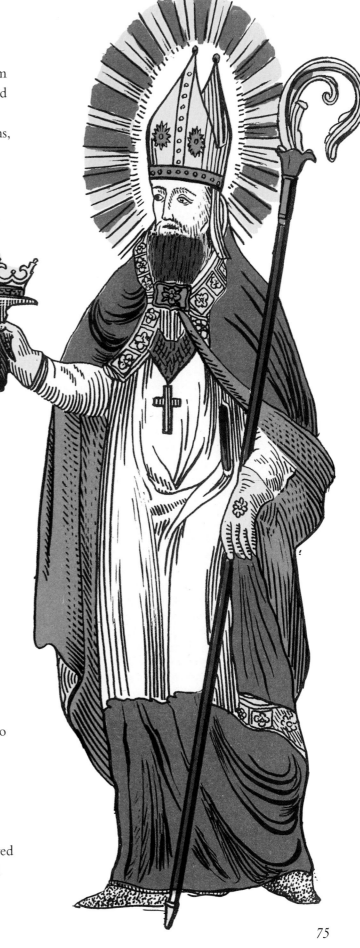

With the aid of some great aristocratic ladies, Vincent de Paul established the Paris foundling hospital and became a legendary figure in the history of children.

description of one way in which babies were taken to these institutions: "A man carries on his back newborn infants in a padded box that can hold three. They stand in their swaddling clothes, breathing air from above. The man stops only to eat his meals and make them suck a bit of milk. When he opens the box, he often finds one baby dead, so he finishes his journey with the two remaining, eager to get rid of his load." These surviving babies arrived at the hospital only half living, and barely one in ten survived. At the beginning of the nineteenth century, the toll of fatalities was so high that an author of the period proposed to have engraved over the hospital doors, "Here, infants are killed at public expense." The asylums and foundling hospitals, with their appalling concentration of sick babies, offered doctors a large field of study.

In the nineteenth century, poverty diminished in France, but societal pressure compelled very young mothers, often servants abused by their master, to deposit their newborns in secret in a foundling hospital "tower." This system, involving a kind of revolving tray, was developed to protect the babies from intemperate weather and preserve the anonymity of the mothers, who would settle the baby in its little

Monsieur Vincent

LEFT: Saint Vincent de Paul. Print. Musée de l'Assistance Publique, Paris

OPPOSITE ABOVE: Abandoned child. 19th century. Print. Musée Carnavalet, Paris

OPPOSITE BELOW: A mother leaving her baby in a foundling hospital's "tower." 19th century. Print

During the sixteenth century, the number of abandoned babies in France grew. According to the thinking of the time, these infants were certainly bastards, the result of illegitimate liaisons. In reality, however, a strong correlation could be seen in Paris between the price of bread and the number of abandonments; in fact, the major motivation was poverty. Parents wanted to give their infants a chance to survive, for at the almshouse babies died like flies within the first few months.

For many centuries, huddled in small baskets, rolled up in rags, left at the entrances to churches and hospitals—or simply in the street—abandoned children left their mark on popular culture in paintings and prints, in books and melodramas. The story of the huge population of foundlings makes up one of the more wrenching pages in history. Such gestures as giving a

crib, pull a bell, and run away, heartbroken. A nun immediately came to get the child. In the early nineteenth century, the authorities found themselves faced with a dilemma: the towers encouraged the abandonment of babies, whose numbers left in the state's care had greatly increased. Yet, if they closed, infanticides would multiply. Finally, the public assistance administration decided to replace the towers with reception offices where anonymity would be respected.

A small ray of light in this vale of tears: the stories of certain mothers, penniless but shrewd, who had their babies brought to the hospital by a midwife accomplice, and then sought work there as a paid wet nurse and had their own infants entrusted to their care. The administration, which was not always fooled, turned a blind eye to such ruses until the mid-nineteenth century. Later, as the earliest aid program for mothers was beginning to take shape, controls became more stringent.

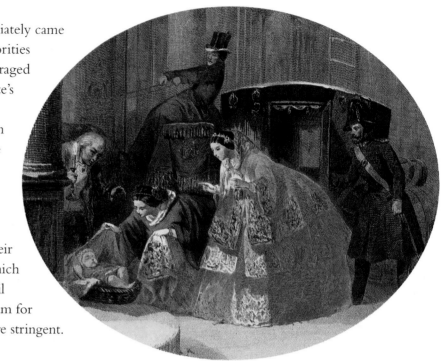

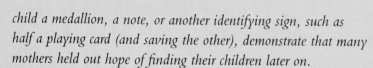

child a medallion, a note, or another identifying sign, such as half a playing card (and saving the other), demonstrate that many mothers held out hope of finding their children later on.

On 29 November 1633, a priest named Vincent de Paul founded the society Daughters of Charity. This order, at first devoted to helping poor people, seven years later was given the responsibility of caring for the abandoned infants of Paris as well. When it was created, the foundling hospital had a good reputation, but faced with an explosion in the number of abandoned babies and a lack of resources, it was quickly overwhelmed and became a place of death. From 1660, an average of 438 foundlings a year were recorded in Paris, and there was a steep climb in the number in the following centuries. Later, abandoned babies were sent to the provinces, and even abroad, under frightful conditions.

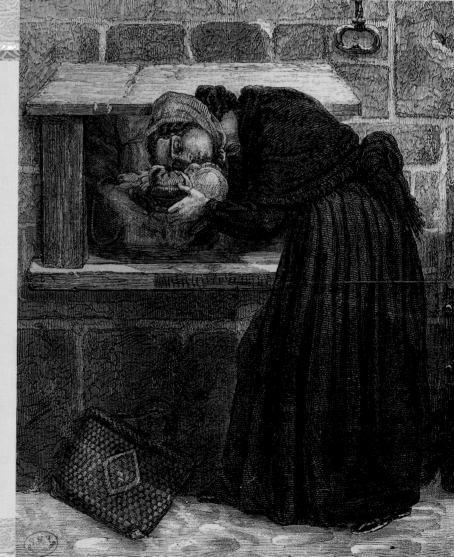

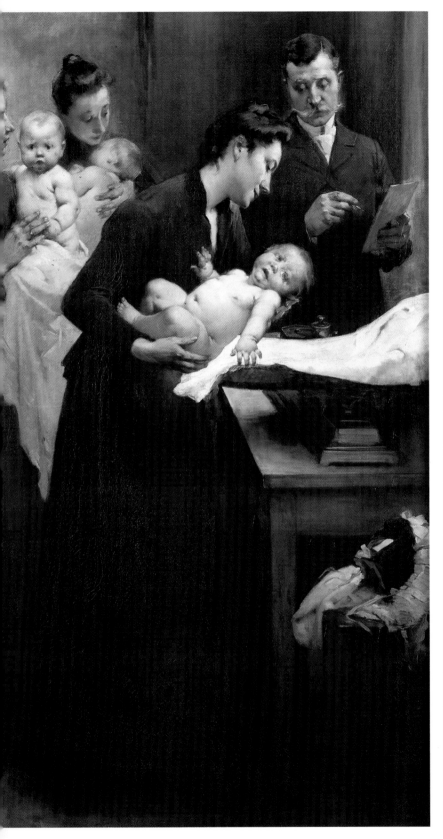
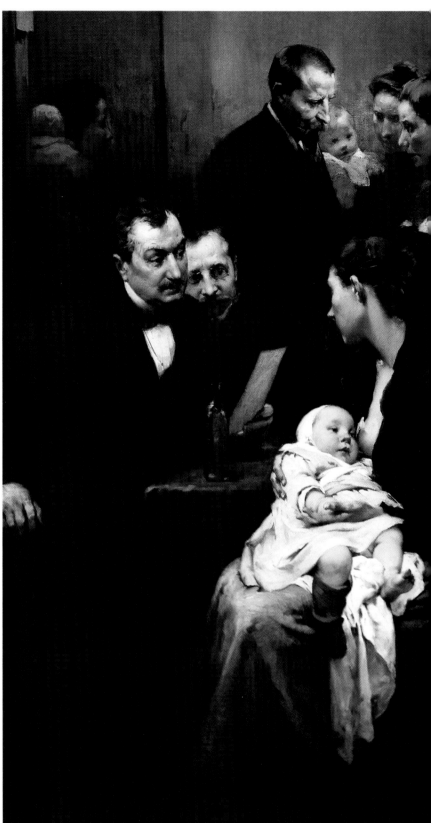

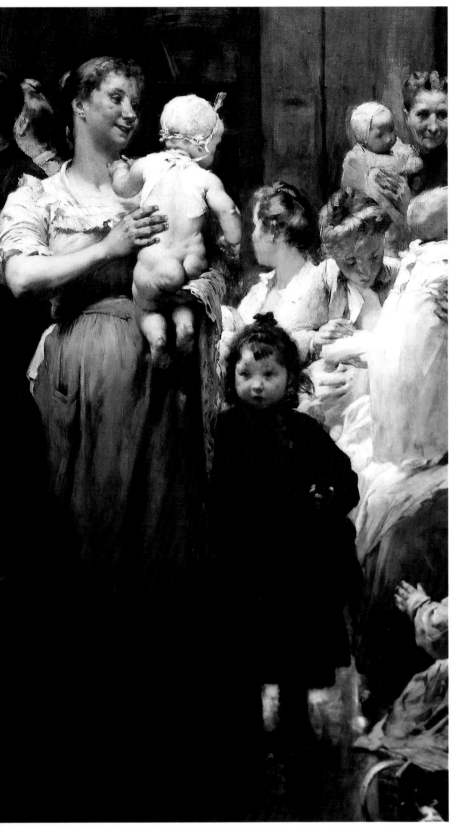
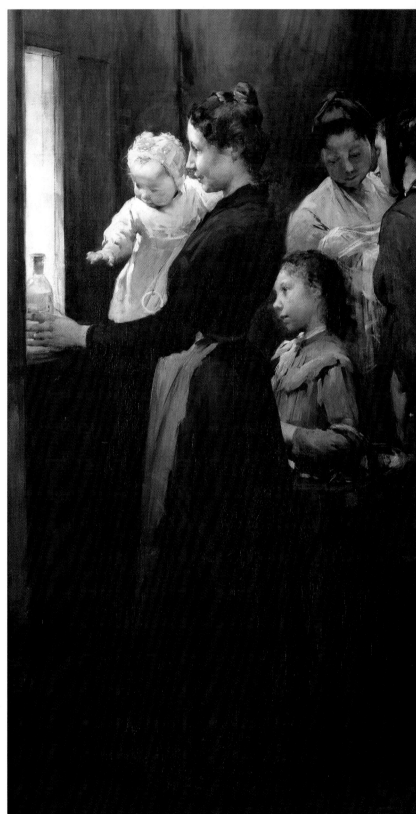

At the end of the nineteenth century, child care had become a science. Although the word pediatrics *did not appear until 1884, caring for children is an age-old concern. The French Dr. Caron said: "Child care is to the health of children as agriculture is to the fertility of the soil."*

PRECEDING PAGES: Jean Geoffroy (1853–1924). *The "Drop of Milk" in Belleville.* Musée de l'Assistance Publique, Paris

BELOW: Center for maternal assistance. 1944. Photograph

OPPOSITE: A baby is weighed. 1909. Photograph

The First Children's Hospitals

The foundling hospital in Paris unintentionally became the greatest center of studies of infant pathology. Pediatrics as well as the study of child care were born during the nineteenth century. The knowledge of ailments that struck infants—measles, tonsillitis, diphtheria, croup, pneumonia, whooping cough, meningitis, scarlet fever, tuberculosis—greatly increased, and their diagnosis grew more accurate.

In 1802, the Paris children's hospital for sick children was founded. It was the first large hospital exclusively for children in the world. A long line of devoted people worked under often difficult conditions throughout the century. Robert Debré gave an account of such a person, one of his instructors, whose name has long since slipped into oblivion: "Arnold Netter had a very unusual appearance. To us, he represented the image of an Old Testament prophet, but a smiling prophet.… Every day, including Sunday and holidays, he was at the hospital, where he arrived before the rest of us. He neglected nothing, forgot not a single child in its little bed, not a single infant in its cradle, leaned over each one smiling like a benevolent grandfather, gently examined the painful area, calmed the small patient, then thought for a long time in silence. He called up from an infallible memory all the texts he had read

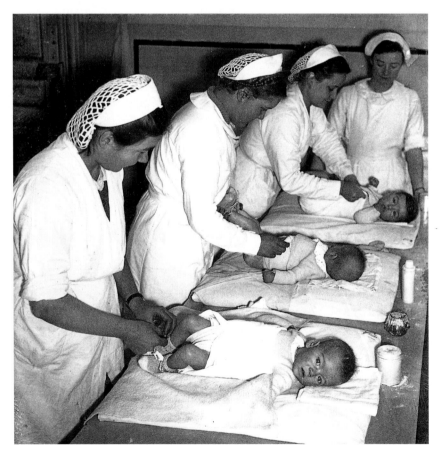

or the cases he had already observed.… His erudition was celebrated. He had read everything and in every language. He knew the history of medicine and the history of illnesses since he saw the first case of encephalitis in Paris in 1915, but not only recent publications came to mind but also the old, picturesque descriptions made by doctors in 1695."

Many such exceptional individuals, some of whom left their names to hospitals, spent time at the Paris children's hospital: Trousseau, Bretonneau, Billard, Parrot, and Laennec. Charles Billard wrote the most important pediatric treatise of the beginning of the nineteenth century. In this work, he described the major stages of psychomotor development of the child. He discussed the way to detect jaundice and defined the average weights and sizes of the infant.

But Billard's book, which inaugurated modern pediatrics, is especially poignant, for it includes a long list of sick babies who died and on whom he subsequently performed autopsies—Caroline, Joseph, Adele, August, Rose, all only a few days or a few months old—abandoned children whose infinitely sad last moments he recounted.

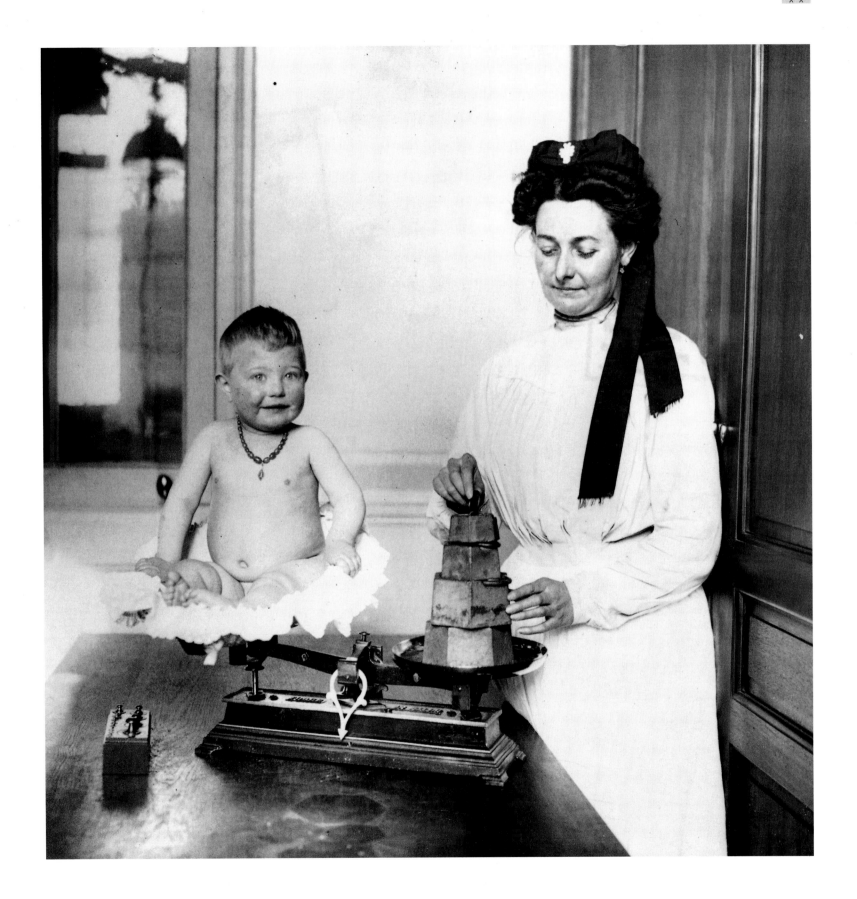

The Invention of the Incubator

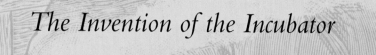

By the eighteenth century, it was well known that it was important to keep premature babies warm. They were given warm-water baths, baths in warm sand, or steam baths to elevate their body temperature. The technique most commonly used to prevent hypothermia in premature babies, or "weak infants," as they were called, consisted of wrapping them in a layer of cotton wool and then in swaddling clothes; for this reason, midwives called these babies "little cottons." They were placed in a cradle with two or three bowls of hot water.

The first incubator appeared in 1857; a cradle made of zinc, it had a double bottom and sides in which hot water could be poured. Another model was tried out in Port-Royal's maternity ward in 1880. Made of wood, it had a glass cover and

was heated with alcohol. These were followed by individual incubators heated by oil, and then those made in earthenware. At first, the babies died of asphyxiation, for these incubators lacked air holes; they were simply glass cages heated from below by bowls of hot water replaced every two or three hours. To prevent the air from drying out, a wet sponge was placed inside. In the 1930s, many metal incubators with glass doors were made that had a tube leading to the open air for ventilation. Gas-heated incubators were tried, but the danger of fire made them impractical. Despite all these inventions, an elderly gentleman, born prematurely in 1914, recounted how he had survived in a shoe box lined with cotton and warmed in the oven, like a dinner roll!

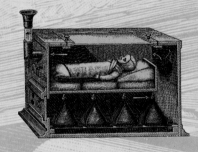

Before the invention of the electric incubator, the most common model used bowls of hot water for heat.

ABOVE: Cross-section of a Tarnier incubator. 19th century. Print

BELOW: The first incubators. 1897, Austria. Print. Bibliothèque Nationale, Paris

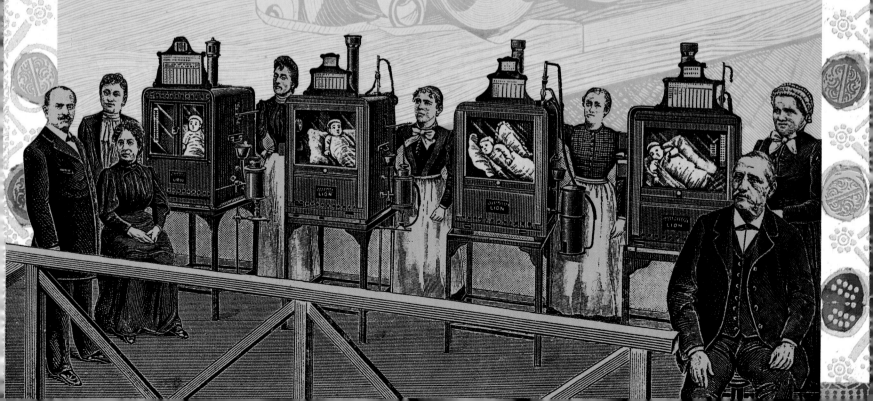

"Drops of Milk"

Among the institutions that played a formative role in infant care and the education of mothers was the first French clinic for babies, founded in 1892 by Dr. Budin in Paris. When this doctor asked mothers how their babies were doing, he had heard too often that the little one had died. This led him to have the mothers bring their children in for free regular check-ups for two years. In this first "school for mothers," a great deal of advice was dispensed, along with sterilized milk. The program proved successful: not a single baby who came to Dr. Budin died.

In 1894, at Fécamp, in Normandy, France, Dr. Dufour created the first "Drop of Milk" clinic, where baskets holding six bottles of pasteurized milk were sold to workers at a modest price. Poor mothers could get them for free. Infant mortality dropped so quickly that wealthier mothers demanded the milk as well.

Other "Drops of Milk" opened up, including one in Belleville founded by Dr. Variot. In exchange for the sterilized milk, mothers were asked to bring their babies in each week for a careful examination; they were monitored with a stethoscope, weighed, and measured. Charts of weights and lengths were established and became institutionalized.

During the 1880s, due to the efforts of Louis Pasteur, medicine advanced to the bacteriological age with the identification of the microbe. After it was discovered that microbes could be killed with carbolic acid, the rules of antiseptics, then of aseptics, finally took hold.

The field of children's medicine also took off, thanks to a favorable political climate. In France, for example, doctors and hygienists sought to reverse a decline in population. New laws offering infant care were enacted. In 1879, the school of medicine in Paris offered the first clinical chair for childhood illnesses. In addition to the advantages of better child care and post-Pasteur hygiene came important discoveries that improved clinical investigations, such as radiography in 1895, and others that led the way to the development of methods of preventive medicine. Infant mortality rates finally receded. The determination to protect infants and educate their mothers that had been manifest among philosophers and doctors at the end of the eighteenth century had made a forceful—and successful—reappearance.

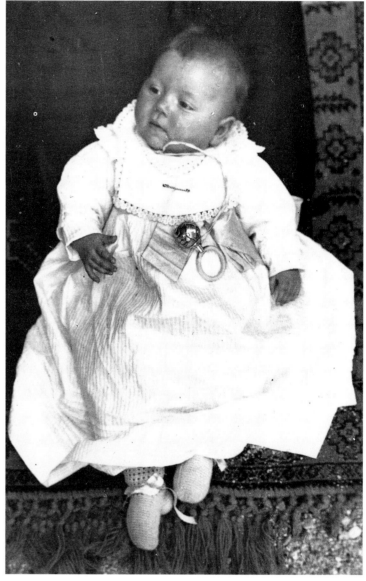

To ease the discomforts of teething, babies have long been given neck-laces, rattles, and other objects to chew on.

ABOVE: Baby with her teething ring. 1895. Photograph

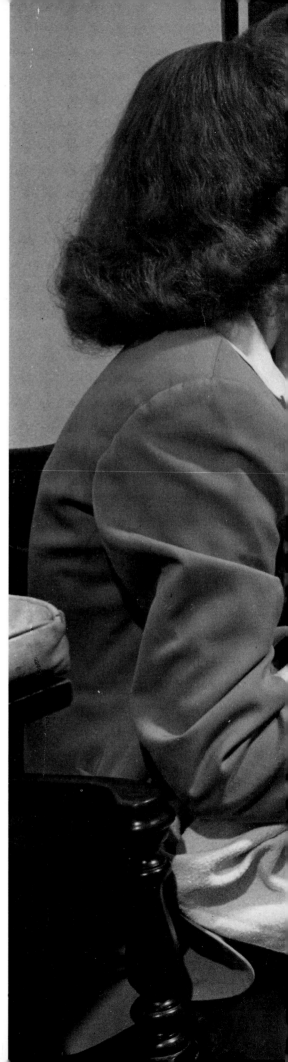

"A doctor's greatest accomplishments were linked to his ability to dispel the specter of a serious illness through a precise diagnosis."

Robert Debré, *L'honneur de vivre*
(The Honor of Living), 1974

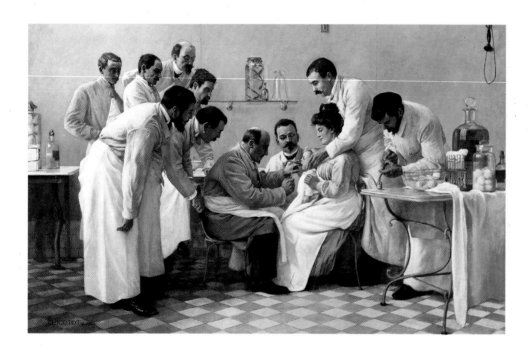

ABOVE: G. Chicotot. *Treating the Diphtheritic Patient.* Musée de l'Assistance Publique, Paris

RIGHT: Wayne Miller/Magnum. Visiting the pediatrician. Photograph

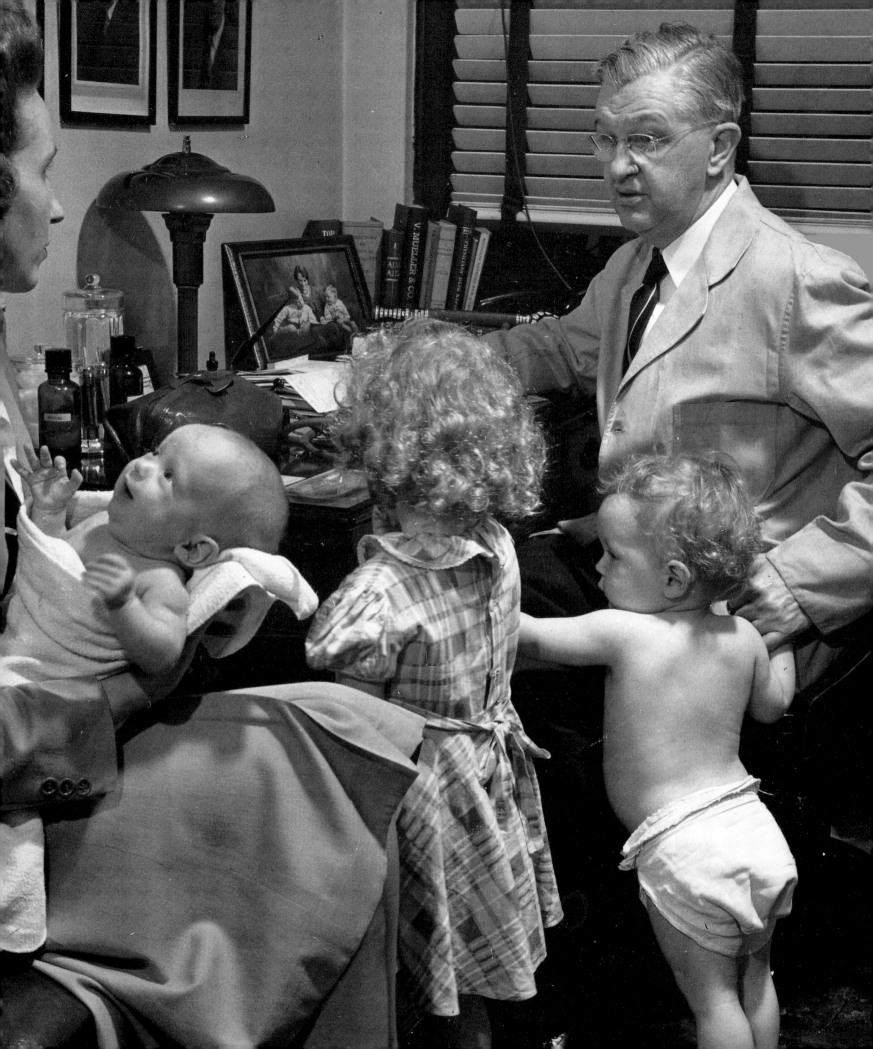

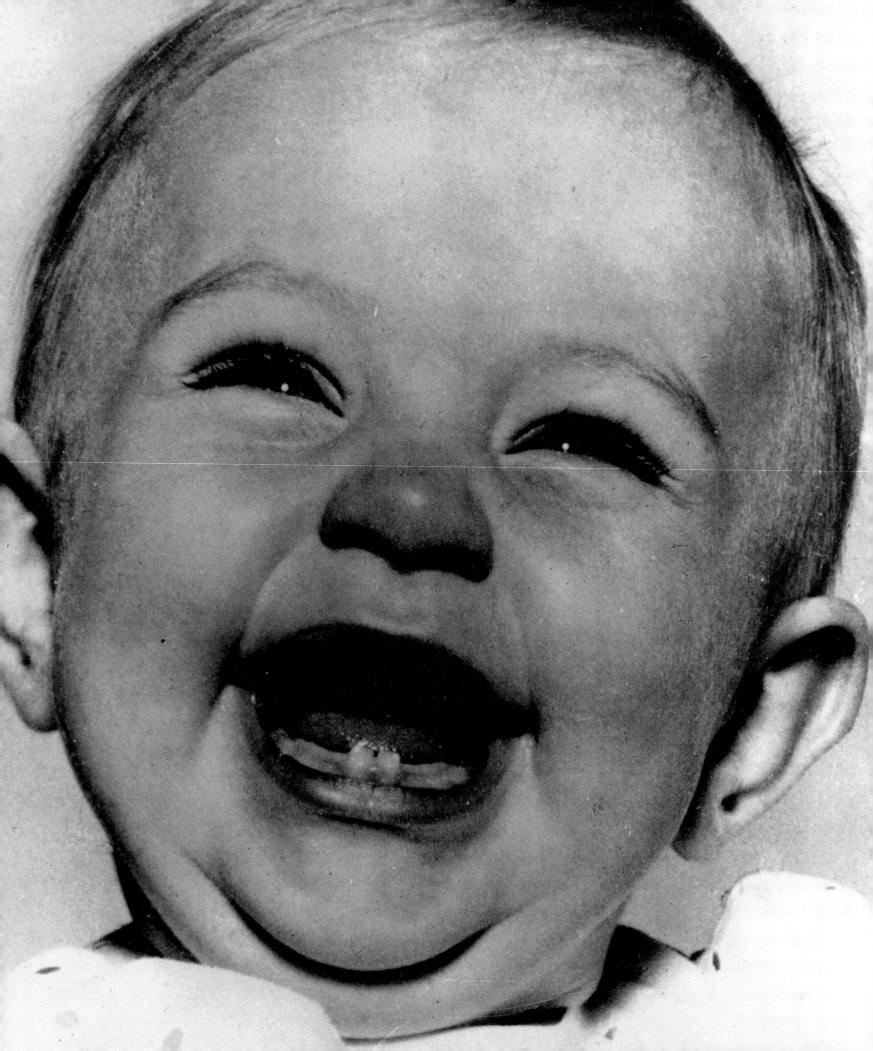

The Giant Steps of Pediatrics

"It is hard to realize today what anguish the appearance of a white sore throat inspired, bringing with it the specter of diphtheria and croup. The abrupt rise in temperature that accompanied a red sore throat brought with it the dread of scarlet fever. Every ear infection brought the fear of complication, then very frequent and very serious, and every abdominal pain the fear of an often fatal appendicitis. A simple headache evoked the possibility of tubercular meningitis, fatal within a few weeks. When a mother said that her baby was losing weight, she imagined some unseen tubercular infection. In the infant, does not severe diarrhea precede infantile cholera, which is often fatal?" recalled the great French pediatrician Robert Debré.

With the rules of hygiene gradually becoming common practice, the development of vaccines and the passage of laws that made them mandatory, the discovery of dietetics and the role of vitamins, the institutionalization of prenatal examinations, the improvement in the comfort and heating of houses, and, especially, the discovery of antibiotics in 1928 by Scottish biologist Sir Alexander Fleming (with industrial production of the drugs beginning in 1943), in a few decades the health of babies made more progress than it had made in the previous millennia. During the years around World War II, the victory against infection appeared to have been won, and biology came to the aid of pediatrics to give doctors previously undreamed-of therapeutic powers. Previously, illnesses had affected babies for long weeks, and their convalescence sometimes took months. Today, they are back to normal in a few days. The period of convalescence has almost entirely disappeared.

Since the end of the nineteenth century, babies have been weighed and measured religiously, and entire chapters have been written on the best way to measure them and on the exact techniques to follow for their hygiene. But early-twentieth-century popular medicine went in the opposite direction: some practitioners and parents felt it was absolutely unnecessary to weigh the baby very often, and they agreed that a daily bath was not critical.

At first, the medical world cast a disapproving eye on such leniency. However, as the wheel turns again, the contemporary trend is to set aside some of the strict rules regarding caring for infants. Now doctors often advise parents to relax and not keep the thermometer always at hand—even if colds and the occasional ear infection punctuate, somewhat too often in the parents' eyes, the first year of their babies' life.

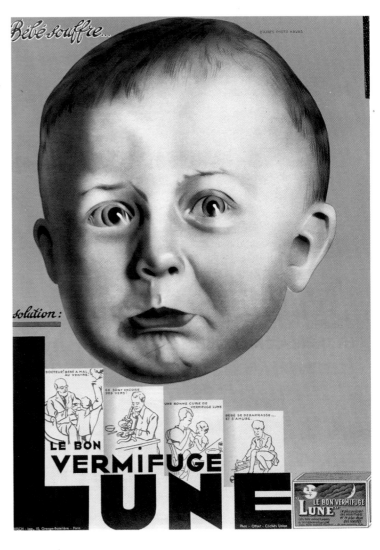

Mercury, iron filings, copper dissolved in acids, absinthe—the appalling remedies for worms of the eighteenth century gave way to more inoffensive treatments.

ABOVE: Advertisement for a worming remedy from *L'Illustration*, 1934

OPPOSITE: Photograph

Feeding

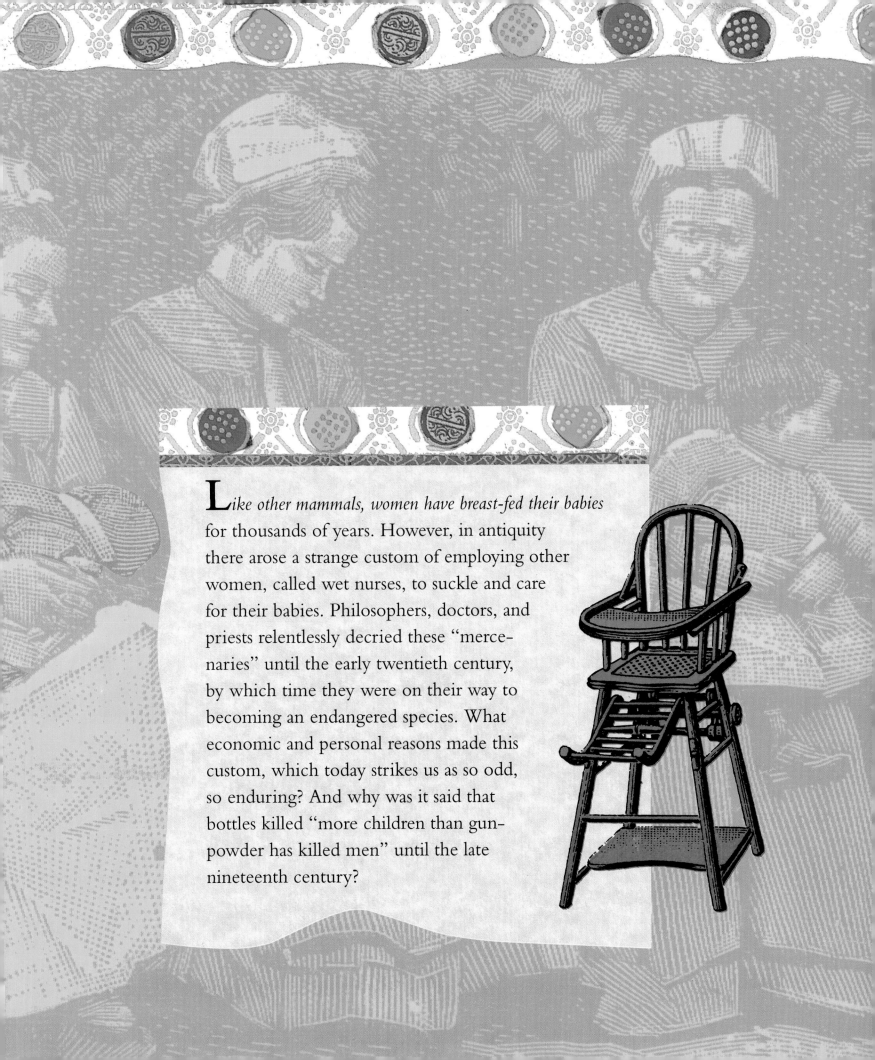

Like other mammals, women have breast-fed their babies for thousands of years. However, in antiquity there arose a strange custom of employing other women, called wet nurses, to suckle and care for their babies. Philosophers, doctors, and priests relentlessly decried these "mercenaries" until the early twentieth century, by which time they were on their way to becoming an endangered species. What economic and personal reasons made this custom, which today strikes us as so odd, so enduring? And why was it said that bottles killed "more children than gunpowder has killed men" until the late nineteenth century?

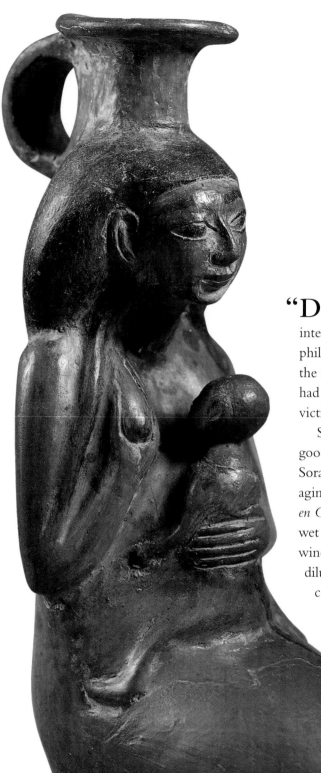

From the Nipple to the Bottle

"**D**o you imagine that nature has given breasts to women as gracious protuberances intended to decorate the chest and not to feed infants?" exclaimed the Roman philosopher Favorinius in the second century. In Rome, breast-feeding served as the subject of stormy debate over many centuries. The Greek moralist Plutarch had already censured "this vile practice of hiring wet nurses and sacrificing tender victims to the greed and avarice of borrowed mothers."

Some doctors, more pragmatic, were content to indicate criteria for selecting a good wet nurse, which had become a status symbol for the wealthy. Roman doctor Soranus of Ephesus condoned the use of these women "so that the mother can avoid aging prematurely from the daily energy that nursing consumes." In his book *L'enfant en Gaule romaine* (The Child in Roman Gaul), Gérard Coulon reported on recipes wet nurses used to increase their milk supply: "Swallow earthworms with a honeyed wine, consume the breasts of animals that produce a large amount of milk or instead dilute the ashes of bat or owl in water and rub the chest with this mixture." If these concoctions proved ineffective, it was advised to appeal to the gods, making votive offerings in the shape of breasts.

The Wet Nurse Market

Several wet nurses took turns breast-feeding the baby of a patrician family, assisted by one woman to watch over the baby, another to rock him, and a third to hold him so that the wet nurse's milk did not get heated up. Wealthy Romans bought slaves who were about to give birth to serve as wet nurses, but parents of the lower classes had to make do with hiring a wet nurse. They went to the market in the Olitorium Forum, where the candidates could be found near what were known as the "lacteal" columns. Hired on contract for about two years, wet nurses were enjoined from having sexual relations and were subject to a fine if they became pregnant. It was, after all, common knowledge that sperm and pregnancy impaired the quality of the milk, which, according to Pliny the Elder, "curdled like a kind of cheese." In addition, these women had to lead a well-ordered life, follow a very strict diet, and do special exercises to stimulate the breast. Soranus advised them to play bowls, lift weights, carry buckets of water, and make beds.

Often accused of negligence, greed, and drunkenness, wet nurses had a poor reputation in ancient times, very different from what one would think based on the evidence left by the children they raised. While mothers and fathers displayed more authority than affection, for the child wet nurses embodied all the tenderness in the world. The bond often lasted a lifetime; numerous stelae dedicated to wet nurses demonstrate a deep attachment. The feeling was often reciprocal, as this epitaph shows: "His wet nurse, sweet as honey, erected this monument to her nursling Valerius Stachyus, who lived eight months and twenty-five days."

Except for the wives of pharaohs, Egyptian women usually nursed their babies themselves. When they had to resort to using animal's milk, they first poured it into a vase in the shape of a mother offering her breast, so that it would be ritually transformed, or "maternalized," before being given to the infant.

OPPOSITE: Egyptian bottle. Musée du Louvre, Paris

Ancient Bottles

Small terra-cotta or glass vessels with slender spouts have been discovered in the tombs of Gallo-Roman two- and three-year-olds. These containers were probably used at weaning to give the children liquids or pap. The only known allusion to these ancestors of the baby bottle comes down to us from the doctor Soranus: "If the child is thirsty after eating, give him some plain water or water with a drop of wine with the artificial nipple; this type of implement allows him to draw out the liquid little by little without any risk, as from a breast."

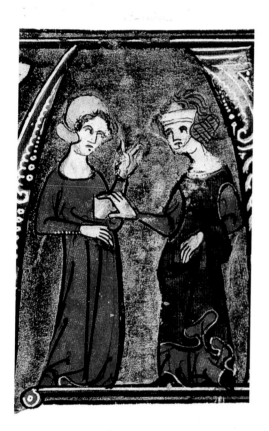

The mother chose her baby's wet nurse with care; before tasting her milk, she felt her breasts, looking for ones that were neither "too big nor too small, too hard nor too soft."

ABOVE: Miniature. 14th century. Bibliothèque Nationale, Paris

OPPOSITE: Miniature. 15th century. Bibliothèque Nationale, Paris

Breast at the Ready

In the Middle Ages, when middle-class babies were feeding, they were often left with their bottoms uncovered or completely nude. Mothers who could often took advantage of feeding time to change their babies or give them a bath. They took the babies' clothes off in front of a fire and spread them out in the heat to dry. The peasants, too busy and perhaps less careful about hygiene, generally fed their babies fully clothed. Any time of day or night—whether she was walking, working, traveling, or sleeping, whether she was inside or out, seated, standing, or lying down—the mother offered the breast as soon as the baby demanded it. The clothing worn by the nursing mother facilitated the baby's immediate satisfaction. Until the fifteenth century, mothers and wet nurses wore dresses with pleats that disguised the vertical slits on the sides through which the breast could easily be slid when required. In the fifteenth century, the style changed; low-necked dresses, over which the breast could be pushed and stay up by itself, proved more useful, keeping the mother's arms free and allowing her to pursue other activities while nursing.

Both the simple peasant and the eminent doctor considered milk to be nothing more than white blood. When a woman became pregnant, she stopped menstruating, for her blood went to nourish the embryo. After birth, this blood rose to the breasts, where it was turned into milk to feed the newborn. Thus, it was understood that the woman continued to transmit to the baby her own physical and moral traits: she actually fashioned the baby. Those who favored mother's milk seized on this weighty argument: the wet nurses could communicate their defects through their milk. This risk, however, did not deter noble families from employing them.

Women of high birth in the Middle Ages devoted themselves to bearing many children close together, on the condition that they would be free from the constraints of nursing them. Given the infant mortality rate, a round dozen children—the average number in these surroundings during this period—was just enough to ensure an heir.

Nonetheless, some noblewomen insisted on nursing their own children no matter the cost. This was the case with Queen Blanche de Castille. It is said that one day, when the queen was absent, a woman of the court gave the future Saint Louis her breast in order to quiet him. Learning of this on her return, Blanche hurled herself on her son in consternation and made him vomit up the foreign milk.

The exclusive privilege of aristocratic families at the beginning of the Middle Ages, the custom of using a wet nurse later extended to the middle class. In the growing cities, women took up a variety of trades. Many of them assisted their husbands as merchants or innkeepers and thus found themselves forced to entrust their babies to the care of other women. In the twelfth century, a veritable trade organization for wet nurses grew into being. By this time, Paris already had placement agencies, and in 1350, a statute regulating the profession was passed.

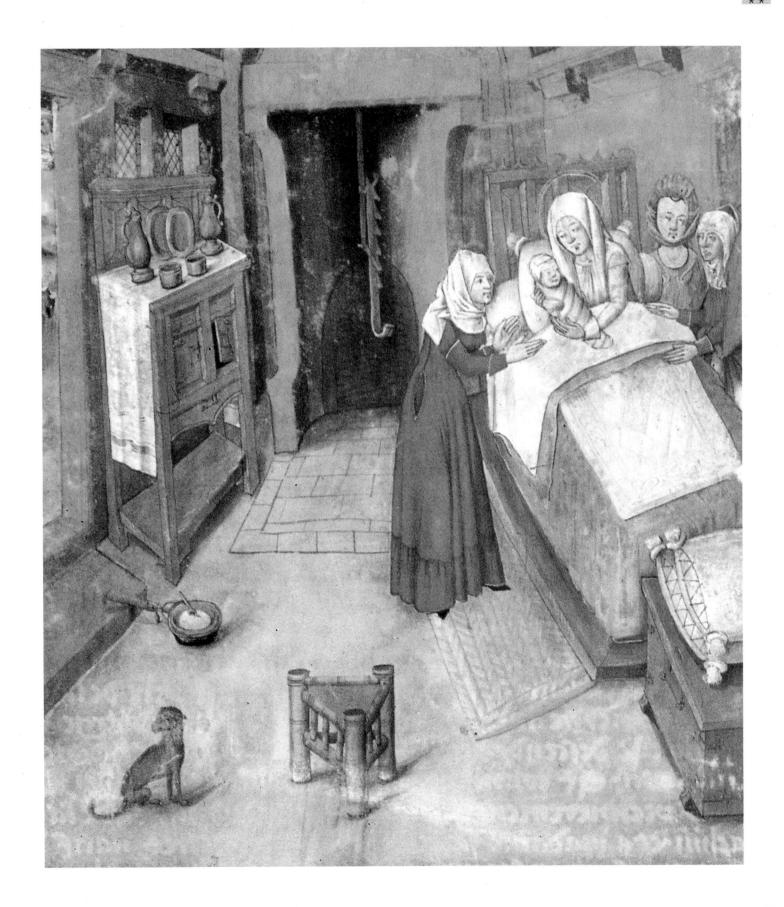

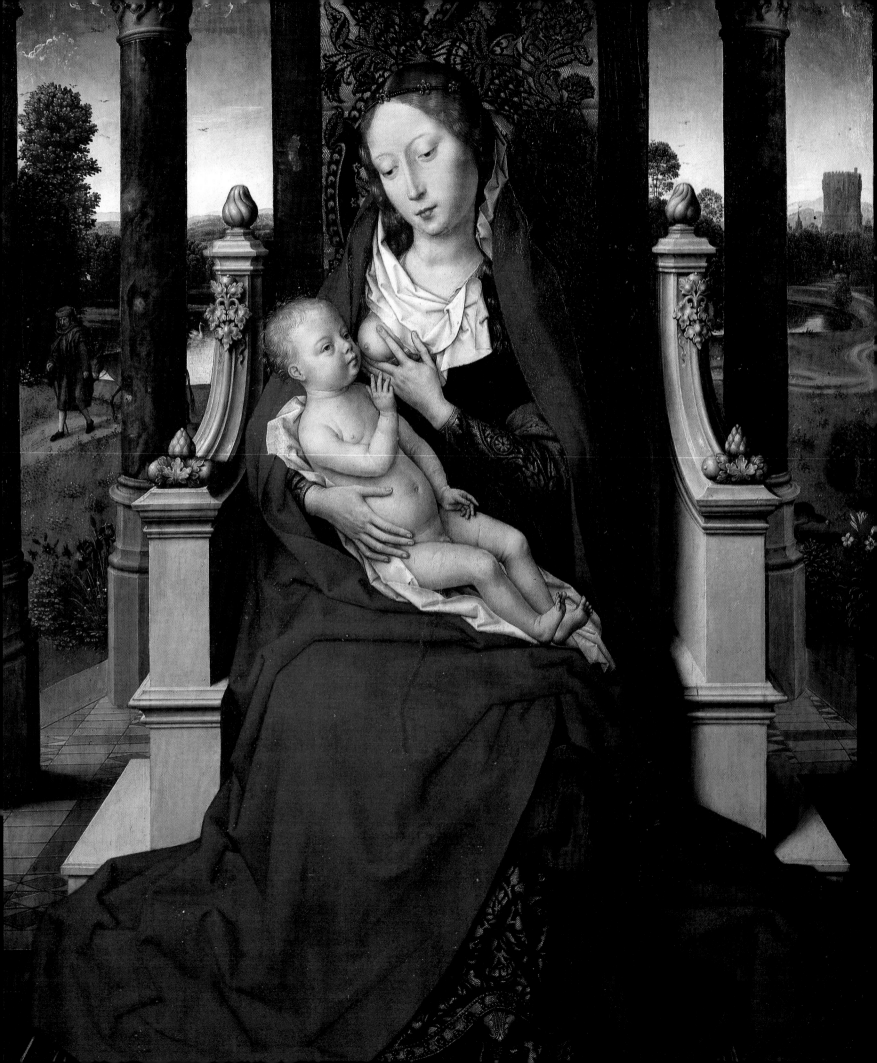

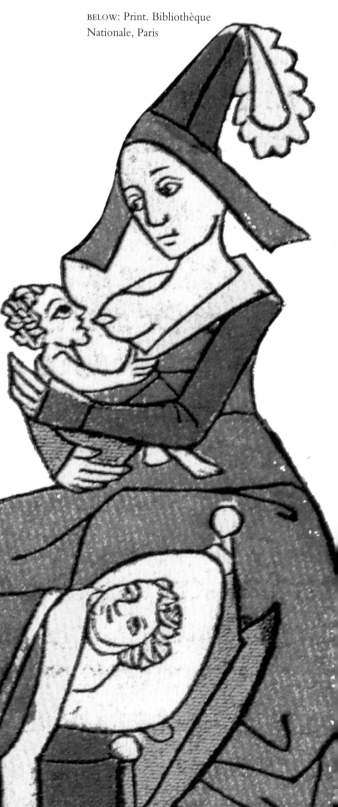

On Milk "Neither Green, nor Red, nor Black"

In the thirteenth century, the Italian doctor Aldobrandino of Siena took inspiration from authors of antiquity to formulate the model for the ideal wet nurse, which was widely adopted. She had to be between twenty-five and thirty years old, as "this is the age when the natural heat is the strongest to give rise to good humors." She had to resemble the mother as much as possible. Her milk had to be "neither too thin, nor too thick, neither green, nor red, nor black" and with a flavor "neither sour, nor bitter, nor salty, but rather sweet." Sixteenth-century French author François Rabelais alluded to the modeling of the baby's nose by the breasts of the wet nurse. Responding to Gargantua's question, "Why does Brother John have such a beautiful nose?" the monk answered, "According to true monastic philosophy, it is because my wet nurse had soft nipples; in suckling, my nose buried itself in them as in butter, where it rose and expanded like soft bread dough. Wet nurses with hard nipples make snub-nosed babies."

The wet nurse had to follow a special diet. She would eat meat with young and tender flesh like that of the baby, such as lamb and kid. She could not have any foods containing onion, garlic, pepper, mint, or basil—that is, ingredients with too strong a flavor. If she did not produce enough milk, she had to eat cabbage, fennel, anise—which "soothe by expelling all wind and stimulating the secretion of milk"—and lettuce, "for the milk in which it abounds."

The wet nurse not only fed her charges, but she changed them, washed them, and dressed them, and she also woke them up in the morning, taught them, and—above all—she loved them. A stronger emotional bond than that between children and their true mothers arose from these daily routines. Sheltered, honored, and generously paid, the resident wet nurse became a major figure in well-off families. Children sent to wet nurses in the country, however, faced many dangers, not the least of which was suffocation. Too poor to provide babies with a cradle and not wanting to place them on the earthen floor, which grew icy after the fire went out, wet nurses brought them into their beds. That way they could nurse them on demand in a pleasantly sleepy state; however, this led to many accidents. At the beginning of the fifteenth century in Florence, a protective device called an *arcuccio* was developed. It was a wooden arch placed over the baby in the adult's bed to prevent him from being crushed. Later on, wet nurses had to use this device by law, under threat of excommunication. Though many infants died while with the wet nurse—statistically more than those nursed by their mothers—at the end of the Middle Ages more and more babies were sent to the country from the cities. For a poor family, this was an unaffordable luxury, so if a poor mother could not feed her baby with her own milk, the bottle sometimes became her only recourse.

In the Middle Ages, pearly white milk symbolized purity. The Virgin Mary's milk became a relic.

OPPOSITE: Hans Memling. *The Virgin Mary Nursing Her Child.* 15th century. Granada cathedral, Spain

BELOW: Print. Bibliothèque Nationale, Paris

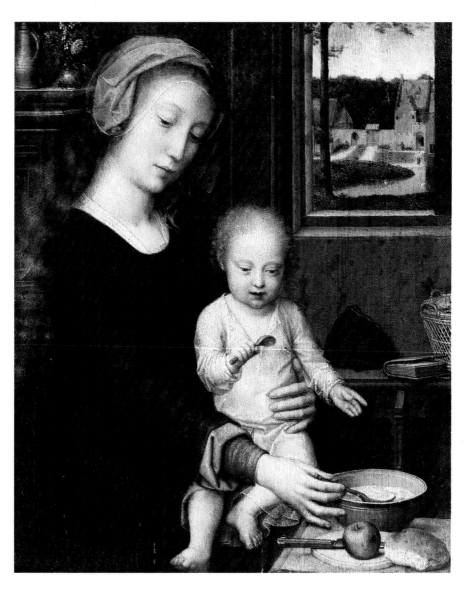

The infant Jesus plays with a small spoon while his mother peacefully feeds him his pap.

ABOVE: Gerard David (1460–1523). *Virgin Mary with the Bowl of Milk.* Musée Réali, Brussels

RIGHT: Adriaen van Ostade. *The Father of the Family.* 1648. Print. Bibliothèque Nationale, Paris

Papa's Pap

In the Middle Ages, from their earliest days infants were fed a thick, soft cereal in addition to milk. Milk was considered to be insufficient nourishment for babies, who were thought to need denser foods to make their bodies more resistant and their flesh firmer. This pap simmered in a small earthen saucepan near the fire, often under the attentive eye of the father, who thus took part in the feeding of the infant. Made of milk, flour, and honey, pap was a luxury item that not every family could offer their babies. With an almost modern concern for dietetics and hygiene, doctors recommended cooking the flour and boiling the water and the milk. They also advised adding a bit of watered-down wine, or wine cooked until the alcohol evaporated, leaving only the tannin, an excellent remedy for diarrhea. Despite these prudent suggestions, doctors fretted over the dangers of feeding a baby a mixed diet too early; many babies died.

The medieval baby was weaned at about the age of two. Most often, the arrival of its next sibling determined the moment of this delicate transition. Every precaution was taken to wean children gradually. The mother or wet nurse gave them the tenderest meats, which she was advised to chew and predigest with her saliva before placing it in the infant's mouth: "They chewed the meat for the baby when he had no teeth, so that he could swallow it without danger and more advantageously." These precautions differed from those taken at the court of Burgundy two centuries later, where the little princes had to be given "very well-done meat very finely minced, such that they will have no problem chewing, and take great care whoever cuts the meat that there are no little bones." All the advice, attentions, and worries centered on babies' food demonstrate the care and affection given them in the Middle Ages.

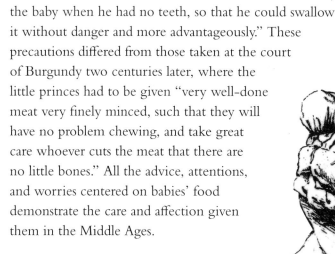

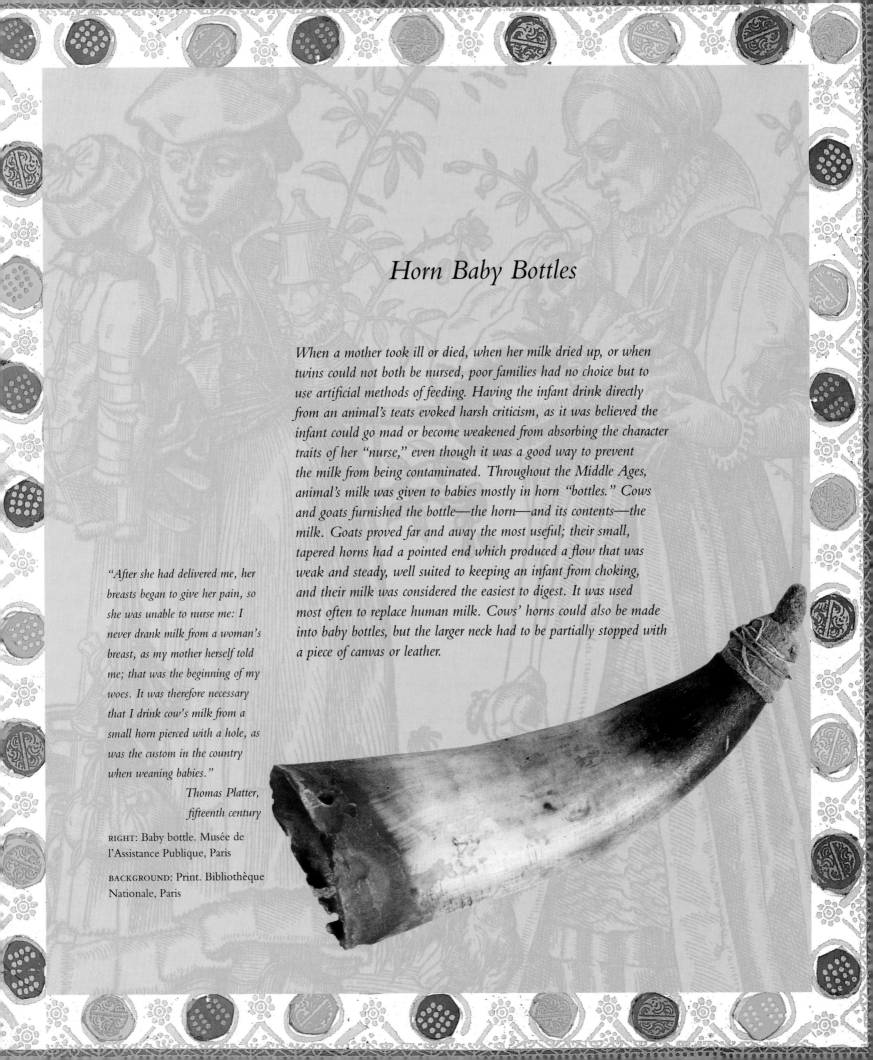

Horn Baby Bottles

When a mother took ill or died, when her milk dried up, or when twins could not both be nursed, poor families had no choice but to use artificial methods of feeding. Having the infant drink directly from an animal's teats evoked harsh criticism, as it was believed the infant could go mad or become weakened from absorbing the character traits of her "nurse," even though it was a good way to prevent the milk from being contaminated. Throughout the Middle Ages, animal's milk was given to babies mostly in horn "bottles." Cows and goats furnished the bottle—the horn—and its contents—the milk. Goats proved far and away the most useful; their small, tapered horns had a pointed end which produced a flow that was weak and steady, well suited to keeping an infant from choking, and their milk was considered the easiest to digest. It was used most often to replace human milk. Cows' horns could also be made into baby bottles, but the larger neck had to be partially stopped with a piece of canvas or leather.

"After she had delivered me, her breasts began to give her pain, so she was unable to nurse me: I never drank milk from a woman's breast, as my mother herself told me; that was the beginning of my woes. It was therefore necessary that I drink cow's milk from a small horn pierced with a hole, as was the custom in the country when weaning babies."

Thomas Platter,
fifteenth century

RIGHT: Baby bottle. Musée de l'Assistance Publique, Paris

BACKGROUND: Print. Bibliothèque Nationale, Paris

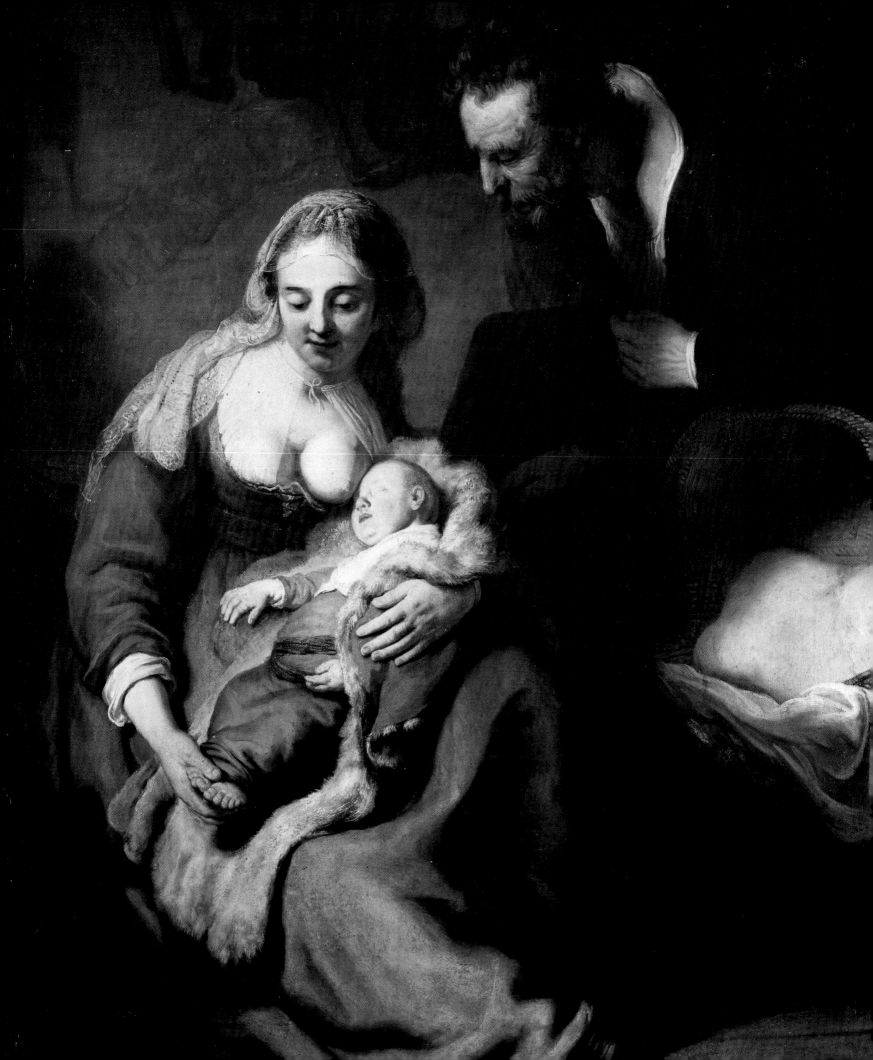

Nurse or Dance

As in the Middle Ages, many sixteenth-century mothers entrusted the task of nursing their children to other women, especially in light of the taboo concerning sexual relations while nursing: sperm made milk spoil, and pregnancy poisoned it. The doctor Laurent Joubert was among the few to rebel against this belief at the time: "The woman I hold dearest in the world," he said, "has nursed all my children, so full of milk is she, and I have not stopped sleeping with her for that reason, and I make love to her as a good husband should to his better half, following the dictates of marriage, and, thank God, our children have been well nourished and are thriving. I give no advice to others that I do not myself follow. Unsatisfied desire is the major threat to milk."

Besides this sexual prohibition, which was barely respected, the evolution of the city woman's way of life led those mothers to call on the services of the wet nurse. A healthy peasant woman offered a happy replacement for the weak, thin, insufficient milk of women of the world exhausted by social demands incompatible with nursing. Their decision not to nurse their children arose from basically frivolous motives: aesthetics, visits and balls, fear of ridicule. "It's just not done," claimed the rules of decorum. "Refined civilization, in whose heart we live, in placing the majority of women of high society under the tyrannical domain of fashion, in subjecting them to the torture of the corset, in often debilitating their digestive organs, in irritating their nervous systems, in making them the victims of those celebrations of fashionable society where they fritter away their existence by going long hours without sleep, by rousing balls, this advanced civilization, has it left all of its mothers the energy to nurse their children well?" In the eighteenth century, the chronicler Louis Sébastien Mercier hastened to reply in the negative.

From the sixteenth to the eighteenth centuries, maternal nursing, practiced less and less in European cities, won the support of the Church, doctors, and philosophers. In desperation, they repeated the theories of classic authors and ransacked their imaginations to come up with new arguments in favor of mothers nursing their babies. It was a sacred duty, dictated by God, the parish priests tried to convince their flocks in the cities and in the villages; theological writings on the subject flourished. In seventeenth-century England and America, the Puritans gave sermons that inveighed against ungodly mothers who tried to avoid their duty.

Mothers, it was said, ran a great risk in going against nature; the milk of the wet nurse could give the baby the most horrible deformities, the most terrible defects. But the mothers themselves were said to face the most terrifying danger: milk that they produced that was not drunk by the infant would back up and spread throughout their body, and this "returned" milk could provoke the worst ills—puerperal fever, apoplexies, and so on—or it could even be diverted and emerge through the navel!

"After the infant is born, a true mother must feed it from her breasts, which are the lovely fountains that a wise and providential Mother Nature has created for this purpose…and what greater pastime could a mother have in this world besides the one she has while nursing her little children, whose amiable babyish talk, their stumbling over the pronunciation of words, their ready and loving laugh, the joyousness they give to the household surpass all the jokers in the world."

Montaigne, Essais
(Essays), 1580

OPPOSITE: Rembrandt. *The Holy Family.* 17th century. Alte Pinakothek, Munich

The Caresses of the Nursling

While nursing was considered a duty, it was also a great satisfaction. "Is there any pastime that can equal that given by an infant who fondles and caresses his nurse while suckling: when with one hand he discovers and touches the other nipple, when he kicks with his feet all those who want to distract him, and at the same time shoots his nurse a thousand little laughs and winks from his disarming eyes?" enthused Laurent Joubert in the sixteenth century. "Good health, merriment, the caresses of the nursling, those are the spectacles, the balls, the entertainments of a good mother," recapitulated another doctor almost two hundred years later.

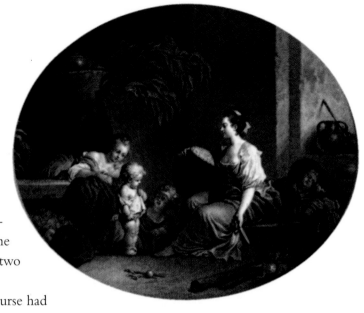

In the late eighteenth century, when the phenomenon of the wet nurse had grown even more widespread in Europe, philosopher and writer Jean-Jacques Rousseau made maternal nursing fashionable in France with his book *L'Emile*. In it, he extolled the ideal family in which blood ties were reinforced by the care given the children. The father, who abandoned his five children for their own good, found it a terrible thing "to share the rights of the mother, or rather, to give them away; to see one's child love another woman more than oneself." By this time, most American women nursed their own children.

"The voice of nature makes itself heard in the hearts of some of our young wives, and they undoubtedly deserve public recognition. Pleasure, charms, rest, they have sacrificed all! But they should let us know if they do not notice the respect that they inspire; if their husbands do not give them enough endearment; if their union be not sweet enough; and if they be not happy enough. Finally, they should let us know if their children, nourished by them, are not healthy enough, strong enough, and more sensitive to good morals."

Prost de Royer,
eighteenth century

LEFT AND ABOVE: N. de Lamay. Prints. 18th century. Bibliothèque Nationale, Paris

OPPOSITE: Edouard Debat-Ponsan. *Before the Ball.* 1886. Musée des Beaux-Arts, Tours

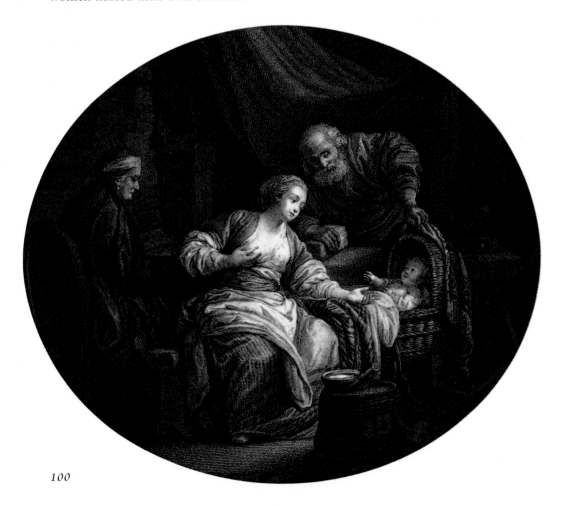

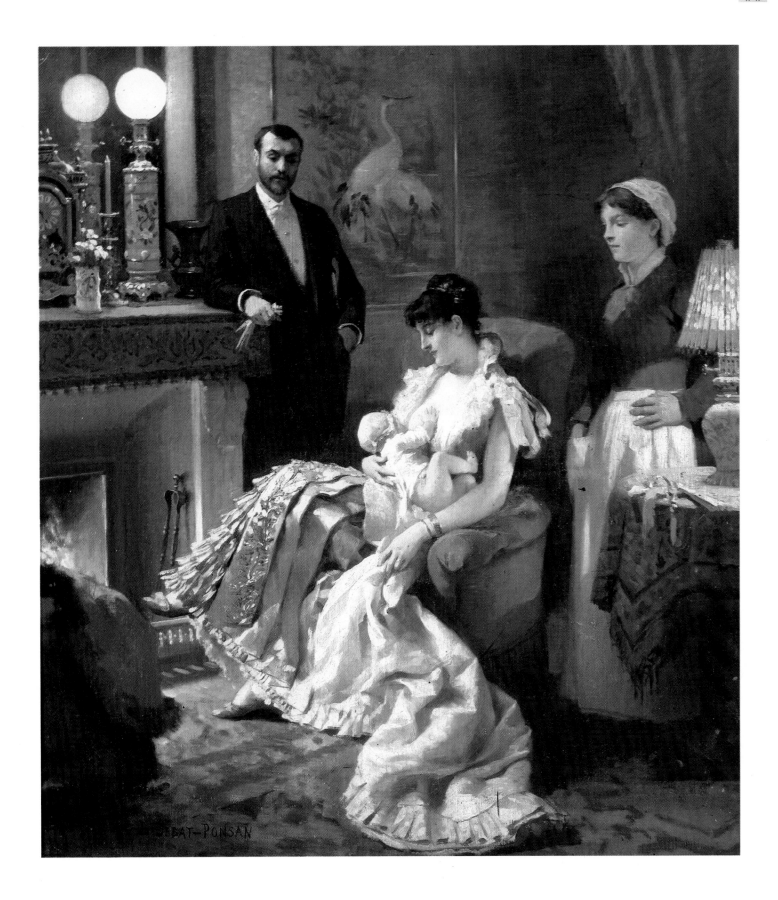

The Great Exodus of the Babies

In the Middle Ages, and up until the sixteenth century, the families that belonged to the highest levels of society—kings, aristocrats, and rich merchants—composed the very great majority of those who employed wet nurses in France. During the seventeenth century, much of the middle class joined their ranks. Finally, in the eighteenth century, a good number of people who lived in the cities, large or small, gave their children over to wet nurses. This practice expanded throughout Europe. Even people from the lower classes took it up, and only those who did not have two pennies to rub together had to forgo it. A police report says that of 21,000 children born in Paris in 1780, barely 1,000 were nursed by their mothers; 1,000 were nursed by wet nurses who came to live in the parents' home; and 19,000 were sent to wet nurses outside the city. The demand was such, and the supply of wet nurses available in and near the city so low, that it became necessary to send children further and further away. Craftsmen's wives, who formed a pool of wet nurses in the city, were among the first to stop nursing their own children so as not to interrupt their work.

In the big European cities of the eighteenth century, most parents found a wet nurse through agencies, run by "recommenders." These agents recruited wet nurses from the country, who were brought to Paris by women who took them into their homes until they received an infant to care for. For a very long time, neither wet nurses nor recommenders were subject to any oversight. However, infant mortality rates were so high in the eighteenth century that officials were spurred to regulate these trades increasingly strictly.

Baskets of Babies

Infants were taken to the wet nurse by people called escorts whose job was to transport the babies in baskets on their backs, in baskets attached to donkeys, or jammed together in open carts like animals. In 1773, a police regulation stated, "It is required that escorts make use of well-built wagons with a plank floor sufficiently provided with new straw and side rails well covered

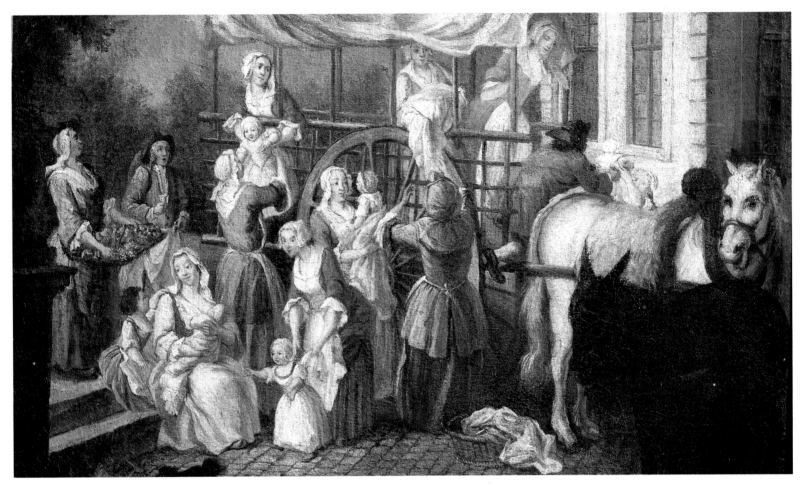

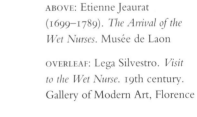

*with close-fitting boards or with straw matting or wicker, and
that they cover their wagon with a sound canvas fastened firmly
with rings and large enough to cover the ends and the sides,
under penalty of a 50-pound fine, dismissal, and even prison.
Under threat of the same penalty, they are forbidden to transport
infants unless there are wet nurses seated on benches in the front
and back of their wagons firmly attached with ropes or straps."*

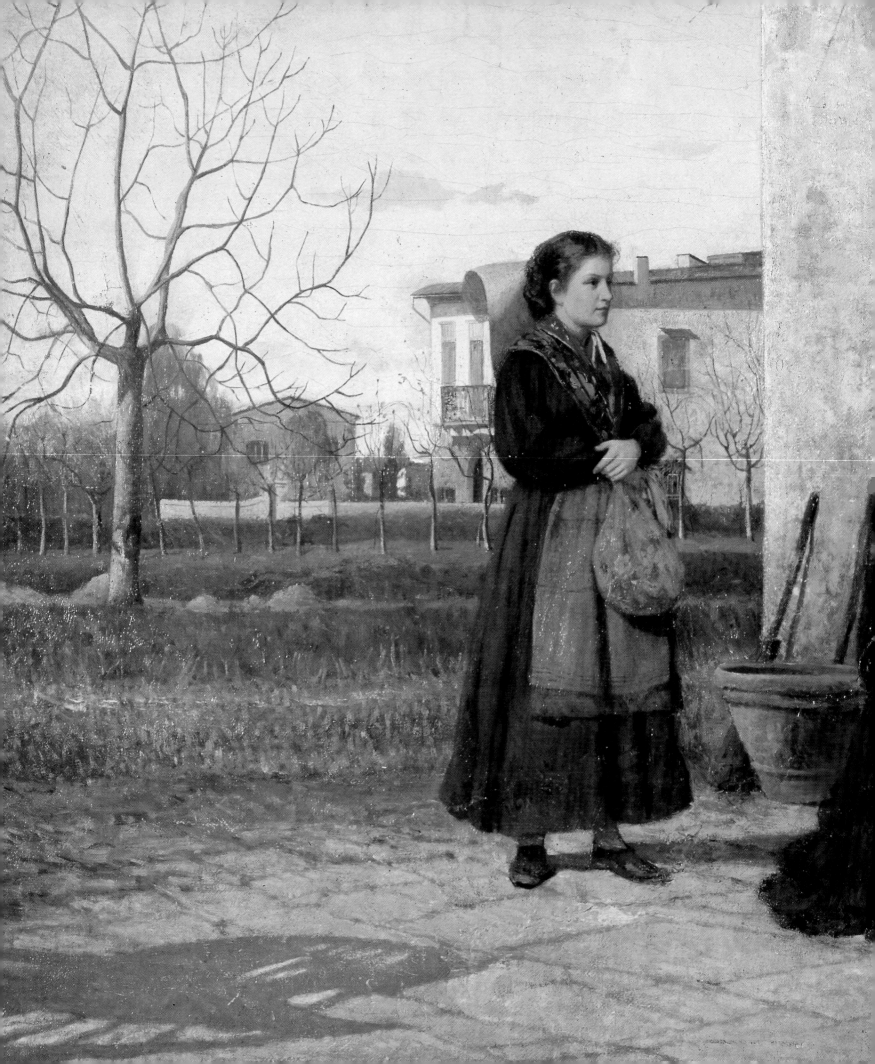

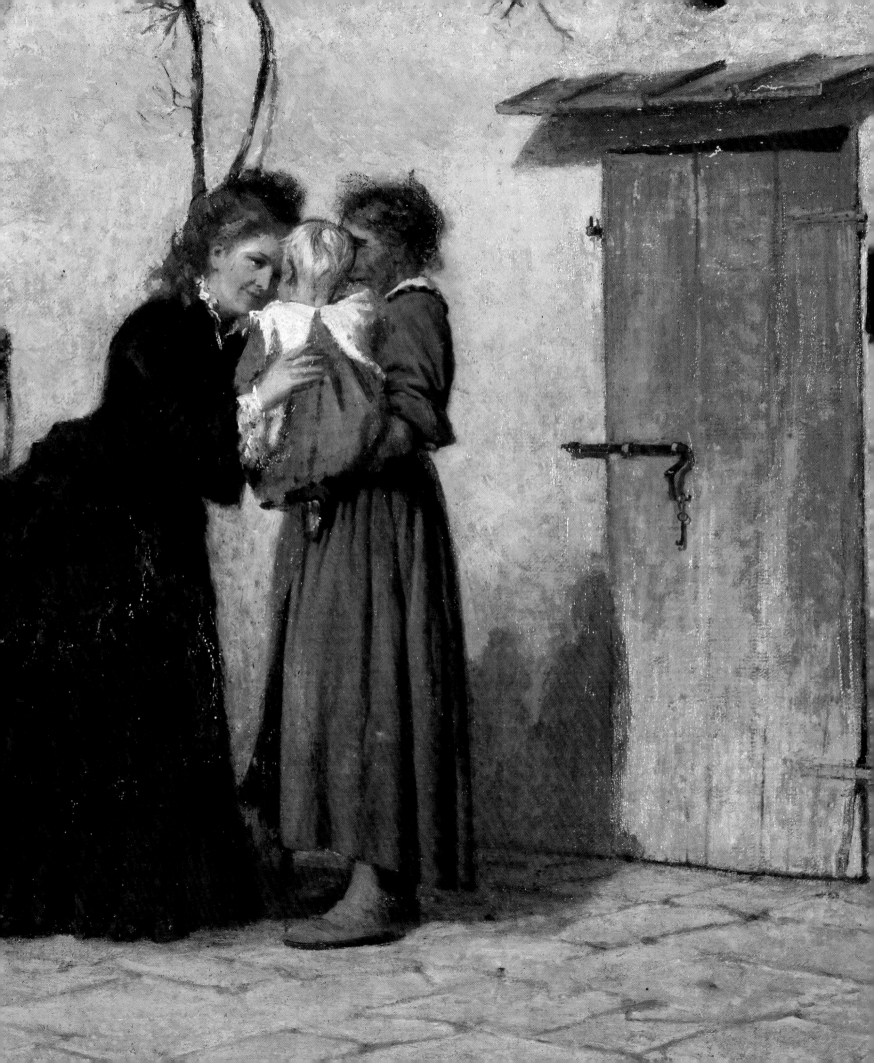

The Code of the Wet Nurses

In the early eighteenth century, a regulation tried to control the trade of the wet nurses in France. Up to that point, wet nurses only had had to obtain a certificate of identity and of morality from their parish priest. In 1769, another regulation ordered the creation of a single, general office of recommenders in Paris. This "Great Office," which replaced a multitude of small ones, operated until the middle of the nineteenth century. Similar offices were created elsewhere in Europe—Versailles, Lyons, Stockholm, and Hamburg. One of the practices in the Great Office during the eighteenth century was to have a doctor sample the milk of the prospective wet nurses, and he would write on their certificates "tasted and approved" or "tasted and rejected."

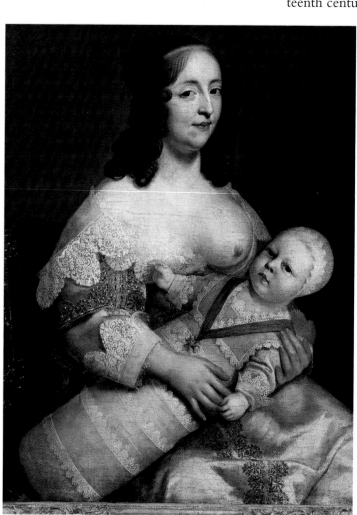

The wet nurses employed by royalty were aristocrats themselves. The haughty Dame Longuet de La Giraudière offers her generous breast to the future Louis XIV.

ABOVE: Louis XIV and his wet nurse. 17th century. Château de Versailles

Despite increased regulation, wet nurses continued to be accused of awful misdeeds, even of letting their small charges die so they could replace them with their own babies while continuing to draw a salary. This terrible picture was painted by the promoters of maternal nursing, who did not take into account the problems encountered by the wet nurses. Fatigue and an increased workload sometimes dried up their milk. When that happened, they added a supplement to the infant's too-meager ration and poured a bit of alcohol in the pap or coated their breast with opium so the baby would permit them to sleep for a few hours.

Many of the babies placed with a wet nurse received few or no visits from their parents. The state of the roads and the length of journeys partly explain this neglect. Yet what should we make of those parents who, told of the death of their child, did not even go to the burial? On the other hand, other parents, who had no news of their children, sent letters to the mayors of their wet nurse's village; in these missives they demonstrate their worry and affection. They might have been the victims of certain wet nurses' negligence or trickery. The wife of a Parisian craftsman cited in the book *Entrer dans la vie* (Entry into Life) by J. Gélis, M. Laget, and M.-F. Morel wrote, "Excuse me for bothering you but you will listen to a mother in the greatest uneasiness over her child who had been given to a wet nurse of the name Guille wife of Holot living in Beaubray. She took him on 18 November 1833. She wrote us on 5 December that my son was ill and since that time I have heard no news of him. I went to the agency every month and never has she acknowledged receiving the money. I beg you, sir, to be so kind as to answer me. You would be doing a great service to a very anxious mother." Many children barely saw their parents before the age of two or three, at which time they moved back into a house where they had never really lived, among strangers to whom they were related.

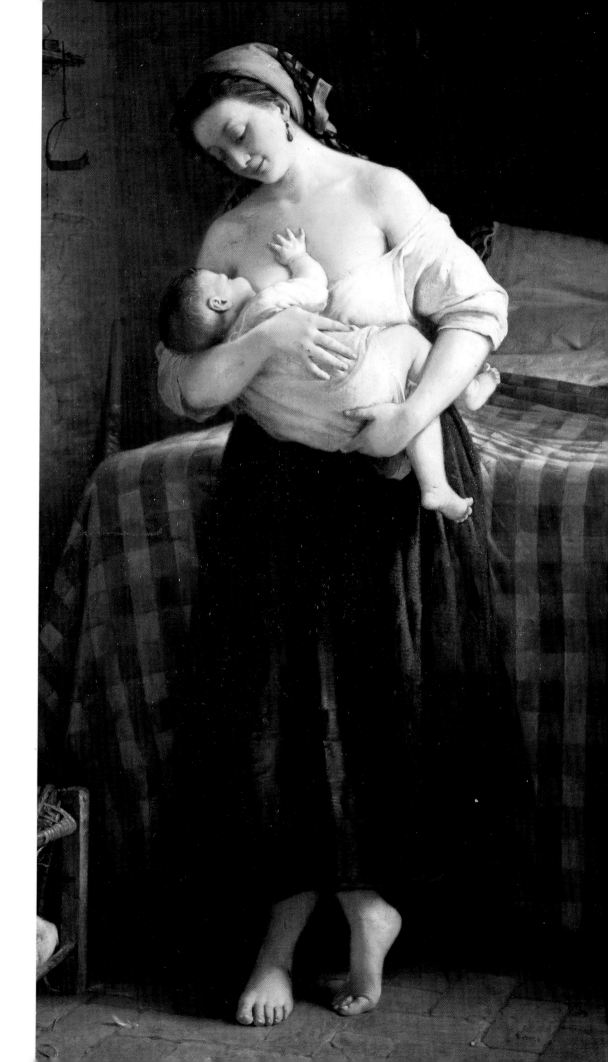

"They are old women who give cow's milk and chewed-up bread. They are drifters lacking husbands, money, and morals who turn the nursing of our children into a horrible business, take in seven or eight infants at a time whom they keep alive briefly with wine, oil, bread, and cheese, whom they beat to death or smother as soon as their cries bother them," accused an eighteenth-century police lieutenant. This extreme depiction of wet nurses makes no allowance for those many who took excellent care of the babies under their protection.

RIGHT: Mattia Preti. *The Wet Nurse.* 19th century. National Gallery, Parma

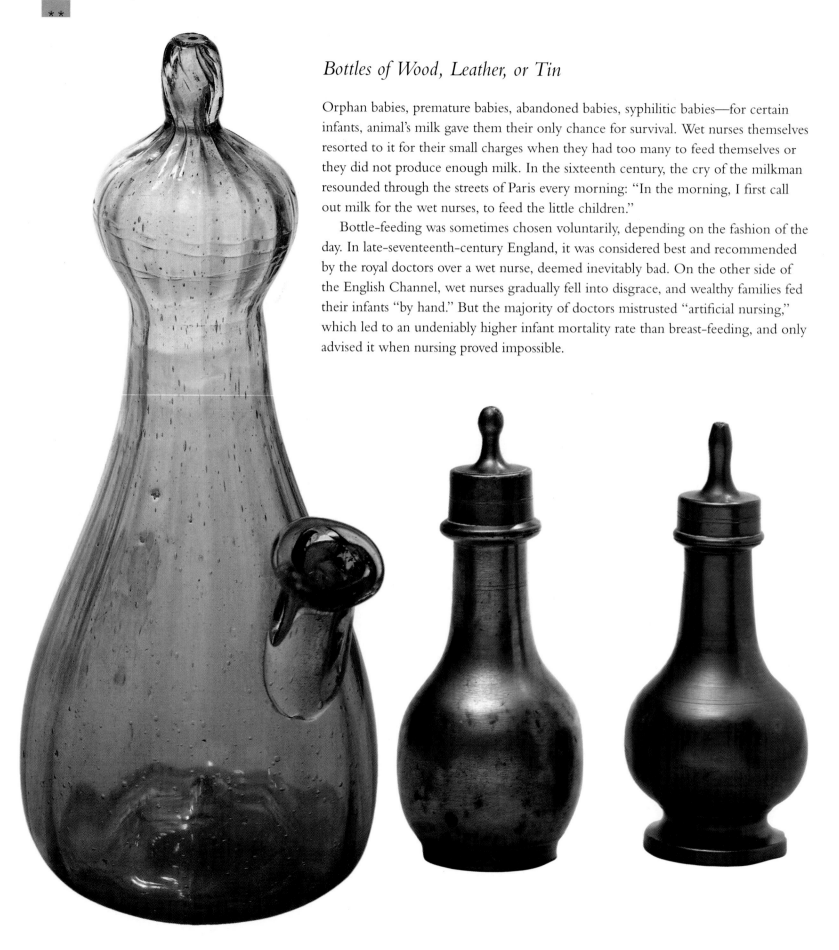

Bottles of Wood, Leather, or Tin

Orphan babies, premature babies, abandoned babies, syphilitic babies—for certain infants, animal's milk gave them their only chance for survival. Wet nurses themselves resorted to it for their small charges when they had too many to feed themselves or they did not produce enough milk. In the sixteenth century, the cry of the milkman resounded through the streets of Paris every morning: "In the morning, I first call out milk for the wet nurses, to feed the little children."

Bottle-feeding was sometimes chosen voluntarily, depending on the fashion of the day. In late-seventeenth-century England, it was considered best and recommended by the royal doctors over a wet nurse, deemed inevitably bad. On the other side of the English Channel, wet nurses gradually fell into disgrace, and wealthy families fed their infants "by hand." But the majority of doctors mistrusted "artificial nursing," which led to an undeniably higher infant mortality rate than breast-feeding, and only advised it when nursing proved impossible.

How could this foreign milk be administered to the baby? There were two solutions: an animal's teat or the bottle. Bottles, some more sophisticated than others, were fashioned from the most diverse materials: ceramics and glass in antiquity; horns in the Middle Ages; wood, leather, or metal in the Renaissance; faience and porcelain in the eighteenth century. Wood and leather soaked up the milk and quickly became dirty and foul-smelling, while glass and porcelain were easily washed. The main challenge was to ensure a steady but weak flow of milk, as close as possible to that obtained from the breast. To partially block an opening that was too large, a sponge or a piece of leather or cloth was used. The nipple was not invented until the end of the sixteenth century, in Sweden. Starting in the seventeenth century, various materials that more closely resembled the female breast were tested for the nipples of bottles: a cow's udder, which rapidly deteriorated, was replaced by cork or leather pierced with holes.

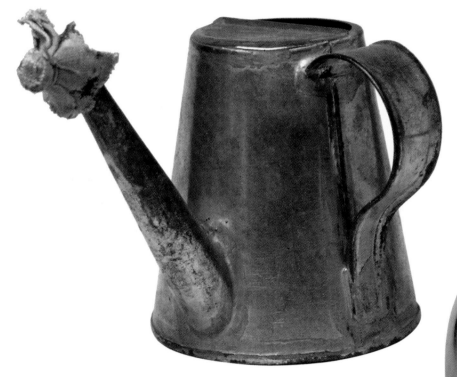

Eighteenth-century glass baby bottles have built-in nipples; they were filled through a spout in the side. Tin baby bottles from the previous century had metal nipples or necks covered with a piece of cloth.

Pap was fed with a small spoon or the finger.

BELOW: Print. 17th century. Bibliothèque Nationale, Paris

OPPOSITE: Carl Böheim. *An Attentive Sister.* 1867. Austrian Gallery, Vienna

Open Beaks

Like medieval babies, those of the seventeenth and eighteenth centuries were given supplementary foods very early on. Mothers gauged their infants' health by their weight and tried to strengthen them by overfeeding them. Until the eighteenth century, many doctors endorsed pap, within certain limits. Ambroise Paré advised starting it in the second week of life; Mauriceau in the third month; Dionis in the fourth. At the time, few doctors, among them Gui Patin, prohibited "this thick and viscous food that we cram into infants." Louis XIII first tasted pap at about a month, and this mixture, very much in favor at the court during the sixteenth and seventeenth centuries, was even served at the table for adults. At this time, ordinary pap was made of flour or bread cooked in water or milk, with the occasional addition of beer or wine. Panade, a variation, was a thick sauce made with flour, bread, or grains mixed with butter, meat broth, or milk, and sometimes eggs. In the sixteenth century, pap was nourishing enough, deficient only in fruits and vegetables, which babies needed for vitamin C. Oddly, in the seventeenth century doctors recommended lightening the mixture by replacing the milk and meat broth with water or beer—thus doing away with vitamins, protein, calcium, and iron. This evolution in the composition of a baby's food contributed to the development of such ailments as rickets.

With their finger or a small spoon, the mother, wet nurse, or father took a bit of pap. They blew on it, chewed it, then placed it in the baby's mouth. The time-honored technique of prechewing—it dates back to antiquity—made it possible for babies to consume even a thick pap; whether recommended or condemned by doctors, this practice is still in use in many third-world countries. It not only serves to crush the small pieces in the food, but it also has the advantages of starting the digestive process by adding adult saliva, and then facilitating the introduction of solid food into the baby's diet at the time of weaning. This method of feeding explains why clean and healthy teeth were one of the criteria for the selection of a wet nurse in the seventeenth century. By the eighteenth century, however, this "indigestible paste" suffered more and more criticism from doctors, who accused it of increasing the newborn's risk of death. In England and France, children were weaned at about two years or earlier, at the time of a new pregnancy, to avoid having "the first child suck the feet of the one on its way." Weaning was started earlier in America, but it was done more gradually.

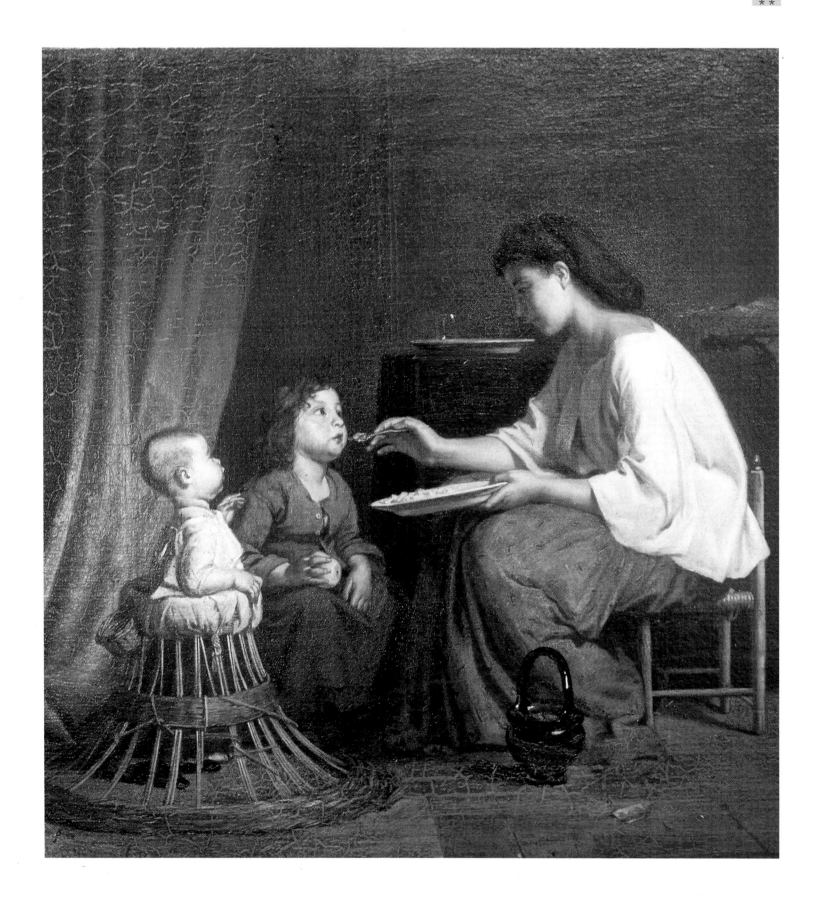

If women's nipples did not stick out enough for the baby to suck from, doctors recommended that the mothers take off their corsets and "titillate the nipple to make it become erect." If it was recalcitrant, they used artificial nipples made from cows' teats, which were recommended until 1830.

BELOW: Breast pump and artificial nipples in ivory. 19th century. Prints

From Witch to Nanny

Since Europe was basically rural until the beginning of the twentieth century, the majority of babies there, despite everything, were nursed by their mothers. In the country, the inability to nurse was considered a major problem. Thus, Françoise Loux reports in her book *Le jeune enfant et son corps dans la médecine traditionnelle* (The Young Child and His Body in Traditional Medicine) that when a woman died in childbirth in Alsace, she was buried with shoes studded with nails so that in the weeks following her death, she could return to nurse her child. The wealthier members of the middle class stopped sending their children to the country. In order to keep their children with the family, as well as for the status it conferred, they preferred to take on a resident wet nurse. This led to the development of a new industry: the on-site wet nurse. On the other hand, workers, craftspeople, and merchants, who lived in crowded conditions in the large cities, continued to send their children to the wet nurse in the country. In Colonial America, some wet nurses—black or white—came to live with wealthy families, especially those with many children.

If more babies died under the care of a wet nurse than with their mother, it was not necessarily due to a lack of tenderness, to ignorance, or to greed. In a truly innovative and unexpected analysis, the English historian Valerie Fildes illuminated the physiological factors in her book *Breasts, Bottles and Babies*. All babies are born

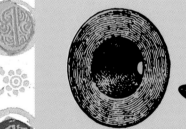
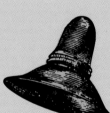
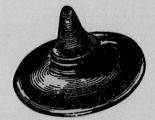
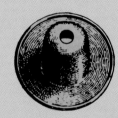

Suckling Implements

Nursing mothers or wet nurses could encounter numerous problems, the most common being engorged breasts. In rural areas, a woman with too much milk got relief by placing on her swollen breast a warm pancake or omelette or a poultice made from milk, soft bread, egg yolk, wine dregs, crushed squash leaves, or, a rare and delicate confection, roses from Provins cooked in red wine. To draw off the milk from painful breasts, the most original methods were to be suckled by a puppy, a woman, or a man. At the end of the nineteenth century, one Frenchman was a celebrated "suckler": "You would come upon him in the roads that led from village to village, always going to one after the other, on his way to childbirths. It has been confirmed that in serious cases he has crossed the borders

of the department of Gard [where he lived]. The professors of the Montpellier medical school have recommended him to their most prominent clients. This suckler was a terribly ugly peasant with a bushy red beard."

The breast pump was—and still is—a less extravagant, more mechanical tool to help relieve swollen breasts. Tubes, plungers, and suction devices with small pumps to draw out the milk—all manner of breast pumps are available. Today, we can choose a manual or electric model. These devices make it possible for the baby to have her mother's milk even when her mother is not there. Indeed, there is no substitute for mother's milk, the only food that is perfectly adapted to the needs of a newborn.

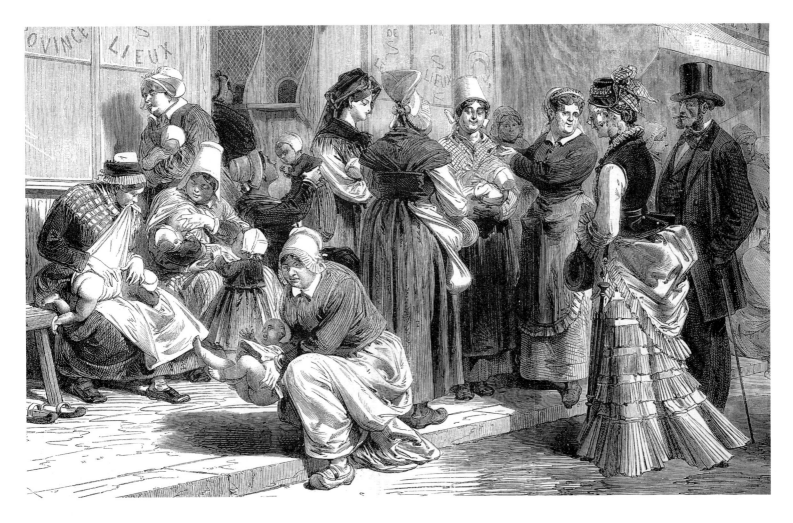

with their mothers' immunities. However, being sent far away into an environment for which they have no built-up defenses and weakened by the distress of separation as well as by a long and difficult journey put them in a highly vulnerable state. In addition, babies not nursed by their mothers do not get colostrum, a high-protein, high-antibody fluid produced by a new mother's breasts; it possesses as-yet-unknown immunizing qualities. Thus, many infants thought to have been suffocated may well have been victims of sudden death or acute infection.

The resident wet nurse came to occupy the top rank among the servants. Her influence was such that she was even accused of taking advantage of the belief that her milk would suffer if she were to be thwarted. Actually, these simple young women often left their own babies back in the country, condemning many of them to waste away: "When you see on the public promenades plump and majestic nurses whose heads are ornamented with a bonnet streaming with long and wide multi-colored ribbons, carrying a baby in her arms, note that more often than not it means that elsewhere is another poor little one who suffers or is already dead," wrote the obstetrician Adolphe Pinard in 1904.

As soon as wet nurses began to be required to pass qualifying examinations, doctors began to suspect them of fraud. Perhaps some women showed only their "reserve" breast, the one the infant never nursed from.

ABOVE: *The Office of the Wet Nurses.* 19th century. Print

OVERLEAF: Léon Lhermitte. *The Noontime Meal.* 1881. Art Gallery and Museum, Burnley Towneley Hall

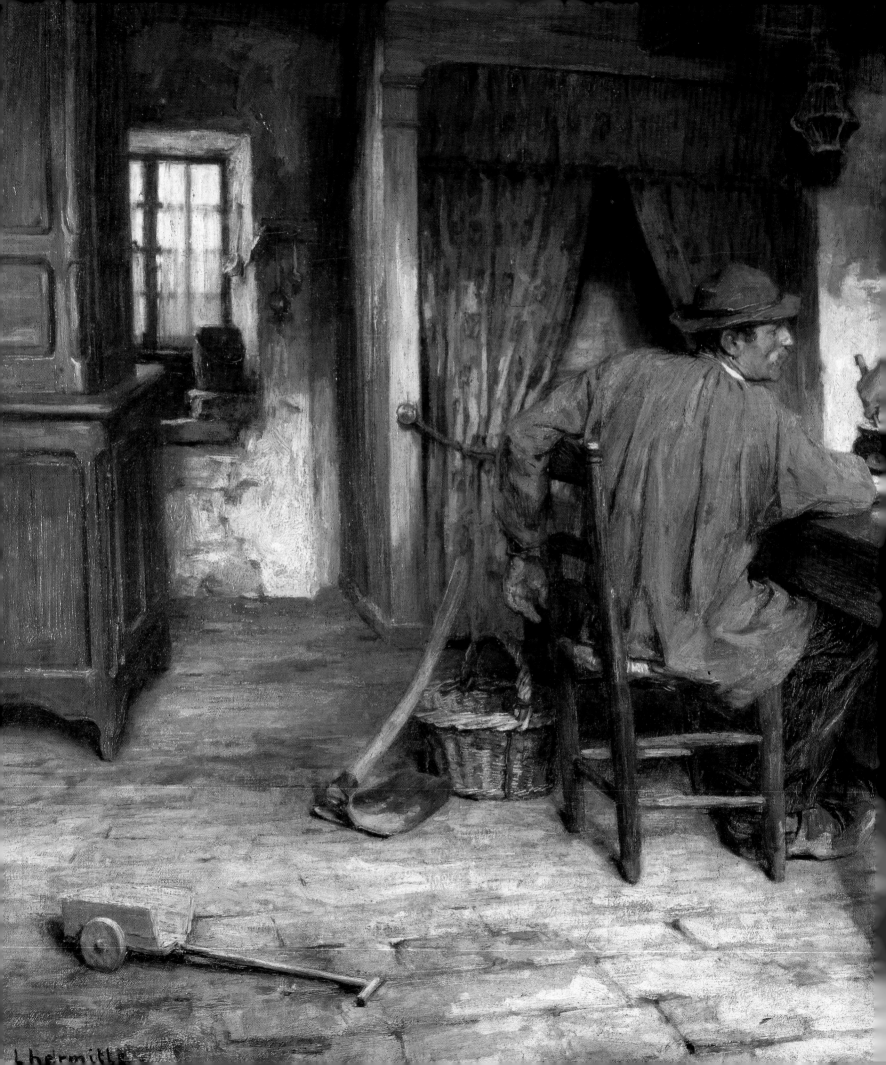

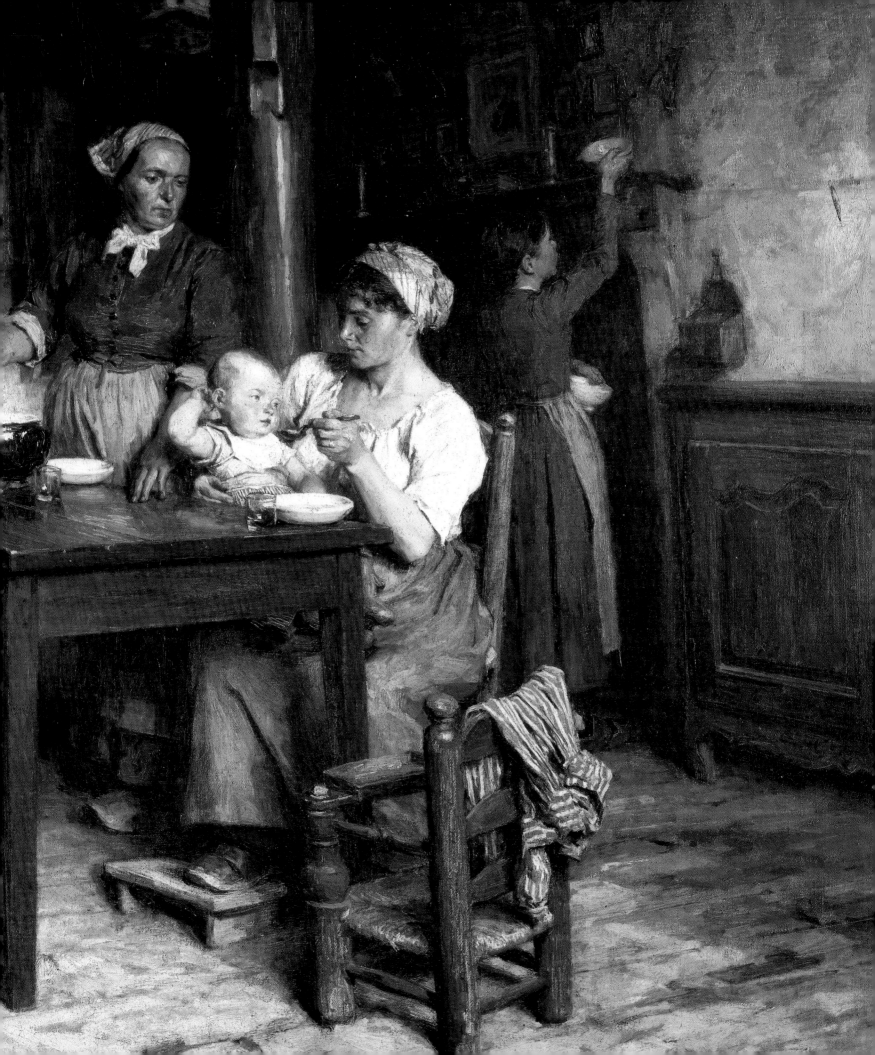

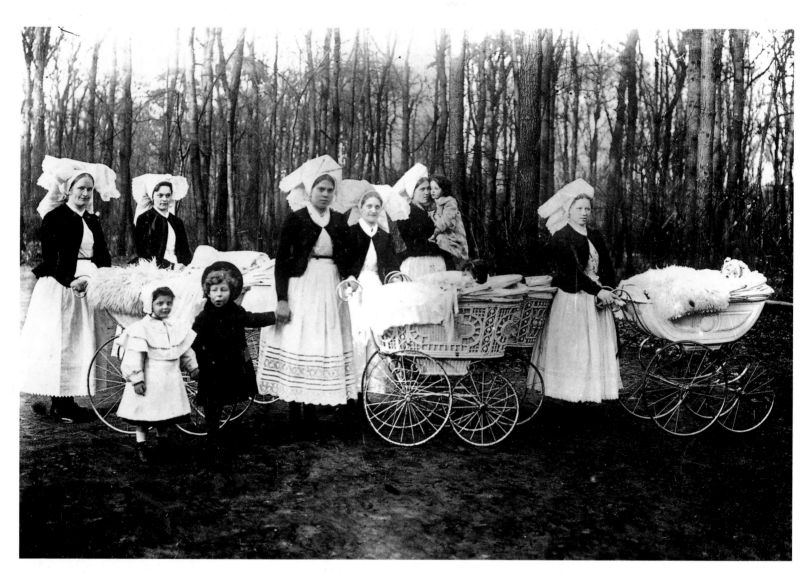

"*The husband of the wet nurse lives in sacrifice; he is seized by an overwhelming desire to embrace his wife. You cannot give in to this desire.*"

Dr. Cassine, Le conseiller de la jeune femme *(Advice to the Young Wife), 1894*

ABOVE: Wet nurses in Germany. c. 1900. Photograph

OPPOSITE: Caricature. 20th century

Overstuffed and Caricatured: The Parisian Nurse

Even when she had a good situation, plenty of food, a comfortable room, and generous wages, the wet nurse was watched closely, distrusted, and inspected; these annoyances left her no privacy. "Several were subject to constipation and did not want to say anything for fear of jeopardizing their status with the parents. It is best, once their deceit has been discovered, to admonish them and compel them to be more open, under threat of being sent away," warned one doctor good-naturedly. One of the most colorful of Parisian social archetypes, nurses populated literature, the theater, and the newspapers. They tended to be represented as fat young geese or older women with their bloom gone rather than as gentle and affectionate women. Of the many songs written about them, one by Yvette Guilbert is called "The Wet Nurse Dry."

"*When on lovely Sundays in May,*

The heart overflowing with glee,

The soldiers will lower their arms

Before the wet nurse and her charms;

They regard with open mouth

A skinny wet nurse poorly endowed

Who walks alone in park and town

With the corners of her mouth turned down

She goes away proper and prim.

Pity her, a wet nurse dry

Who's lost her assets of days gone by,

So woefully flat is her chest

That you can't see the hint of a breast;

Don't even think of looking there

If you dread space that's not meant to be bare.

She turns yellow and withers away,

The wet nurse dry."

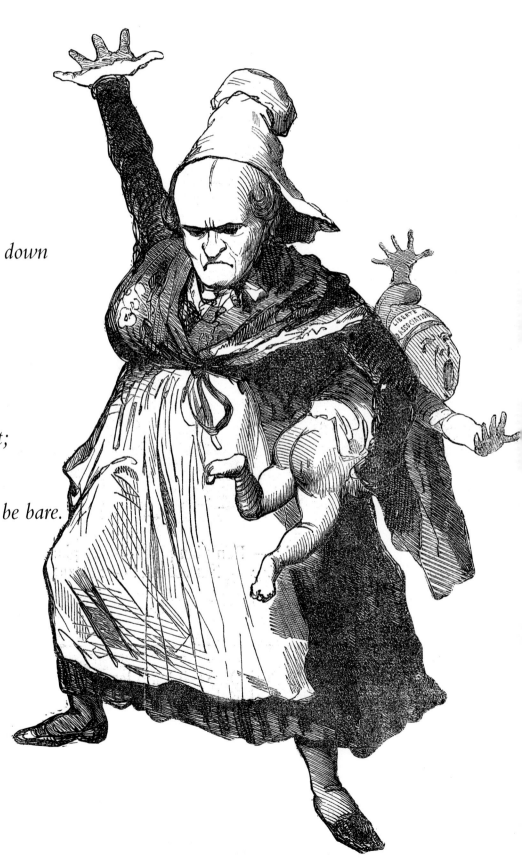

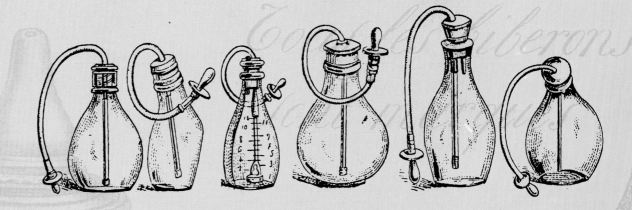

ABOVE: Various models of bottles with tubes.

Poisonous Bottles, Murderous Nipples

Even though the bottle with a tube—a breeding ground for germs—was particularly deadly, it was immensely successful. The slightest suck would bring milk to the baby, even without tipping the bottle. This suited a great many wet nurses, who could thus let a baby feed on her own. These fatal models were not outlawed until 1910.

ABOVE: Various models of bottles with tubes.

BELOW: English advertisement. Early 20th century

BACKGROUND: Advertisement for the bottles of Madame veuve Breton

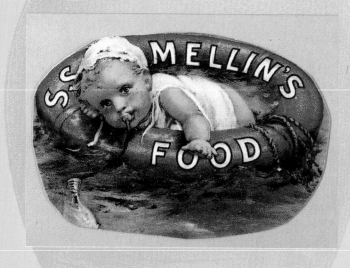

"When a mother brings you a pale and waxen baby with flaccid flesh and who, after having had diarrhea for some time, already has hollow eyes and a pinched nose, you need not ask how the child was fed, for you have seen the effect of the bottle," wrote two doctors in 1889. Over the course of time, the baby bottle underwent numerous transformations, but never so many as in the nineteenth century. Yet, despite the explosion of technical advances, bottles were attacked by doctors, who accused them, with justification, of causing deadly gastrointestinal disturbances in infants. Labeled "instruments of death" in the 1870s, by about 1890 they were called the "Perfect Nourisher," the name of one of the well-known models. In between, great improvements were made: pasteurization was discovered, the shapes of the bottles were simplified, and their necks were enlarged.

In verse, a stream of handbills attacked the bottle with a tube, and concluded by boasting of the Perfect Nourisher's advantages:

In this delightful image
A lazy wet nurse
Stretches out, relaxed and sleepy.
Nearby, her infant,
Left alone with his nourishment,
Thrashes about in a fit.
He still holds, o travesty,
The long tube he heedlessly
Sucked; and Sickness comes quick
To take his tummy in its grip.
It's the cholera microbe
That leaves him contorted.
But here's a person new
In the foreground of this view,
Deeply absorbed in her brew.
We can tell that his mother
Has happily discovered
The use of the Perfect Nourisher.
She dreads not the germ
That swarms and brings harm
To so many babies all over the world.
To her cherished dependent
She gives a smart present.
A bottle that cannot be soiled.

Despite the indictment of the medical world, bottle-feeding became more popular at the end of the nineteenth century, and the number of French infants placed

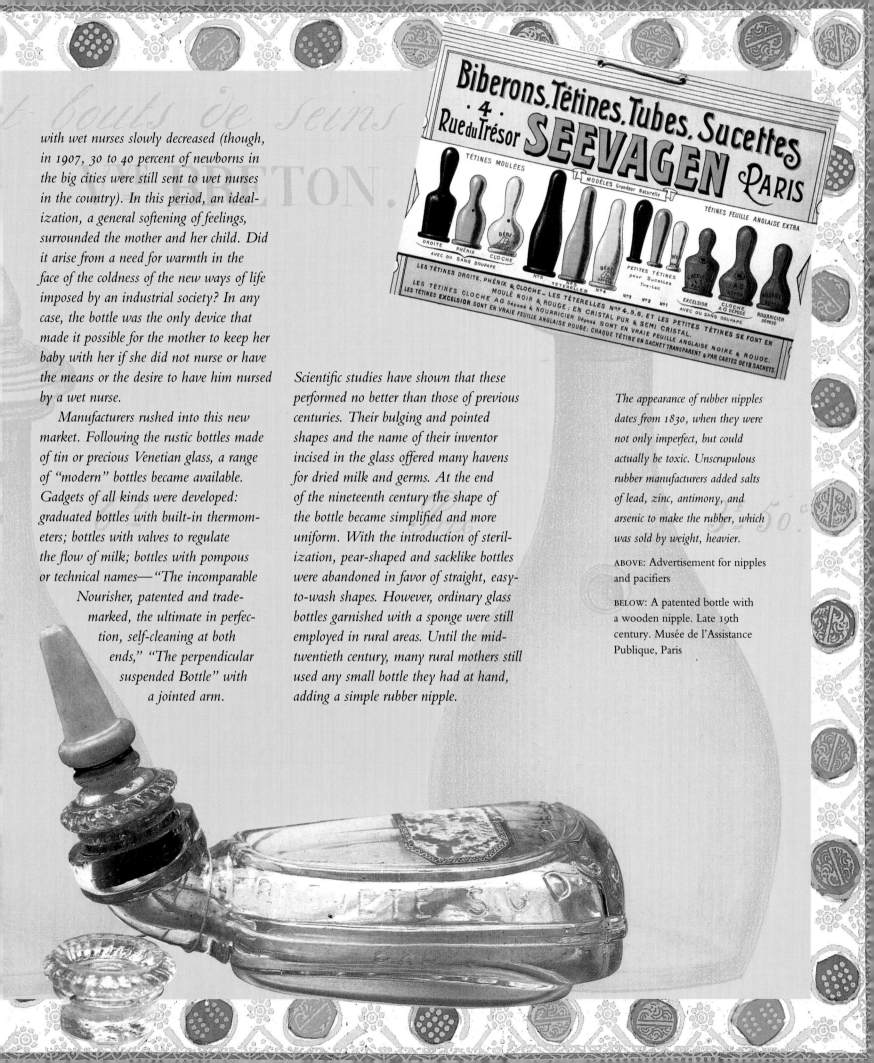

with wet nurses slowly decreased (though, in 1907, 30 to 40 percent of newborns in the big cities were still sent to wet nurses in the country). In this period, an idealization, a general softening of feelings, surrounded the mother and her child. Did it arise from a need for warmth in the face of the coldness of the new ways of life imposed by an industrial society? In any case, the bottle was the only device that made it possible for the mother to keep her baby with her if she did not nurse or have the means or the desire to have him nursed by a wet nurse.

Manufacturers rushed into this new market. Following the rustic bottles made of tin or precious Venetian glass, a range of "modern" bottles became available. Gadgets of all kinds were developed: graduated bottles with built-in thermometers; bottles with valves to regulate the flow of milk; bottles with pompous or technical names—"The incomparable Nourisher, patented and trademarked, the ultimate in perfection, self-cleaning at both ends," "The perpendicular suspended Bottle" with a jointed arm.

Scientific studies have shown that these performed no better than those of previous centuries. Their bulging and pointed shapes and the name of their inventor incised in the glass offered many havens for dried milk and germs. At the end of the nineteenth century the shape of the bottle became simplified and more uniform. With the introduction of sterilization, pear-shaped and sacklike bottles were abandoned in favor of straight, easy-to-wash shapes. However, ordinary glass bottles garnished with a sponge were still employed in rural areas. Until the mid-twentieth century, many rural mothers still used any small bottle they had at hand, adding a simple rubber nipple.

The appearance of rubber nipples dates from 1830, when they were not only imperfect, but could actually be toxic. Unscrupulous rubber manufacturers added salts of lead, zinc, antimony, and arsenic to make the rubber, which was sold by weight, heavier.

ABOVE: Advertisement for nipples and pacifiers

BELOW: A patented bottle with a wooden nipple. Late 19th century. Musée de l'Assistance Publique, Paris

In 1881, a stable of donkeys was set up at the Foundling Hospital to feed syphilitic babies. The donkeys, in no danger of contracting syphilis, could each nurse two infants a day. The babies were placed on the knees of women seated on stools in such a way that they could squeeze the animals' teats to help draw out the milk.

RIGHT: *The Parrot Baby Farm*, from *L'Illustration*. 1887. Print

"It is normal in the place where I live to see the women of the village call on goats for help when they cannot nurse their children from their own breasts; and at this very moment I have two who have not tasted woman's milk for more than eight days. The goats are always ready to come nurse these infants, and recognizing their cries, they come running to them: if they are asked to nurse a baby other than their own, they refuse; and the infant reacts the same way to another goat."

Montaigne,
Essais *(Essays)*

OPPOSITE: Postcard. 20th century

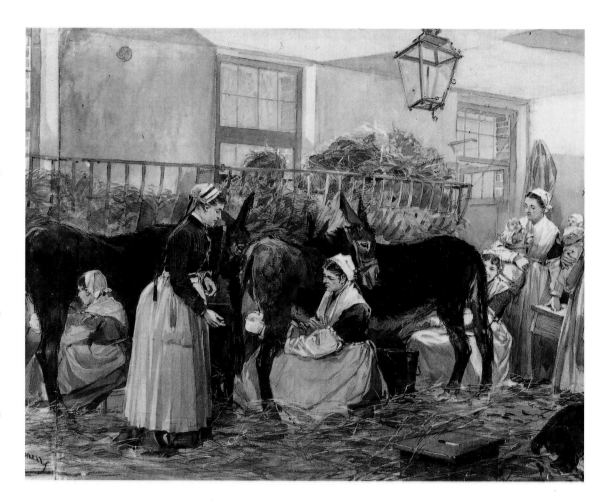

Hairy Wet Nurses

In the nineteenth century, the bottle had acquired such a bad reputation that some doctors advised feeding babies directly from animals' teats. This was the case with babies whose mothers were too weak or ill to nurse them, as well as infants who had acquired contagious illnesses such as syphilis. Born in 1823, Victor Hugo's son Léopold could not be nursed by his sick mother nor by the many wet nurses who were then tried. The family finally bought a goat that succeeded in nursing the child. Doctors preferred a donkey's milk; its composition most closely approached that of human milk, so newborns digested it easily. Despite its reputation for stubbornness and the thickness of its teats, the donkey readily accepted its role as wet nurse for human infants. However, its large size and limited milk production made it difficult for this long-eared wet nurse to catch on, especially in cities. The much smaller goat was easier to keep. One doctor claimed that goats grew attached to the babies they nursed. He described, as in a fairy tale, goats that came running at the least cry of their adopted children, and then lifted the blanket with their horns and straddled the cradle to offer their teats.

The Milk Traffic

Such outlandish techniques for nursing the baby were meant to avoid at all costs the poisonous bottle. If it was true that the unsanitariness of bottles and their nipples were often at fault, what could be said of the milk that the babies drank? Those who lived in the country near a farm where the cows were healthy and who drank the milk when it was very fresh had the opportunity to drink a product of good quality. But those in the cities who could only afford cheap milk had to ingest a liquid that bore only a passing acquaintance with milk. Its transport posed all sorts of problems. The collection of milk in poorly washed cans and its conveyance by wagon or railroad with no refrigeration offered ideal conditions for the proliferation of microorganisms. Besides facing these dangers, babies often had to drink an adulterated mixture; it was common to mix milk with water to make it go further. In order to return to it the look and taste of pure milk, a variety of ingredients were added, enumerated by Marie-Claude Delahaye in her book *Tétons tétines* (Teats and Nipples): coloring agents, such as carbonized carrots, grilled onions, caramel, marigold petals, and lily stamens; thickeners, such as whitewash, plaster, white clay, and starch. Finally, to replace the cream that had been removed, emulsions of almonds or animal brains were dissolved in the liquid.

Until the beginning of the twentieth century, the medical establishment fought over the superiority of raw versus boiled milk. Before Pasteur's work, the question was presented with less urgency, and milk was often given raw, although several doctors had already deduced its dangers, especially during hot weather. After the discovery of microorganisms in 1878, milk was supposed to be boiled before being given to babies. However, that did not always happen. The power of inertia bred

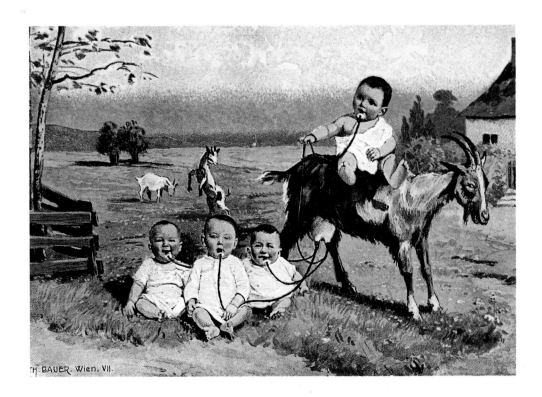

H. BAUER. Wien, VII.

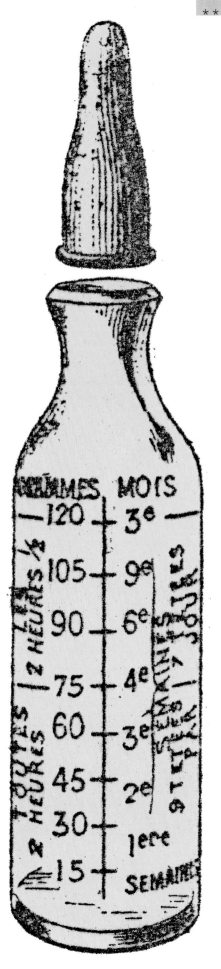

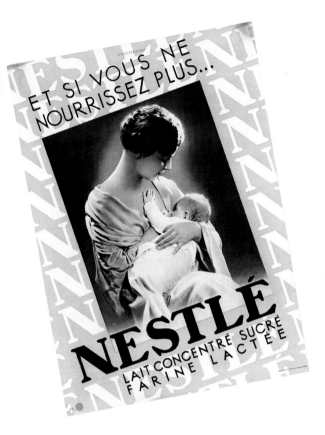

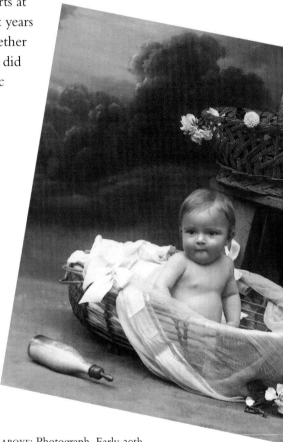

by habit, mistrust toward new techniques, the cost of sterilized milk, and the stubborn resistance of some doctors who continued to favor raw milk all promoted the drinking of unboiled milk. In 1885, the French Commission for Hygiene and Infancy once more forbade the use of boiled milk. Finally, in the first decade of the twentieth century, the majority of medical professionals advised boiling milk. They waited until 1910, however, to suggest that the nipple of the bottle be boiled as well.

With sterilized milk and cleaner nipples, bottle-feeding finally became safe. Infants could stay in their families and be raised by their mothers and fathers. The doctors discovered that highly nutritious kinds of milk did not sit well with newborns. They advised diluting cow's milk with sugared water, in various proportions according to the baby's age. The first efforts at infant formula, which appeared in the last years of the nineteenth century, were not altogether successful: babies could digest it, but they did not grow. Milky, enzymatic, or phosphatic powders followed, and successful infant formulas were not developed until some thirty years later. The first experiments with powdered milk took place in the mid-nineteenth century, but it did not become popular in Europe until after World War II, with the arrival of the Americans. It then became very fashionable.

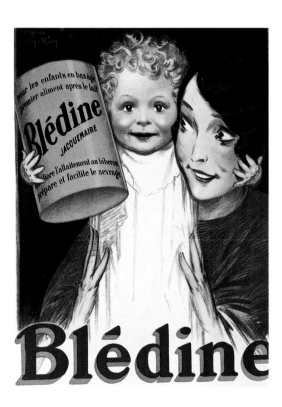

Its canned and freeze-dried forms made fresh milk outmoded. Mothers found it more modern—and safer—to use these products, and suddenly nursing seemed backward. The supporters of the new dried milks asserted, "The woman is not a pantry."

LEFT AND OPPOSITE: Advertisements. 20th century

ABOVE: Photograph. Early 20th century

OVERLEAF: Henri Manuel. Young mothers. c. 1915. Photograph

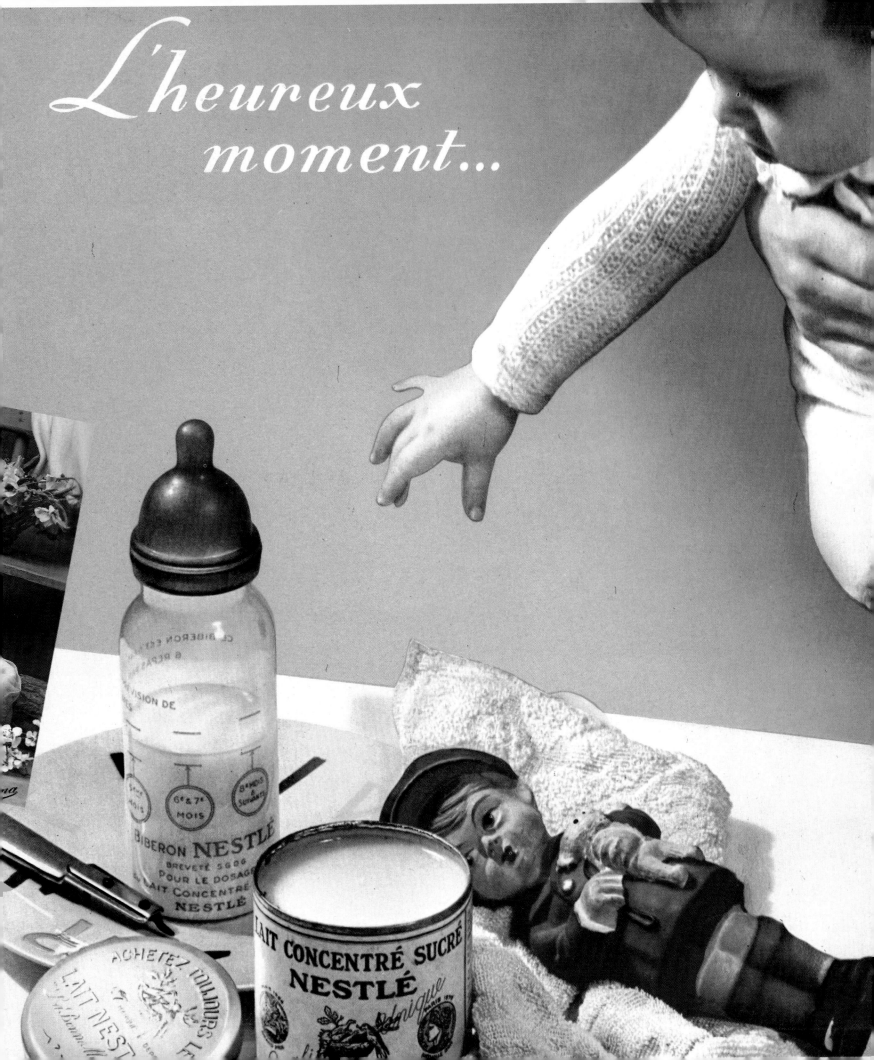

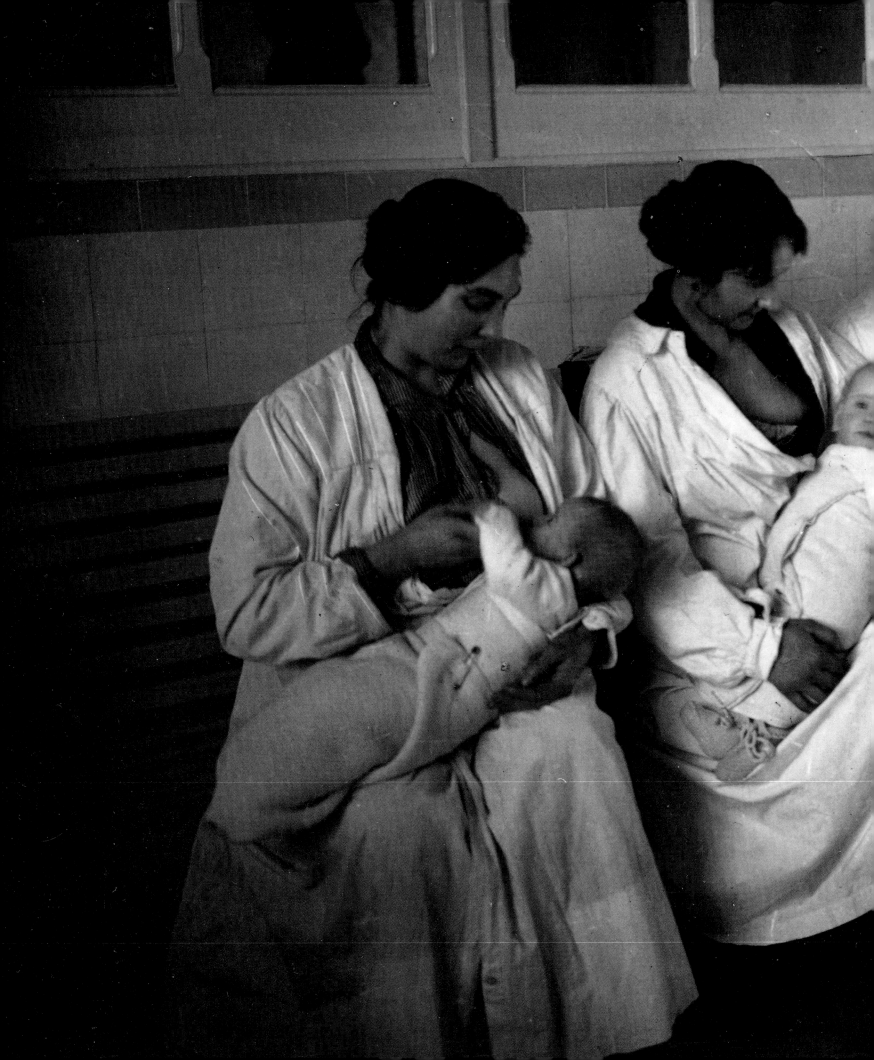

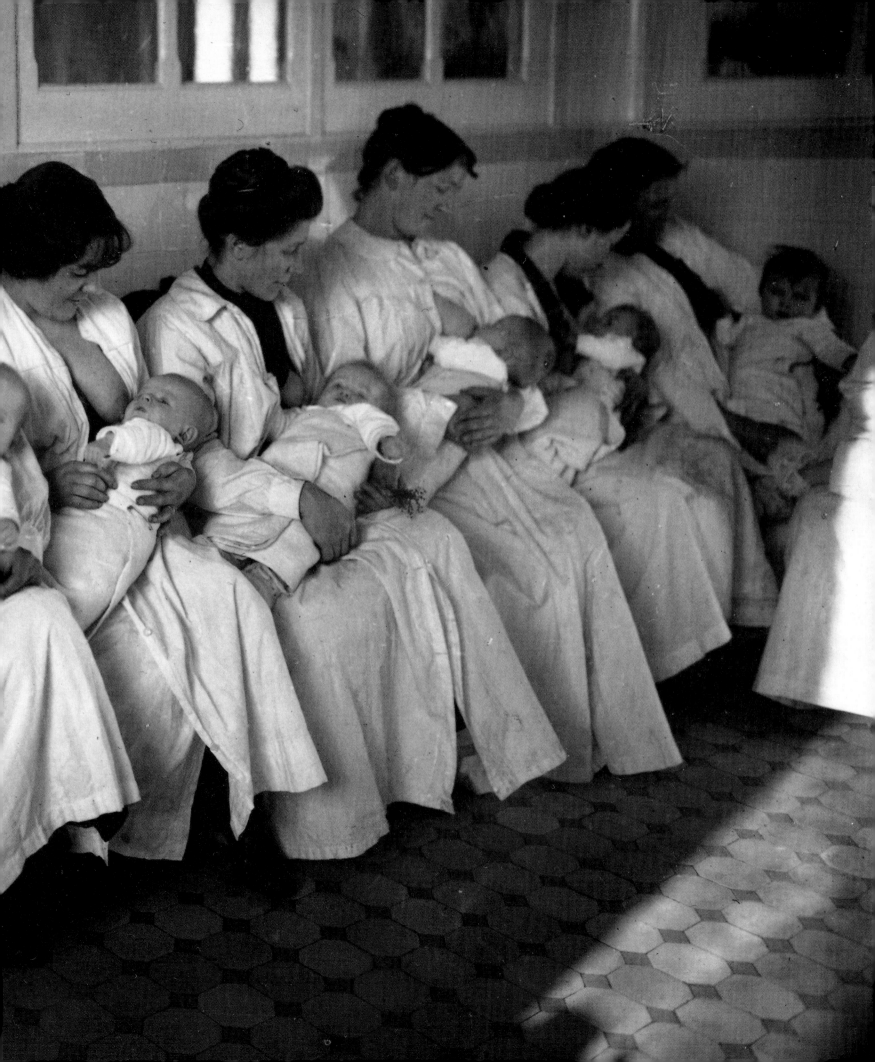

From Pap to Little Jar

Until the end of the nineteenth century, babies continued to be raised in traditional ways. At three or four months, they were given pap made with lard and cabbage, wine, and sometimes alcohol. In order to immunize them against certain illnesses, pious images of the protector saints reduced to powder were added to the broth. What foods with vitamins did these people have at their disposal? An apple was one of the rare desserts they could offer to their baby. No bananas—or kiwis—were available at the time; until World War I, how many children had eaten an orange on any day other than Christmas? In reality, even if the traditional paps continued to be attacked by doctors because they were hard to digest, they were surely prepared with the greatest possible care, made with good meal, watched while on the fire, and kept hot in the coals.

In the late nineteenth century, some sensible doctors advised using recipes based on tradition: starting at the age of five months, introduce some thin pap made with whole-wheat flour or the soft part of bread dried and ground to a powder. They also proposed other ingredients: tapioca, potato starch, cream of barley, the ground meal called racahout, rusk, and oatmeal. Toward twelve months, they agreed to crusts of bread soaked in meat juice, a chop bone to suck on, and scrambled eggs. It is interesting to note that not a single mention is made of vegetables or stewed fruit.

Solids given to babies changed little from the seventeenth century to the first decades of the twentieth. Not until the beginnings of the consumer society, with the arrival of new foods from other continents, technical revolutions in packaging, and the intervention of dietitians in the feeding of babies did parents' choices become more varied. Ready-to-mix cereals, baby food in little jars, crackers—the public has at its disposition a parade of products to feed this hungry little person who was once called a simple "alimentary canal."

Plastic bib, colorful highchair, special spoon: the modern tools to help parents with that delightful but sometimes messy task of feeding the baby.

LEFT: Nestlé advertisement
OPPOSITE: Photograph. 1951

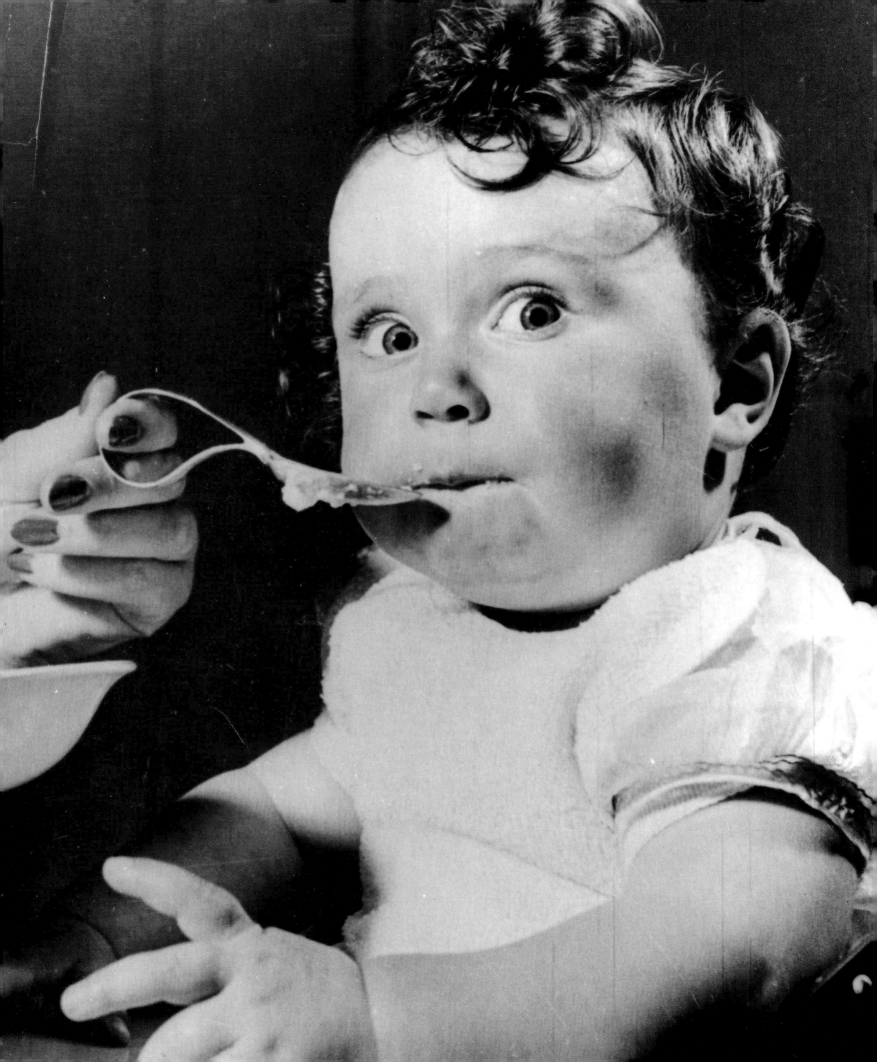

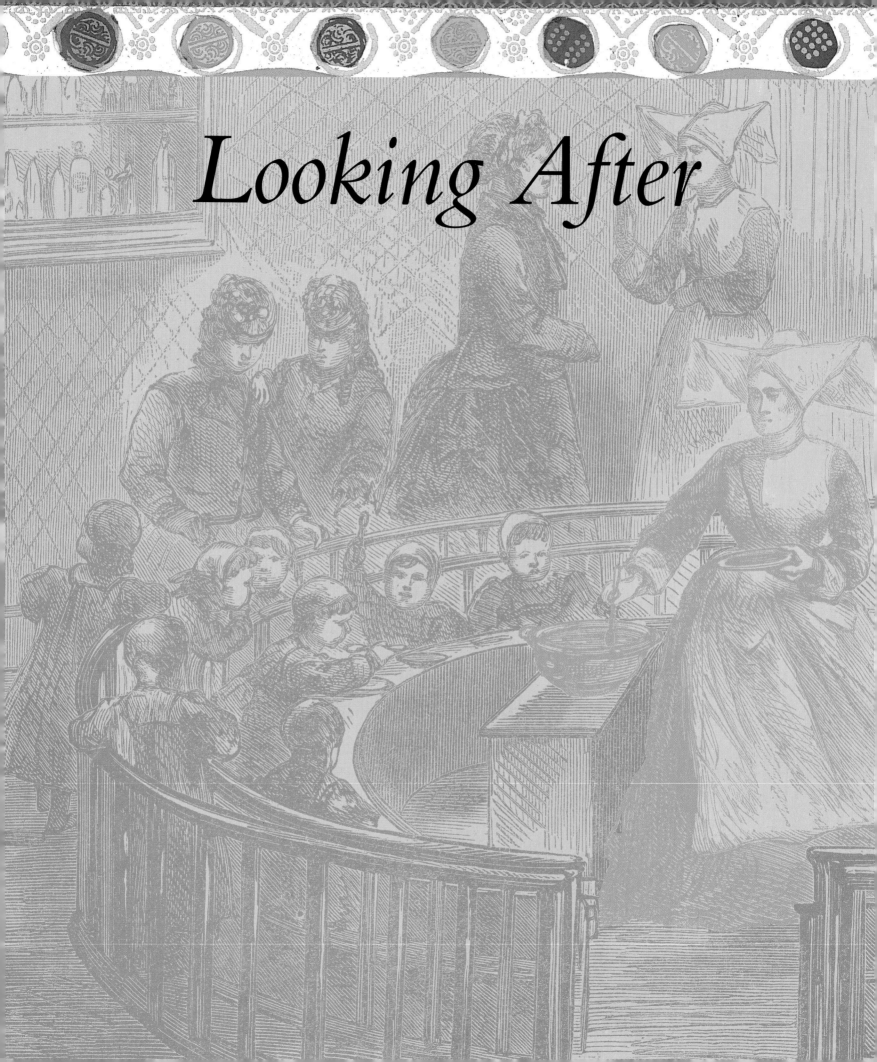

Looking After

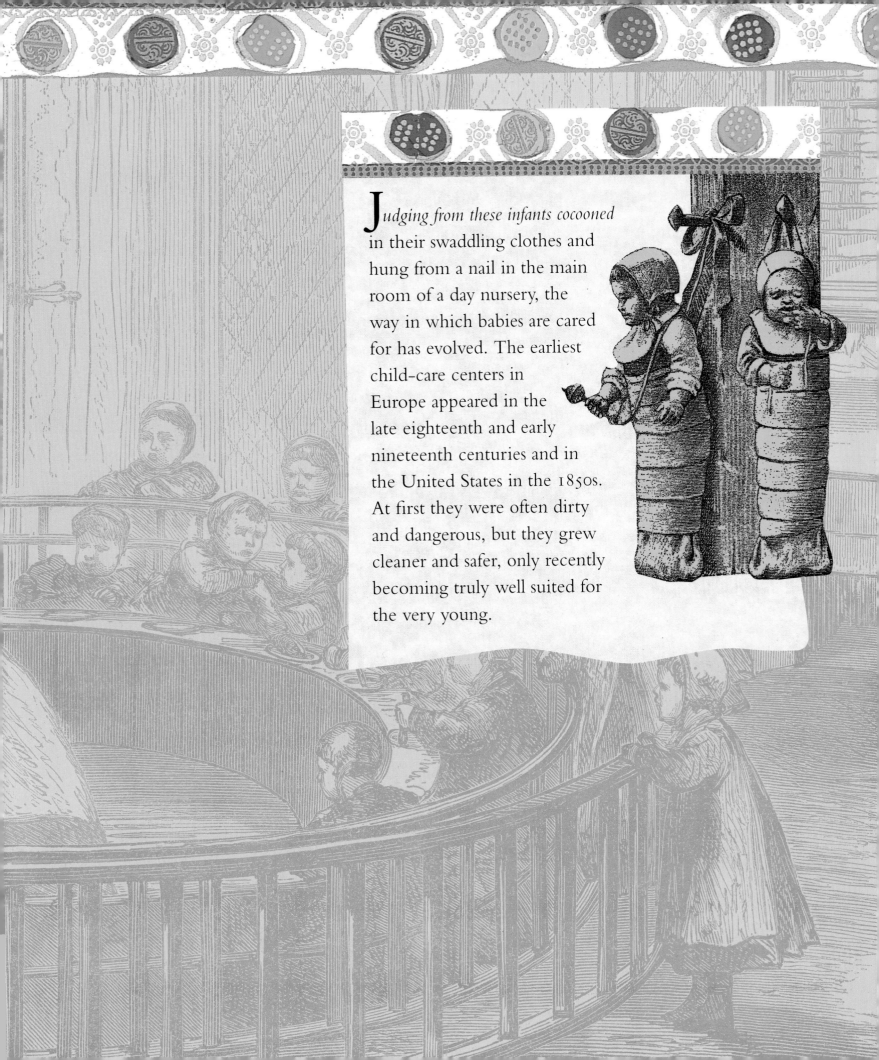

Judging *from these infants cocooned* in their swaddling clothes and hung from a nail in the main room of a day nursery, the way in which babies are cared for has evolved. The earliest child-care centers in Europe appeared in the late eighteenth and early nineteenth centuries and in the United States in the 1850s. At first they were often dirty and dangerous, but they grew cleaner and safer, only recently becoming truly well suited for the very young.

The Pioneering Day Nurseries

"These poor infants still damp from their mothers' tears are so doomed to an early death that the large vehicle they ride in is known as a 'purgatory' in the countryside."
J.-B. Firmin Marbeau, 1866

BELOW: *The Departure of the Wet Nurses.* 19th century. Print. Musée de l'Assistance Publique, Paris

OPPOSITE: Angelo Dall'Oca Bianca (1858–1930). *The Piazza delle Erbe.* Gallery of Modern Art, Genoa

For centuries, most infants were either lugged about by their peasant mothers, who took them to the fields with them in wicker baskets, or left in the care of a grandmother or an older—though not necessarily much older—sister. This form of child care was not ideal, as it sometimes happened that babies who had begun to walk would end up drowned in a pond or the farm's well. Women who lived and worked in the cities had no alternative: they could not possibly nurse their babies for a year or two and be home to watch them when they started to move around and explore. Their only choice was to send their children to a wet nurse. Wealthy families could hire a resident nurse, but no other system of watching children near the parents' house existed.

It should be noted, however, that in the eighteenth and nineteenth centuries, city air was foul—tuberculosis, among other illnesses, took a heavy toll—and a child was often better off in the country. Families of modest means often made great financial sacrifices to send their infants away to a place where the air was good. Even if the babies were breast-fed by wet nurses in the city, they would have had to receive a bottle of cow's milk at night, and giving them cow's milk in the city was generally as good as giving them

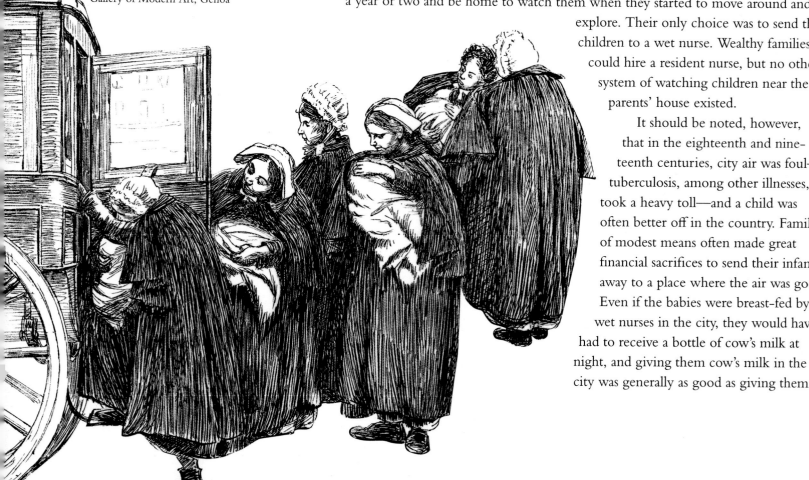

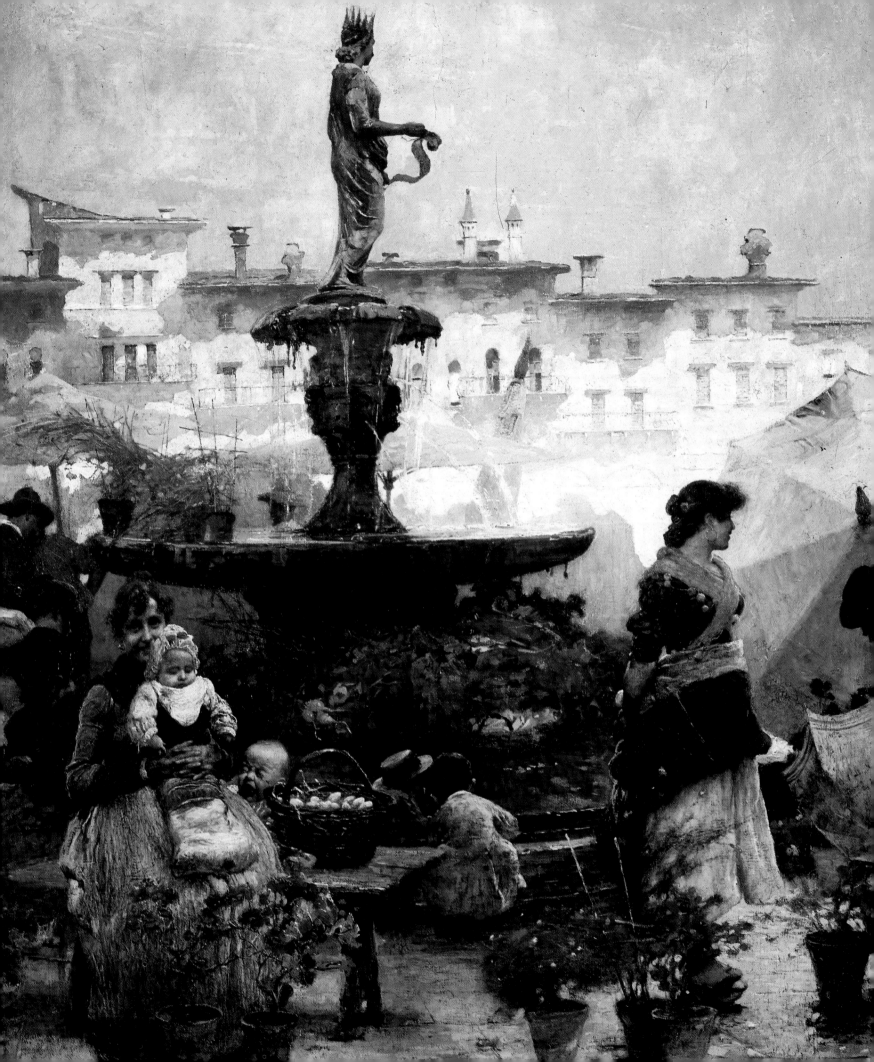

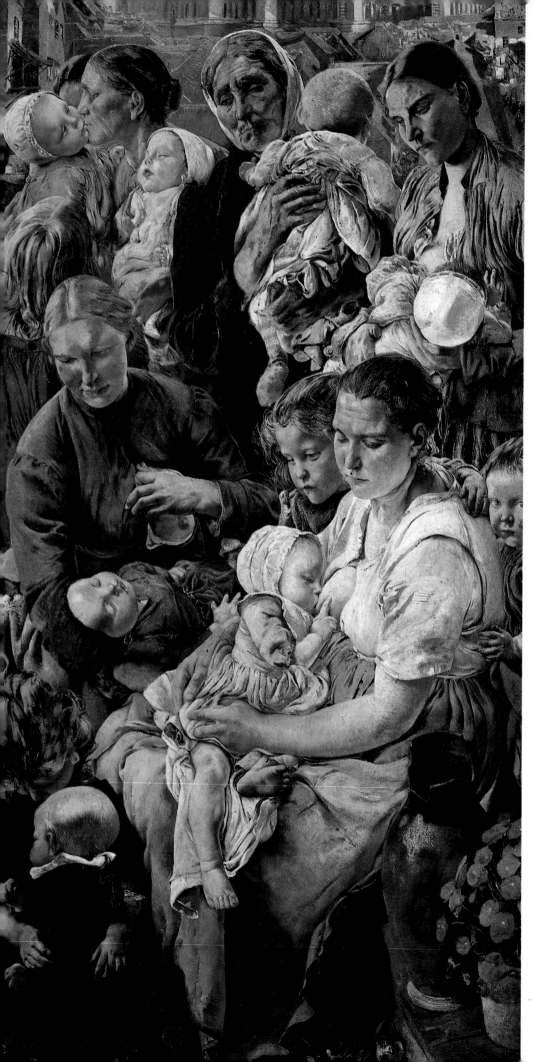

"She rises before five o'clock, dresses the baby, prepares his little bundle, runs to the nursery, runs to work; at nine o'clock, she comes back to eat lunch and nurse her child; at two o'clock, she returns once more; at eight o'clock, she rushes up, takes her child and his dirty laundry for the day, goes home to put the poor thing to bed and wash his laundry so it will be dry the next day; and every day she must start all over again!"

J.-B. Firmin Marbeau, 1863

poison. Better, after all, to send the baby to live with a peasant wet nurse who owned a cow. Many have criticized the parents who sent their babies to live far away, but the fact is that they did not have much of a choice. And how can one say that they did not suffer heart-wrenching pain when their babies left them? They knew they would hear no news of them for a very long time, as the majority of wet nurses were illiterate.

The day nursery, or child-care center, was something new. An attempt at one had been made at the end of the eighteenth century, under the aegis of an aristocrat, Madame de Pastoret. It consisted of twelve cradles set in a row in two large, well-heated rooms in Paris. The babies were placed under the care of a Sister of Charity aided by a mother. Their mothers came once or twice during the day to feed their children and took them back at night. The emergence of the true child-care center took another half century.

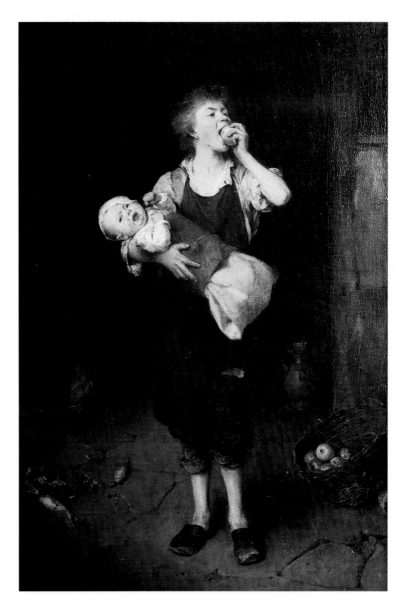

Day Care for the Workers' Children

"We gave it the name where Jesus was born, to signify that it did not restrict itself to the concerns of the body. The nursery extends its services only to families in need and those who are deserving; it does not accept children whose mothers behave badly, nor whose mothers work at home, nor sick children."

In 1844, Jean-Baptiste Firmin Marbeau conceived the first day nursery (also called a crèche) in France, next door to the administrative building of the First Arrondissement in Paris, with an enthusiasm equal to that of his contemporary philanthropists. These early establishments, intended to care for children during their mothers' work hours, took only breast-fed babies: their goal was to support maternal nursing in the "needy" classes. The mothers had to nurse their babies twice during the day. Between their visits, the babies were fed with cow's milk

ABOVE: Ludwig Knaus. *The Shoemaker Baby Watcher.* 1861. Municipal Museum, Gmünd, Swabia

OPPOSITE: Léon Frédéric (1856–1940). *The Age of the Worker.* Musée d'Orsay, Paris

OVERLEAF: Gaetano Chierici (1838–1920). *A Mother's Joys.* Gallery of Modern Art, Florence

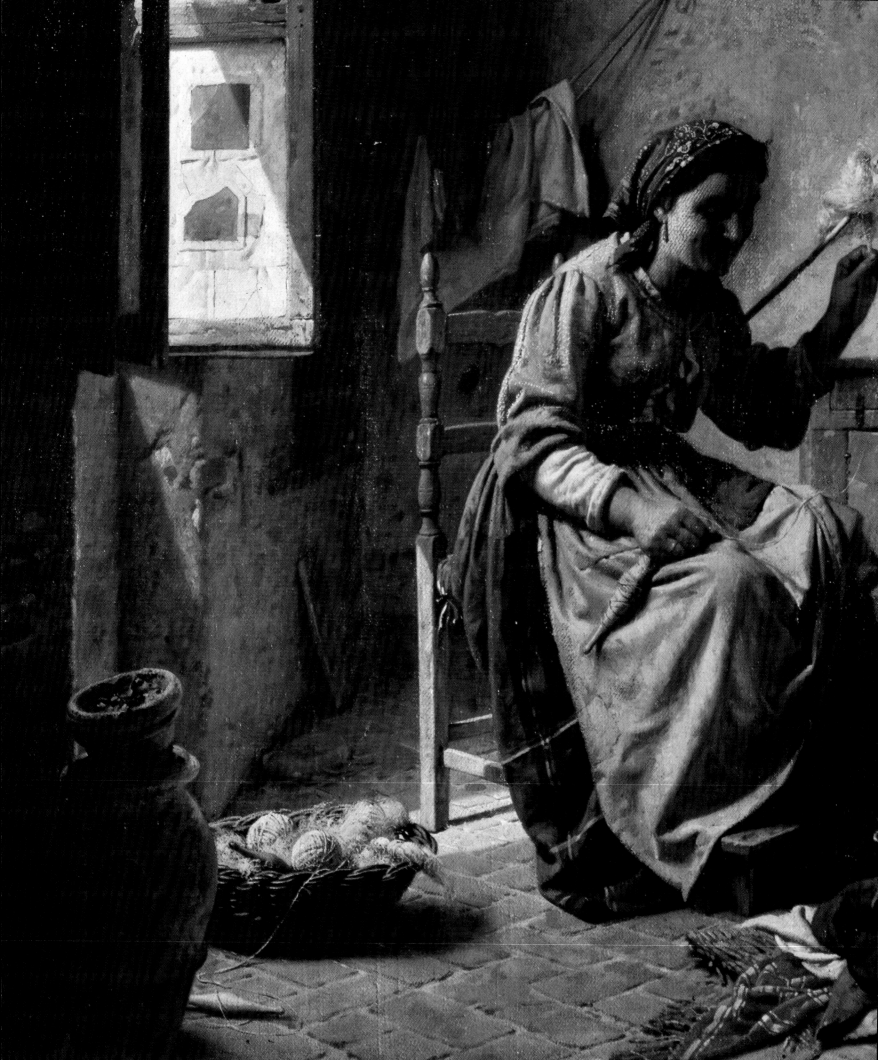

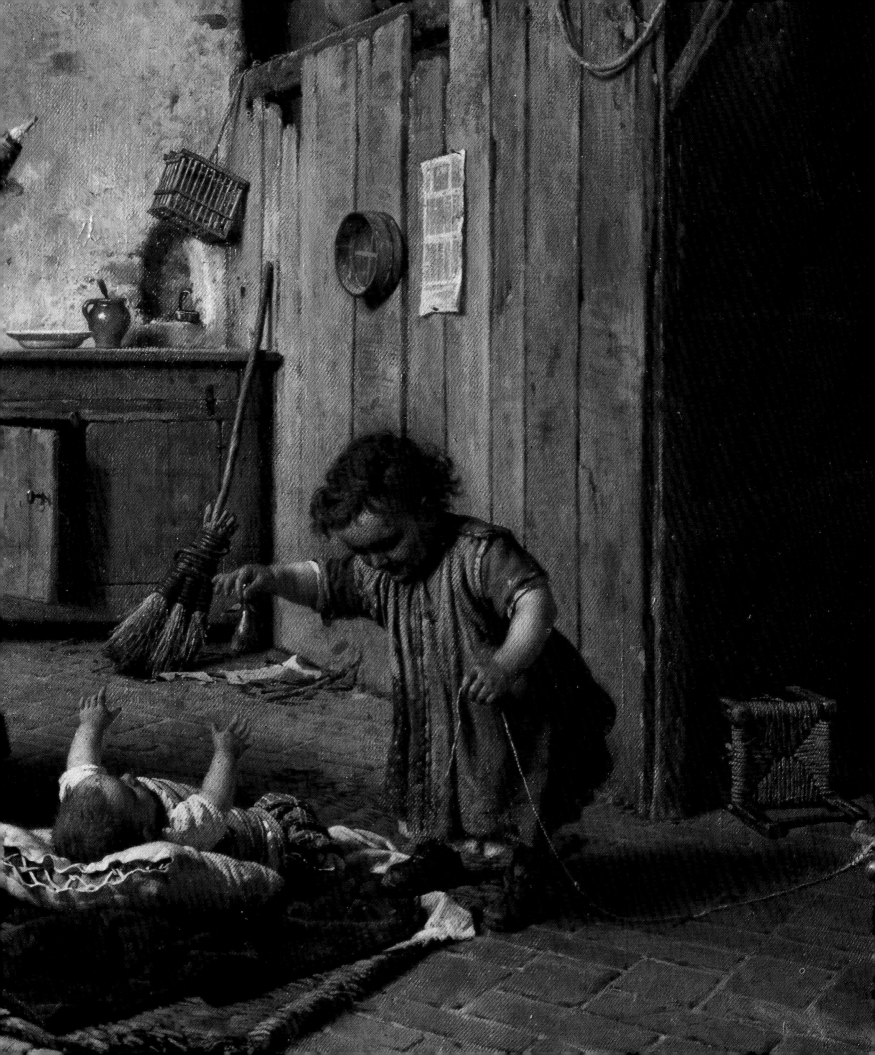

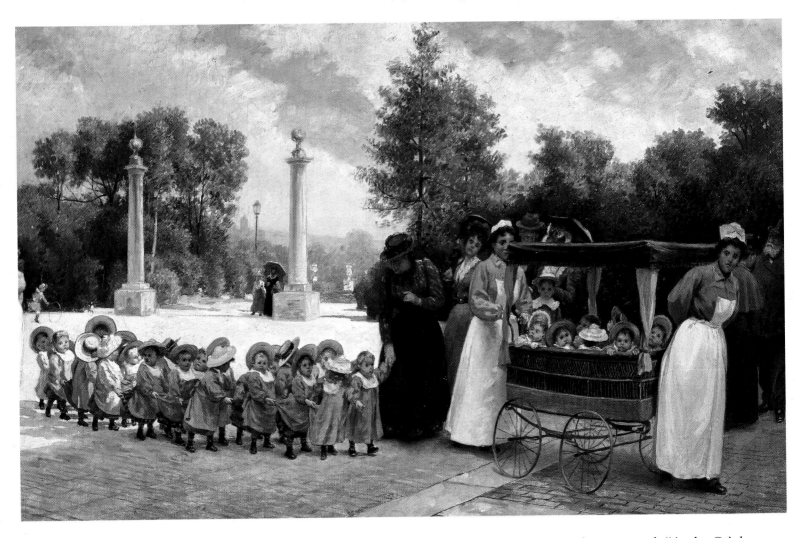

In the nineteenth century, doctors said that the nursery should be well ventilated. Meanwhile, taking the children for a walk became part of the routine.

ABOVE: Timoléon Lobrichon (1831–1914). *The Children's Walk.* Roy Miles Gallery, London

diluted with hot water and oatmeal. Firmin Marbeau asserted, "At the Crèche you see puny children gain strength in a few days of good care and good nourishment; little rascals become tractable in a few weeks; imbeciles, or near imbeciles, become cured in a few months; such is the powerful effect of a good upbringing from the earliest age." With a touching solicitude, he evoked the fate of the older children: "The brother or sister who had been appointed caretakers by necessity can now go to school." Finally, he concluded in a ringing hymn of praise, "The Crèche does a great deal of good at very little expense; let us spur ourselves to spread the idea. It says to the poor mother: Entrust your infant to me and work in tranquility; he will be cared for like a child of the rich. It says to the government: Establish many Crèches, and you will have less need of hospitals and prisons. It says to civilization: Rejoice! the divine Crèche will be your cradle; the Crèche of the poor people will bring you a new assurance of peace, of union, of love, and of progress." Nonetheless, the number of nurseries grew only gradually for more than a century.

"A Mass of Babies"

A physician at the Children's Hospital, Dr. Variot, explained sadly why the "agglomeration" of babies in the French child-care centers called pouponnières was ill advised. "This charming expression, pouponnière, calls to mind the image of wholesome establishments, well situated in the open air, with a choice staff of wet nurses or nannies to care for babies who are brought up together in the best hygienic conditions. The idea of founding and running such institutions is attractive at first glance to charitable people who take a particular interest in the earliest stages of childhood. How many times have I been consulted by charitable but inexperienced ladies who dreamed of founding pouponnières but were completely unaware of all the difficulties that would trap them later on. To my great regret, I must have dispelled a great many illusions by simply observing that the collective raising of infants was not natural and was not without its dangers; that it was preferable to keep the child with her mother or, if that is not possible, that it was better to entrust her to the good care of another woman."

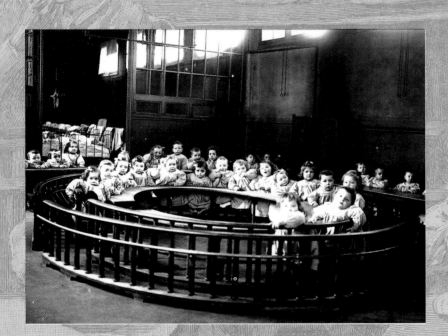

Unlike a day nursery, where the children returned to their parents every evening, in the French pouponnière they would be cared for both day and night.

ABOVE: A pouponnière with its area for baby traffic. 20th century. Photograph

BACKGROUND: The Foundlings' Lunch. 19th century. Print

In wealthy families, the governess, with impeccable references and an immaculate apron and hairdo, took care of the children and reigned over the nursery.

BELOW: Norman Rockwell. *The Nanny*. Cover illustration for the *Saturday Evening Post*, 1936

Squalid Nurseries

In the United States, the first day nurseries were operated by private charities, and at first, French day nurseries were opened by private benefactors, protectors of childhood, or those who worried about a population decline because of the high infant mortality rate (after wars, children would become the focus of attention). About twenty years after the first forays into this area, the French government granted subsidies to those opening day nurseries, before setting up such institutions itself. This drew severe criticism from the medical establishment, which objected to the centers' lack of hygiene and incompetent and insufficient staffs. It should be mentioned, however, that most nurseries were founded in industrial areas that suffered from poor living conditions.

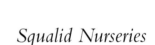

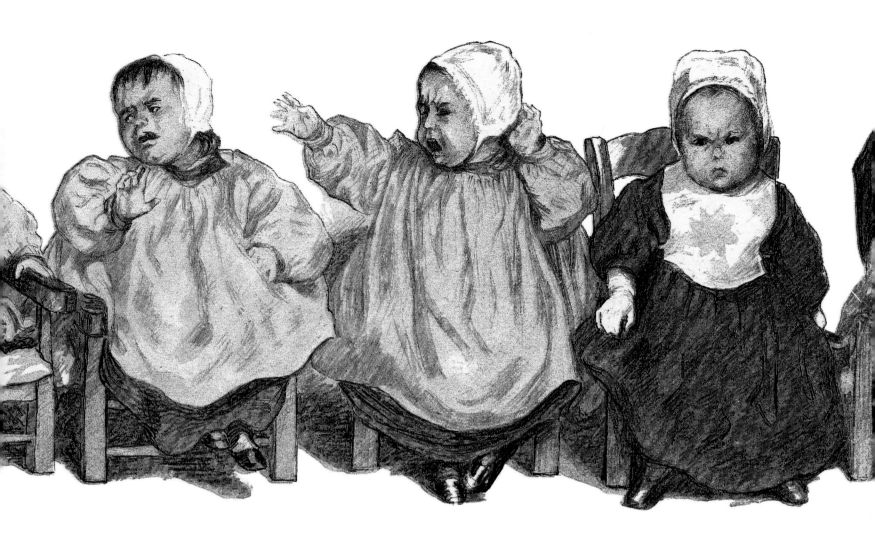

Some philanthropic employers made an attempt to include baby rooms in their factories where the children of workers could be watched and nursed, but the mothers, who might work up to fifteen hours a day, had a hard time producing sufficient milk. Doctors condemned these institutions because the babies' closeness to each other led to increased risks of contagion and because of their high prices. The good doctor Variot, who attacked nurseries and baby rooms at the beginning of the twentieth century from a full knowledge of his subject, undoubtedly was the one individual who did the most to improve them. He explained how dangerous it was to crowd babies together. "It should not surprise us," he declared, "that these establishments too often become breeding grounds for [disease]. Few are the mothers who do not say, 'He was fine when I left him at the nursery to go to work; look at the state he is in when they returned him to me.'"

Numerous complaints arose concerning certain establishments. The newspaper *Le Matin* repeated some of them in its issue of 28 March 1916: "At right is a mushroom bed, that is, from the beginning of the year to the end, piles of horse manure with pestilential mustiness. At left are heaps of sludge used by the immediate neighbors of commercial plant nurseries, from which myriads of flies swarm in summer, surviving all the efforts of the exterminators." Throughout his life, Variot

The backs of babies' smocks were passed over the backs of their little chairs until the babies were able to hold themselves up well enough to stay seated on their own. All wear canvas bonnets, an article of clothing that disappeared in the course of the twentieth century.

ABOVE: *Foundlings.* 19th century. Print

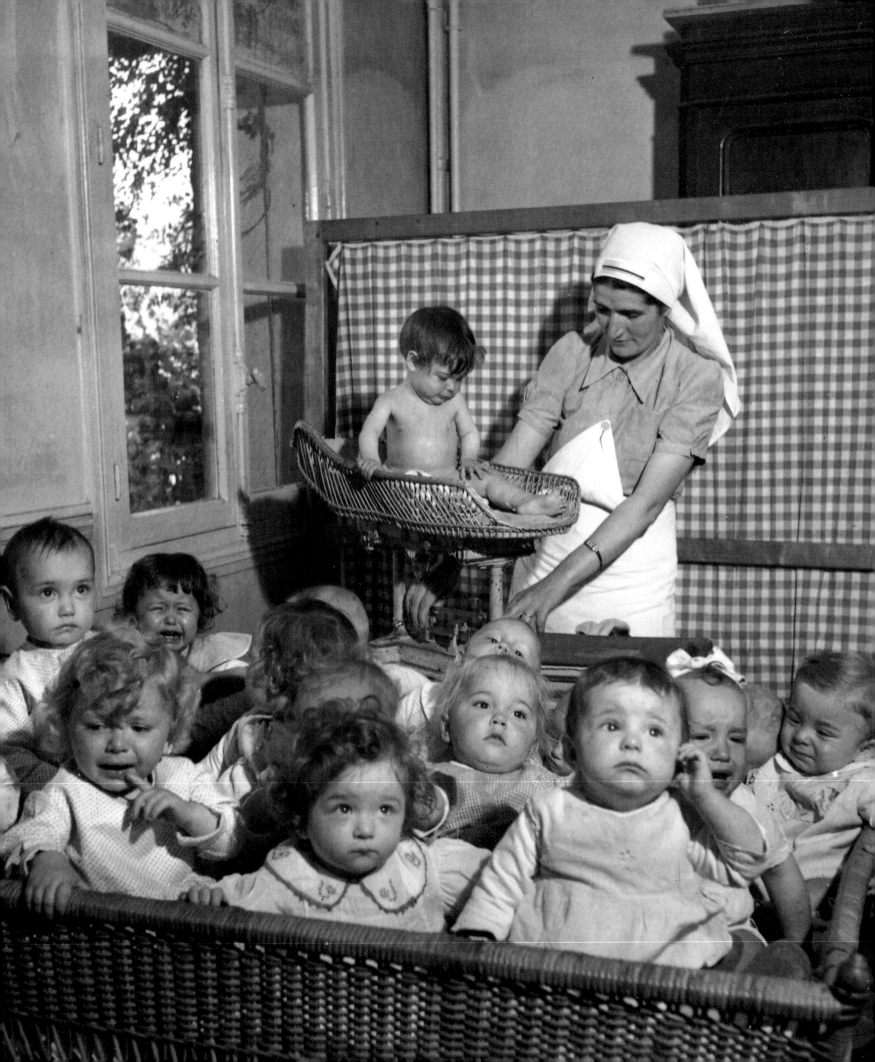

fought to improve the fate of babies. A doctor at the children's hospital in Paris at the beginning of the century, he was responsible for the nursery for bottle-fed infants. After World War II, he evoked his memories of that period: "I endeavored to improve this service, set up in old, unhealthy buildings, but without great success, I confess. Nonetheless, I managed to have built one tiled room just for preparing baby bottles. Up to then the bottles were prepared in a small kitchen that also served as a bathroom and a changing room. The poor arrangements and the inadequacy of our hospital nurseries in Paris, with an insufficient number of people to care for the babies, was all the more regrettable in that the Germans, well before the war, did not shrink from any expense to arrange hygienically and comfortably the establishments where babies were brought together.... French doctors returning from Germany expressed astonishment at the wonderful organization of these services."

Sterilized Nurseries

Day nurseries proved to be complex and difficult to run. In addition, they continued to be criticized not only by doctors but also by various moralists who accused them of weakening family bonds and turning mothers from their duty. After 1880, in France the central government and local administrators wanted to regulate these institutions, which they partially underwrote. Many elected representatives wished to regain control of this realm, which the Catholic charitable organizations had long dominated. They wanted to transform the nurseries into instruments for spreading to the working classes the new rules of Pasteurian hygiene, which, at the end of the nineteenth century, had become a real passion. Gradually, local communities, aided by the central government, opened nurseries, taking them over from private charity. Quickly recognized as public utilities,

"Thanks to these excellent conditions of hygiene, thanks to the instruction our nurses receive, and thanks to good sterilized milk, we have achieved genuine resurrections among babies with stunted development," enthused Dr. Variot.

OPPOSITE: Robert Doisneau. Photograph

BELOW: Detail of a postcard

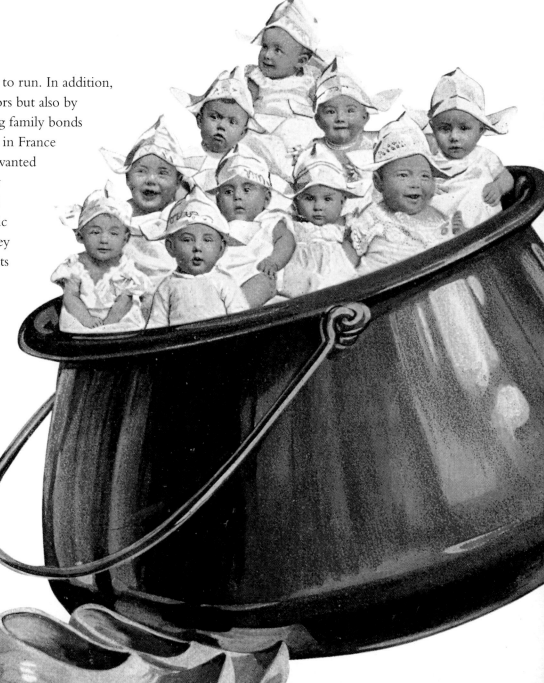

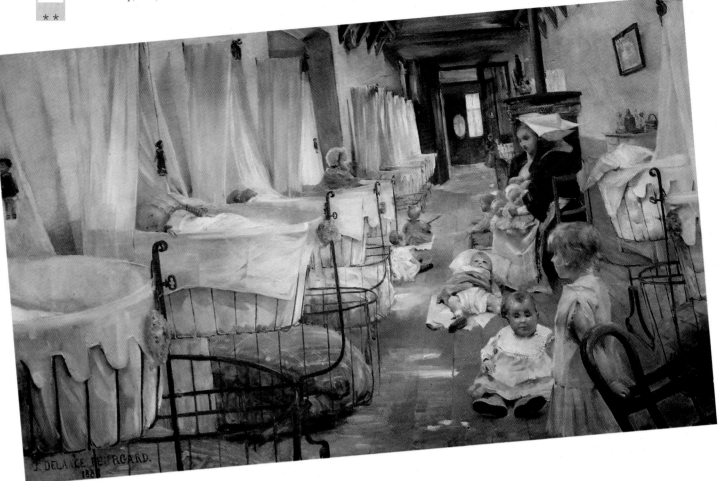

A wide chasm lay between the ideal and the actual nursery. A study published by a doctor in 1902 indicated that a third of all French nurseries did not have a bathroom, and one of them did not even have running water. However, the evolution of modern comforts, the development of vaccines against childhood diseases, and the progress made in dietetics gradually improved the quality of life in these facilities.

ABOVE: Julie Delance-Feurgard (1859–1892). *The Cradles.* Musée des Beaux-Arts, Brest

OPPOSITE: Robert Doisneau. Photograph

they finally made it possible for mothers to keep their babies at home instead of sending them far away to a wet nurse. Given the slow rate of growth in the number of nurseries, however, the institution of the wet nurse did not disappear in France until the 1930s. In the 1960s, French nurseries went too far in the direction of hygiene. The people who ran them became obsessed with cleanliness, at the expense of such functions as greeting and establishing good relations with the children. The children were passed over a counter like parcels. This practice persisted in certain establishments until 1972. The children were weighed, then placed in a cradle alone, without any toys. They saw nothing of the world but the whiteness of the walls, the curtains, and the staff uniforms.

In the 1970s, it all changed: twenty years of research on child development wrought a transformation of the child-care centers. Today, toys, plastic pools, fountains, seesaws, drums, colored mobiles, walls decorated with lively paintings, and mirrors for making faces in still do not prevent diehards from comparing putting babies in nurseries to the industrial raising of chickens. Without endorsing any particular point of view, it must be said that a warm and friendly caretaker who gives children a simple cardboard hut to play in could make them as happy as they'd be with an orgy of carefully conceived developmental toys.

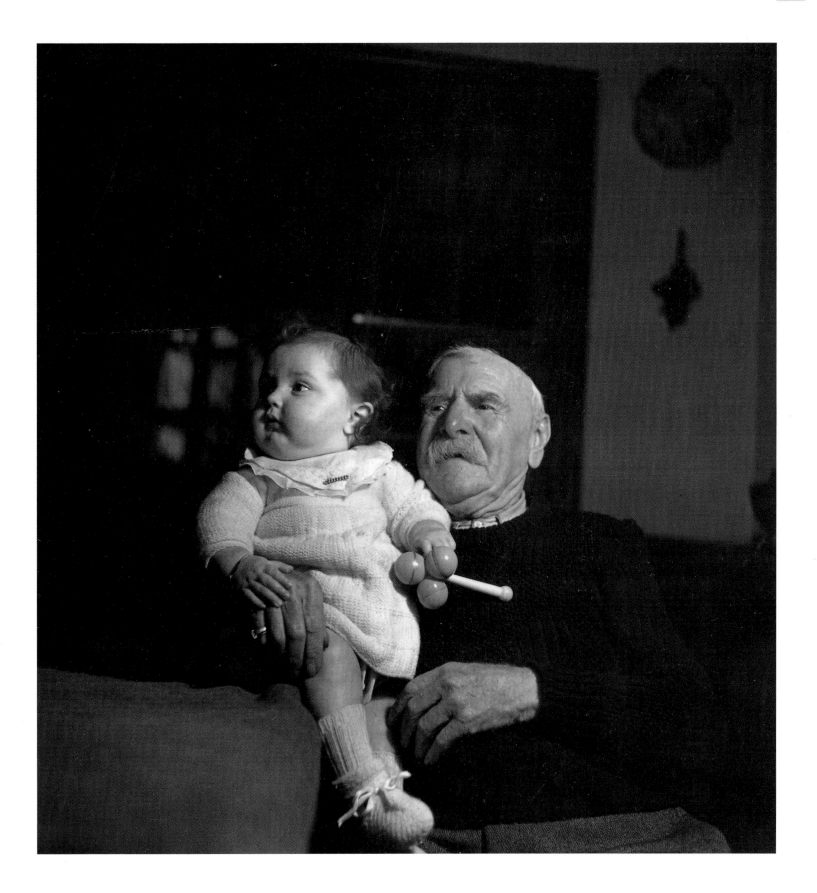

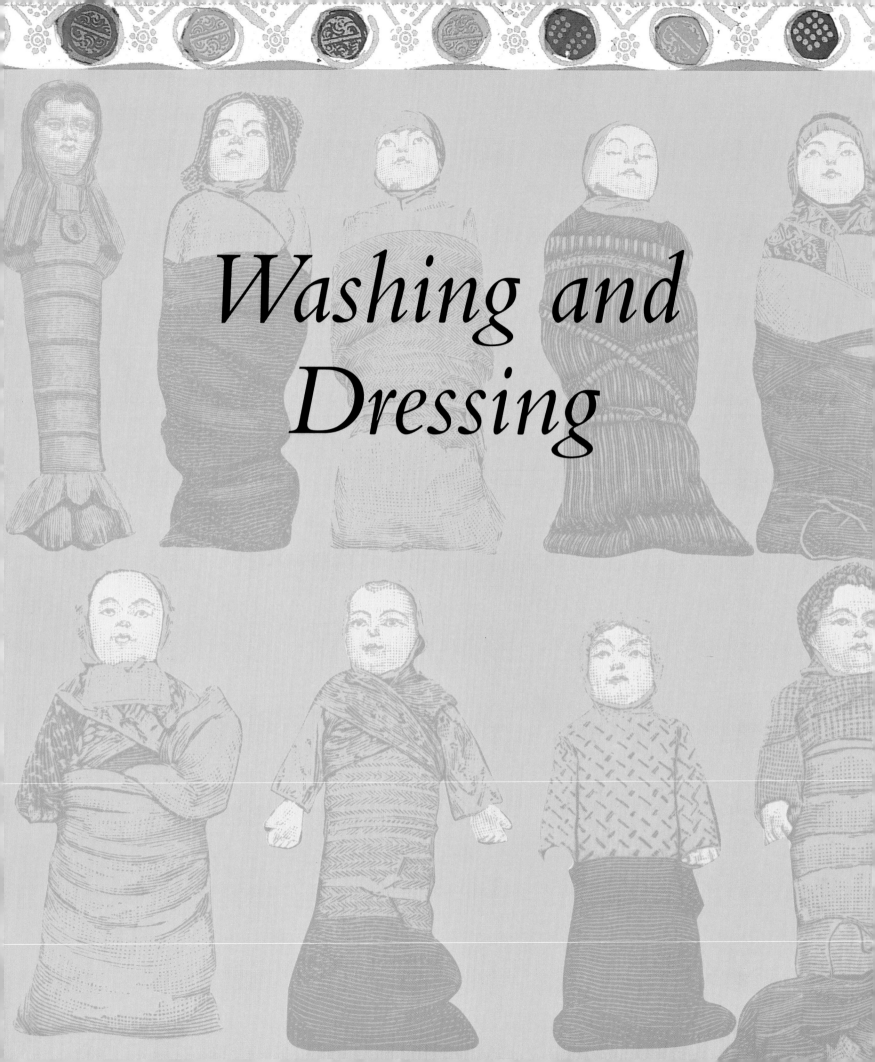

Washing and Dressing

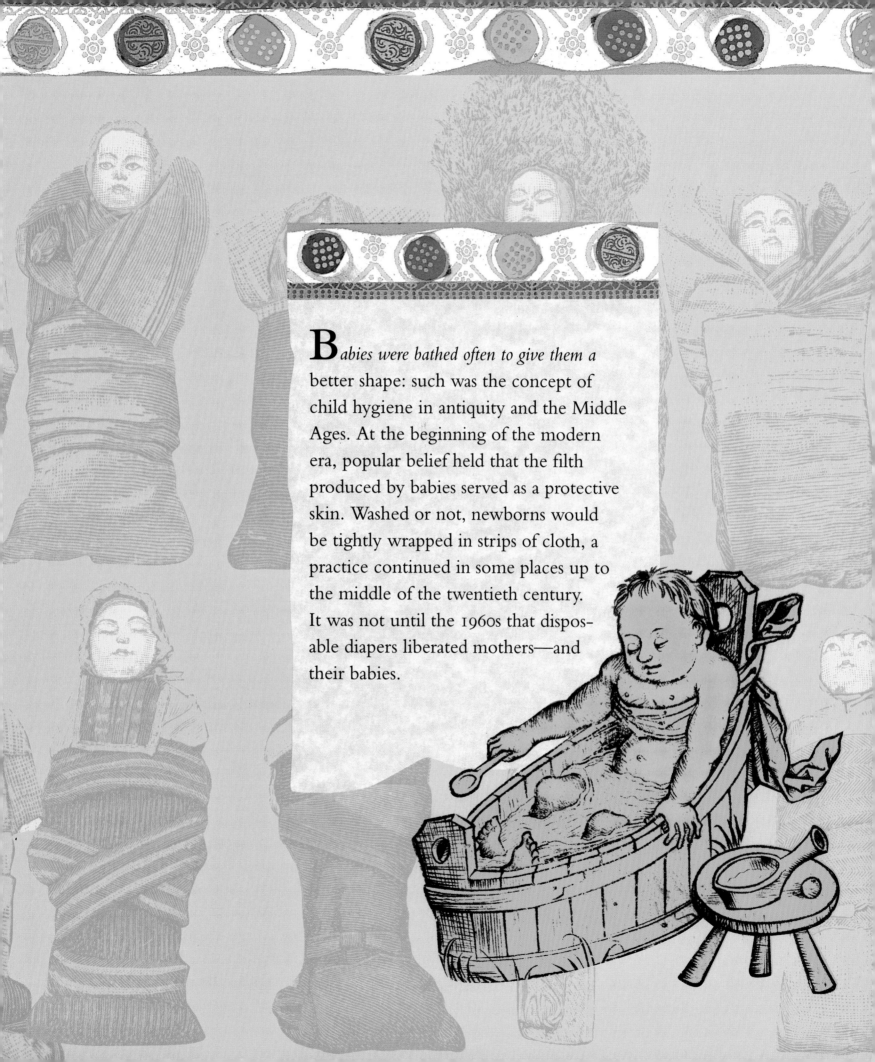

Babies were bathed often to give them a better shape: such was the concept of child hygiene in antiquity and the Middle Ages. At the beginning of the modern era, popular belief held that the filth produced by babies served as a protective skin. Washed or not, newborns would be tightly wrapped in strips of cloth, a practice continued in some places up to the middle of the twentieth century. It was not until the 1960s that disposable diapers liberated mothers—and their babies.

Molded, Powdered, and Tied with String

"As we think that swaddling clothes serve to make the body firm and to prevent deformities, we advise taking off the bands when the body is already fairly firm and there is no longer any fear of any parts being deformed. However, the bands should not be removed without a transition, nor all at once, for any sudden passage to the opposite state takes the sensibility by surprise."

Soranus of Ephesus,
Gynecology

RIGHT: Ex-voto. Gallo-Roman. Musée des Antiquités Nationales, Saint-Germain-en-Laye

OPPOSITE: Master of Uttenheim. *The Birth of the Virgin Mary.* 15th century. National Museum of Germany, Nuremberg

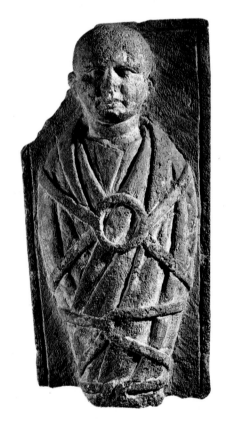

Moments *after his* arrival in the world, the newborn was plunged in the cold water of a stream before being placed on a shield, next to a lance. If he died following such handling, it meant he was unworthy to become a valorous warrior. In ancient Greece, the citizens of Sparta thus winnowed out the babies worth raising. Several centuries later, Roman mothers and wet nurses washed their babies in warm water, sometimes more than three times a day, according to the doctor Soranus of Ephesus. He advised giving only one bath a day, for fear that the infants would grow soft. The goal of all this bathing was not so much to rid babies of dirt as to "sculpt" them; bathtime was an ideal opportunity to shape their small bodies, still extremely moist, malleable as wax, and spongy "as sea foam," according to the doctors of antiquity. A program of daily exercises and massage assured that, as adults, they would conform to the Roman standards of beauty.

The nurse pulled a baby from the bath by her ankles and held her upside down to give her spinal column a nice curve. Out of the bath, for centuries the baby would be shaped by being swaddled in bands of woolen cloth. The bands' width and arrangement depended on the sex of the child. Boys would be wrapped tightly in overlapping thin bands to make their backs well shaped; girls' bands would be arranged to help them develop firm breasts and flared hips. If the baby's body had solidified sufficiently after the fortieth day in this wrapping, it was gradually freed from its bands and clothed in a simple soft tunic.

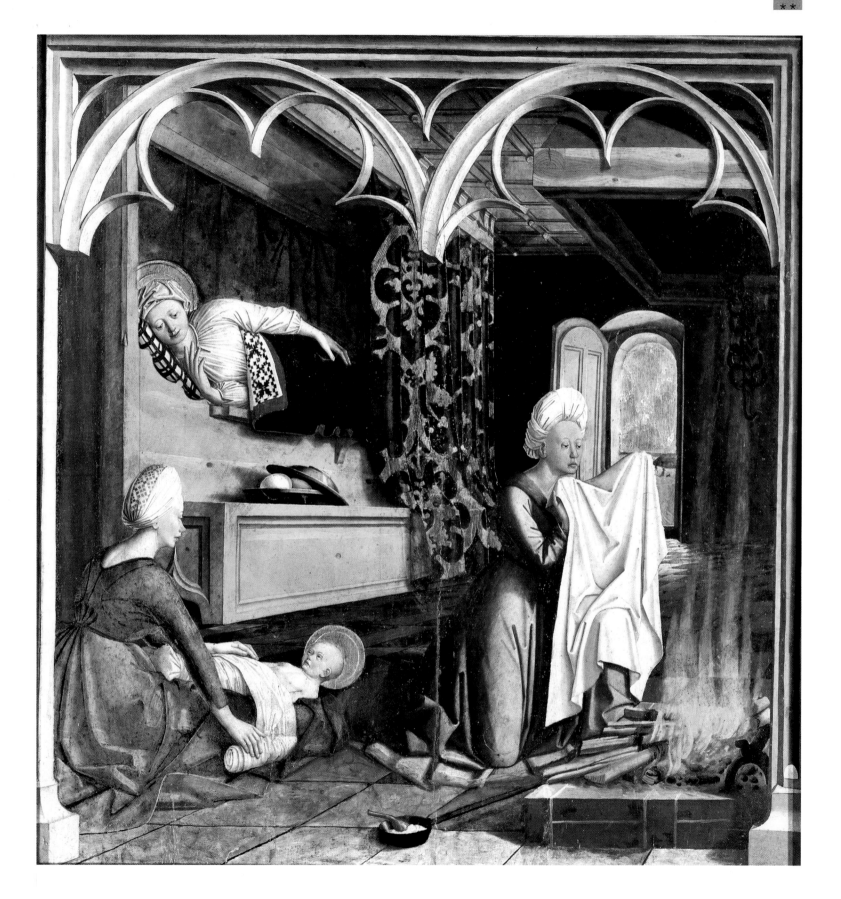

BELOW: Miniature. 15th century. Bibliothèque Nationale, Paris

The Messes of the Middle Ages

In one of the rooms of a medieval castle, servants and nurses bustled about: one poured hot water into a copper tub in which a sheet had been placed to protect the newborn from the hard and cold metal surface; before the fireplace another heated the large white sheets in which the baby would be wrapped and dried as soon as she came out of the bath. One nurse tested the water to be sure it was lukewarm before placing the baby in the tub. In the months following birth, this ceremony of the bath would be repeated often, for both the pleasure and well-being of the infant. In the twelfth century, the poems of Marie de France mentioned seven daily changes followed by seven baths! While the aristocratic and royal families of the Middle Ages let their children enjoy the pleasures of water, what of the peasants and workers? Their babies undoubtedly were bathed but rarely, in wooden laundry tubs. Frequent bathing was the privilege of the upper classes of the Middle Ages, faithful to the practices of antiquity. Later, by the seventeenth and eighteenth centuries, babies rarely experienced the joys of the bath.

In the French bedroom, at the end of the canopied bed stood the *layette*, a small sculpted wooden box that contained piles of the baby's white linens, or swaddling

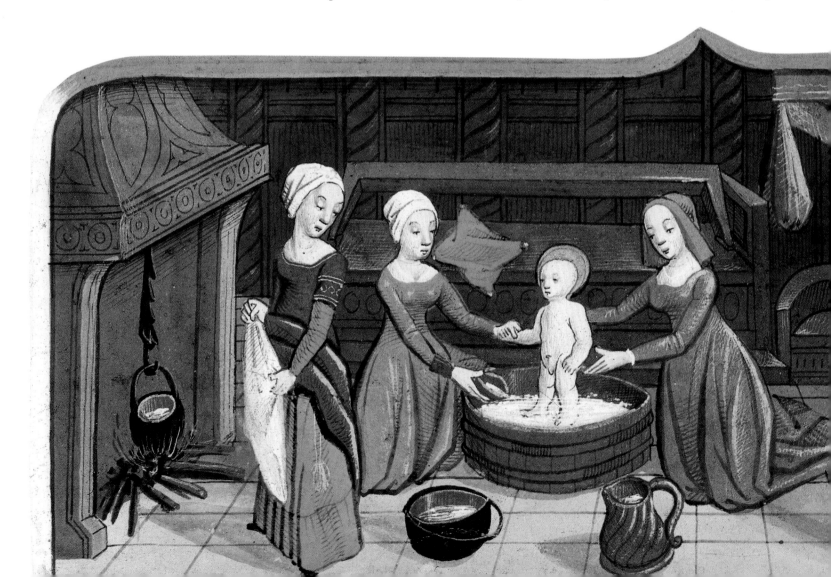

bands, carefully folded. Once the child was sated by the nipple, washed, and relaxed by the bath, the nurse set her on the paved floor on top of two layers of cloth to dress her. Always attentive to the infant's well-being, she placed a cushion under the baby's head so that it would be comfortably raised. The two layers of cloth were a sheet of fine white linen—the equivalent of today's diaper, intended to keep the baby clean—on top of a woolen swaddling cloth of scarlet red. Warm and soft, this fabric took the place of clothing. The nurse folded the cloths between the baby's legs and around her chest and then adjusted the linen sheet around her head, like a hood. Then she took a long band of cloth, often scarlet, which she unrolled and slid under the baby's shoulders and crossed over, with a deft and practiced hand, down to the ankles, where she knotted together the two ends of the band. Quickly wrapped, the baby would be unwrapped even more quickly to be fed and changed. Infant peasants were swaddled, just like the wealthy children; however, the cloths were not linen and wool but hemp, and the outer layer and bands were not bright red but brown, the natural color of hemp.

During the day, medieval babies had many opportunities to move and kick freely; their swaddling clothes were taken off often. For feeding, changing, and baths, the wet nurse or mother left infants nude, especially in the summertime. During warm weather and after the baby had grown larger, only the baby's bottom half would be

Medieval manuscripts described the first bath after birth, which was given by the midwife in a wooden tub. Babies considered too weak to be washed were simply rubbed with salt or wine.

BELOW: Woman preparing a bath in a tub. 16th century. Musée Unterlinden, Colmar

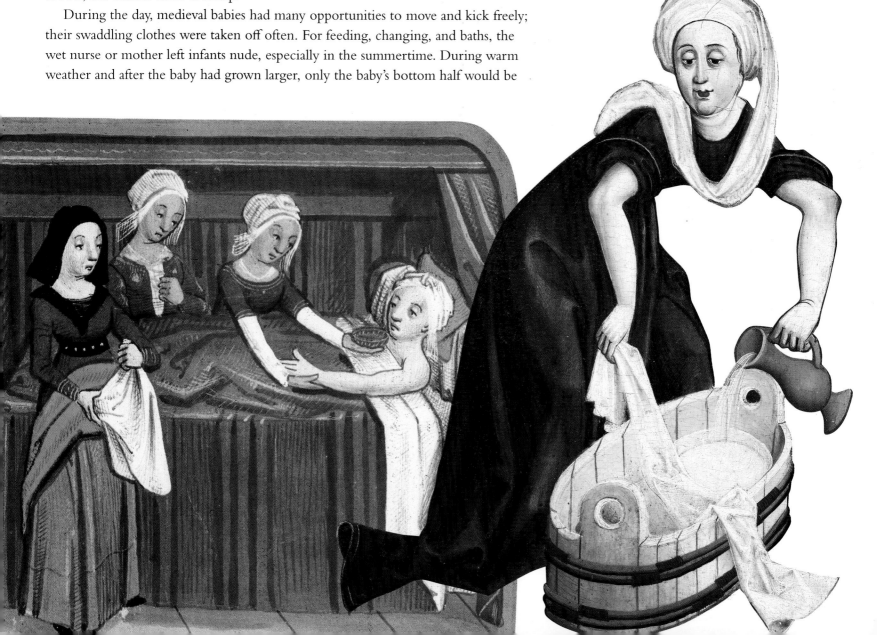

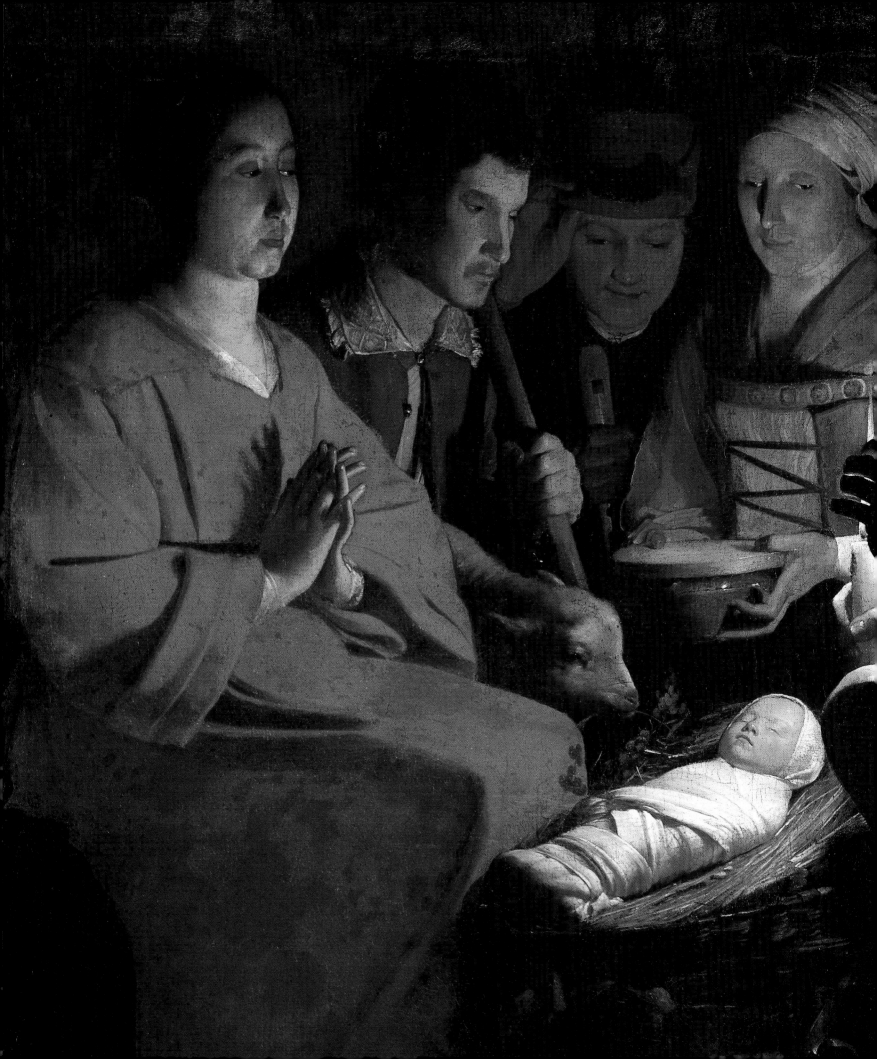

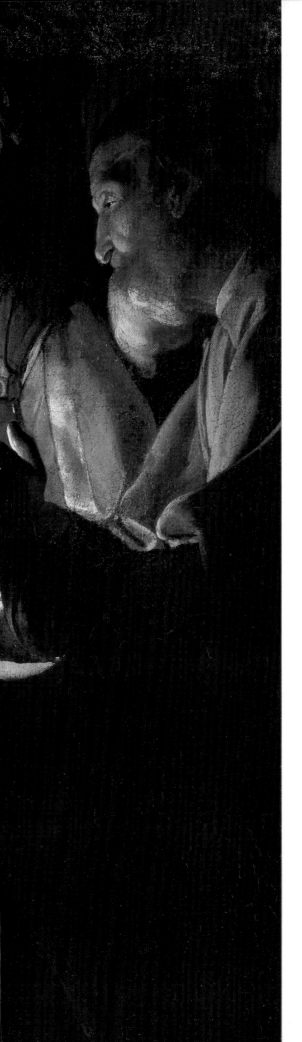

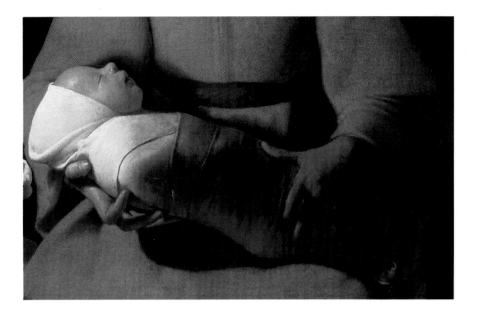

swaddled, leaving her arms free. This more flexible outfit served as the perfect transition to the small dress or blouse to which babies graduated at about one year of age. Under this large blouse that fell to the ground, they wore nothing, not even a diaper. In the Middle Ages, there were no chamber pots; a handful of hot ashes thrown over the baby's excrement allowed it to be easily swept away on the floors of packed earth or tile.

The Indispensable Shell

"The infant had to be wrapped in swaddling clothes in order to give his small body the right shape, which is the most decent and convenient for humans, and to have him grow used to standing on his two feet; for, without that, he would walk perhaps on all fours, like most of the other animals." Mauriceau, the seventeenth-century doctor, here echoed popular thought, which since antiquity feared that the still-soft body of the baby could become deformed. Shared by doctors until the eighteenth century, this belief remained firmly rooted in rural areas until the twentieth century. The midwife would wrap the baby in stiff swaddling clothes and pack him into a narrow cradle, beginning the process of giving him shape. As in the Middle Ages,

Babies were swaddled differently in different countries. In Italy, the band was wound in a spiral and knotted at the ankles.

LEFT: Georges de La Tour (1593–1652). *The Adoration of the Shepherds*. Musée du Louvre, Paris

ABOVE: Georges de La Tour. *The Newborn*. Musée des Beaux-Arts, Rennes

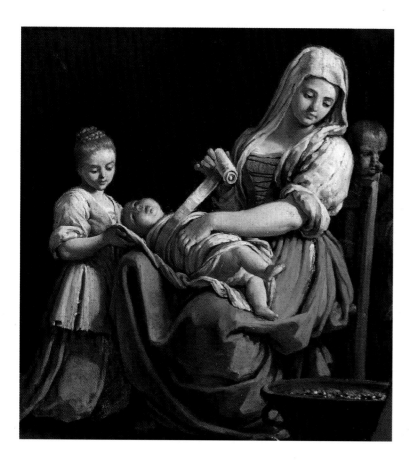

the seventeenth-century nurse carefully pressed the baby's arms against his body and crossed pieces of linen, which served as diapers, and the wool swaddling clothes over the baby's chest and stomach. She would have already placed pieces of linen under his arms to absorb excess sweat. Then she brought his legs together, making them as parallel as possible before enclosing them in the swaddling cloth. Finally, she sealed the envelope with a long band of canvas that wrapped the small body tightly from the soles of the feet to the shoulders. The head and its fragile fontanel—the opening at the top of the skull—also had to be protected and supported. Over a basic head covering kept on night and day, the baby wore a cotton bonnet or a wool cap, depending on the season, often hidden beneath a mobcap or, later, a lace bonnet. During the first days of life, another cap placed on top was tied on to the swaddling clothes on each side above the shoulders. All this material kept the baby's head straight until he was capable of supporting it alone. However, this well-wrapped package, nicely compact, was hardly elegant; there were fancy swaddling cloths for special occasions, made of gold or silk cloth, muslin, or lace, which hid a rich baby's swaddling clothes. On certain days, even the head wrappings were hidden under miniature versions of adult clothing. After a month to six weeks, the arms were left free during the day, but certainly not at night. After eight months, the baby finally wore her first dress, composed of a petticoat with whalebone stays and an apron sewn on.

Raise children following the rules of nature, which makes all things well: that was the line of conduct promoted by Rousseau and his followers in the second half of the eighteenth century. When it came to dressing babies, he urged the immediate end to that "extravagant and barbaric practice" of swaddling clothes. It was better, he said, to be guided by animals and uncivilized peoples. Many others had made this point

"Their first sounds you say are cries? I well believe it: you thwart them from their birth; the first gifts they receive from you are fetters, the first treatments they experience are torments. They cry from the hurt you cause them: thus pinioned, you would cry even louder than they."

Jean-Jacques Rousseau,
L'Emile, *1762*

ABOVE: Gambarini (1680–1725). *Winter.* Pinacoteca Nazionale, Bologna

RIGHT: Infant's undershirt. 18th century. Musée des Arts et Traditions Populaires, Paris

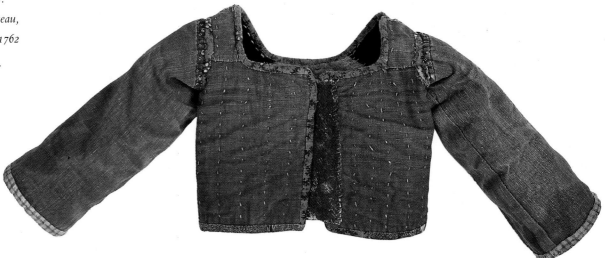

over the centuries. In antiquity, Pliny the Elder had already burst out against this distressing custom: "The infant is no sooner delivered from his prison than he is confined once more; this king of the animals, hands and feet bound, cries and wails; and his life begins in punishment." During the Middle Ages and the Renaissance, many expressed concern over the problems brought on by swaddling clothes that were wrapped too tightly.

Starting in the mid-eighteenth century, doctors and philosophers harshly condemned the whole ensemble of practices attributed to wet nurses, particularly that of swaddling clothes. "Watching them enclosing, tying up, and packaging the baby, one is led to believe that they were wrapping a small pack of wares for sale in another hemisphere," fumed Leroy, a doctor in the Paris school of medicine in 1772. These women were accused of resorting to this style of dress for their small charges because of laziness and neglect. Babies wrapped in swaddling clothes remained quiet; the wet nurses could put them in their cradles, where they rested without moving, or even hang them from a nail to avoid accidents caused by animals while they worked in the fields. An infant wrapped in swaddling clothes was also easier to carry than a wriggling baby; baby carriages and strollers did not exist at the time. In addition, well-wrapped swaddling clothes retained the baby's excrement, so

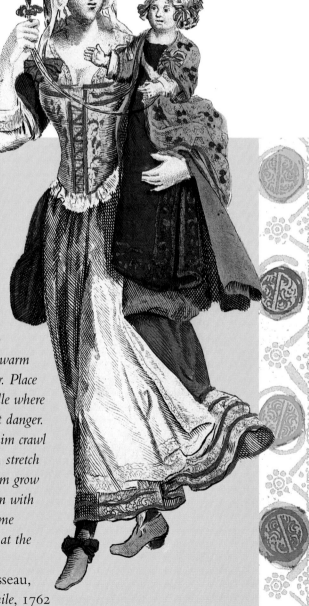

This baby in a dress has reached the age where she is no longer swaddled, a custom harshly criticized by Jean-Jacques Rousseau.

BELOW: Colored print. 18th century. Bibliothèque Nationale, Paris

According to Jean-Jacques

"Countries where they swaddle babies are those that abound in hunchbacks, the lame, the knock-kneed, the rickety, in all manner of deformed people. For fear that the body will become deformed through freedom of movement, they hasten to deform them by putting them under pressure. They are deliberately made crippled in an effort to prevent them from crippling themselves.... Where does this senseless practice come from? From an unnatural practice. Since mothers, despising their primary obligation, no longer wanted to nurse their babies, they had to entrust them to mercenary women who, finding themselves mothers to strange children for whom nature has given them no natural feelings, have sought only to spare themselves trouble. A baby left free needs to be watched constantly; but when he is well tied up, he can be thrown into a corner and left to cry heedlessly.... When the child breathes freely as he emerges from his wrappings, do not let anyone give him others that will continue to constrict him.

No more tight caps, no more bands, no more swaddling clothes; simply ample, flowing fabrics that leave all his limbs free and are neither too heavy to restrict their movements nor too warm to keep them from feeling the air. Place him in a large, well-padded cradle where he can move at will and without danger. When he becomes stronger, let him crawl about the room; let him develop, stretch his small limbs, you will see them grow stronger every day. Compare him with a well-swaddled infant of the same age, and you will be astonished at the difference in their progress."

Jean-Jacques Rousseau,
L'Emile, 1762

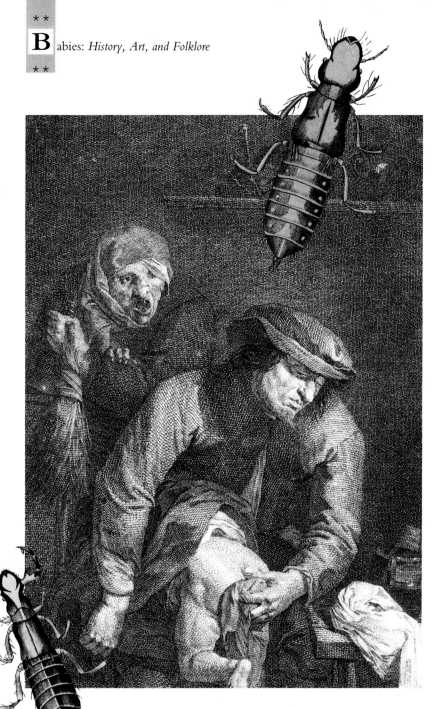

the baby did not need to be changed and cleaned so often.

Doctors of the time claimed to have seen numerous babies come back from the wet nurse deformed, twisted, hunchbacked, mutilated by swaddling clothes in which they had been practically "entombed." They were convinced that swaddling clothes, far from preventing deformities, facilitated them. Certain authors went so far as to maintain that swaddling clothes were a major cause of the population decline. The battle launched against swaddling clothes in the second half of the eighteenth century managed to modify the clothing of the wealthy classes and urban dwellers, but in the country, babies continued to be encased like sausages for more than another century.

The Virtues of Filth

The future king of France Louis XIII took his first bath at the age of seven. During his first year, his head had been rubbed at six weeks, his face washed with fresh butter and sweet almond oil at two months, and his hair combed for the first time just before his first birthday because his head itched. In the seventeenth century, royal babies were hardly any cleaner than common ones, despite the presence of a nurse whose sole function was to regularly change the little dauphin. The frequent baths of the Middle Ages had vanished; in this period, babies had to wait a long time to sample the pleasures of the water. The wealthy classes did not return to daily baths until the end of the eighteenth century. In lower-class and rural settings, baths for babies, like those for adults, remained infrequent until the middle of the twentieth century.

What had been a pleasure in the past now brought fear: fear of seeing the body dissolve in the bath; fear of contracting illnesses, in this period of raging epidemics, by swallowing some water; and, above all, fear of losing that protective envelope so essential to babies—the layer of filth that covered them. This layer was thought to be particularly beneficial for the fragile small head, which it strengthened while protecting the fontanel. Under the woolen bonnet, the head covering had not been removed since birth in order to keep the cranium safe from the cold and protect it from deformities. The layer of dirt was part of the body, like the fingernails and hair, which eventually come off naturally; any outside interference with the baby's body risked mutilating it, depriving it of part of its vital energy.

Fleas were long considered to be beneficial to infants—they were thought to relieve them of their tainted humors.

ABOVE: Parents and children. 17th century. Print

OPPOSITE: Erich Meinhold. Midwife bathing a newborn. 1931. Photograph

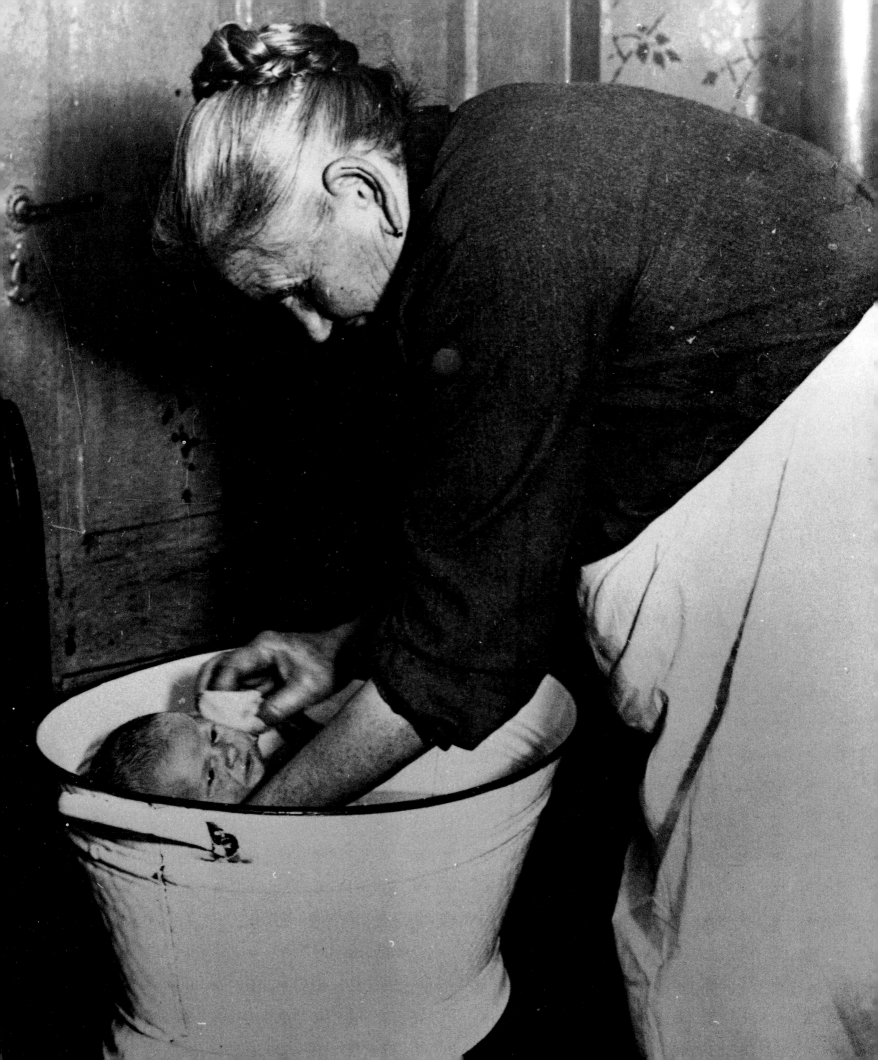

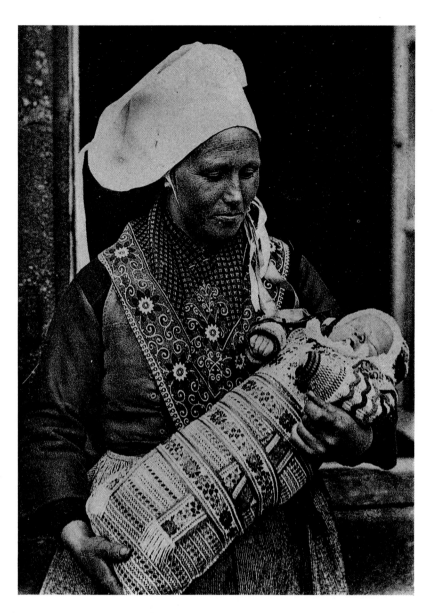

Tedious to put on, this type of swaddling clothes makes changing the infant difficult. At best changed once or twice a day, the baby ends up stagnating in her filth for many hours.

ABOVE: Photograph

The Virtues of Urine

Very rarely washed, seventeenth- and eighteenth-century babies were infrequently changed. When the mother or the nurse unwrapped the swaddling clothes to clean the baby, she often did no more than wipe her bottom, using neither soap nor water. Then she powdered it with the dust of worm-eaten wood, the baby powder of the past, to absorb moisture. She stretched the swaddling cloth, soaked with urine, in front of the fire before rewrapping the infant in yesterday's dry cloth. Urine was long thought to possess disinfecting qualities, especially for the baby's bottom. These beliefs in the benefits of uncleanliness explain why the lower classes and rural populations did not follow the lessons of hygiene preached by eighteenth-century moralists and doctors. At the end of the nineteenth century, one of these claimed that three-quarters of the children sent to wet nurses came back without having had a single bath. The women of the country long remained convinced of the virtues of a layer of filth for their babies, some of them until the early twentieth century. This faith is revealed in many proverbs, among them, "The dirtier children are, the healthier they are" and "The excrement of the infant is never repulsive."

Even in the most informed settings, no one was aware of the prophylactic value of good hygiene until the end of the eighteenth century. Only then did doctors begin to discover that cleanliness was one of the conditions of good health. They went so far as to advise that babies be washed from time to time and that the cloths used as diapers be changed as soon as they were wetted or dirtied. This practical advice, however, did not take root in the popular mind before the twentieth century.

The campaign against the layer of filth in the 1750s was undertaken for the sake of not only health but also public morality. In the wake of Rousseau, who extolled a reinvigorating cold bath starting in the first months of life, in the nineteenth century cleanliness was exalted as a moral value: its aim was not simply to be clean but to become hardy. At the beginning of the twentieth century, the invention of kitchen stoves and gas burners allowed well-off families to bathe their children easily in warm water. While water games and bath toys have been endorsed by psychologists for only the last few decades or so, mothers have long taken advantage of this moment of intimacy with their infants.

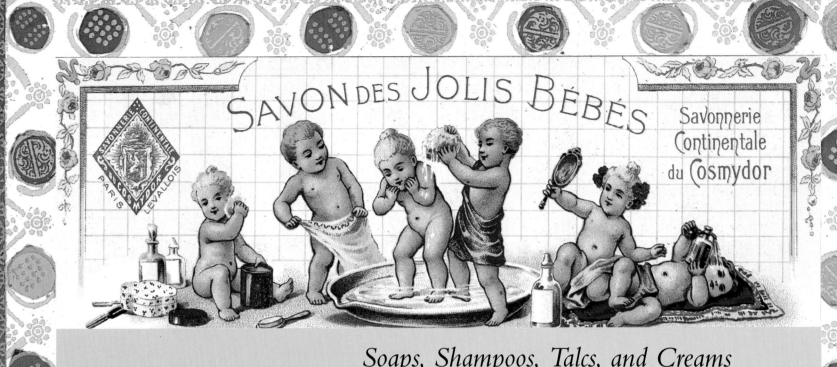

SAVON DES JOLIS BÉBÉS

Savonnerie
Continentale
du Cosmydor

Soaps, Shampoos, Talcs, and Creams

Shampoo was invented by the English. At the end of the nineteenth century, it consisted of soft soap boiled in water with soda crystals added.

ABOVE: Advertisement

BELOW: Photograph

Before the development of the numerous soaps, creams, and shampoos available today to cleanse and soothe babies' skin and wash their hair, recipes and potions of varying effectiveness already existed. At the end of the sixteenth century, Guillemeau advised bathing babies'

thighs and bottoms with rosewater and plantain. For irritated bottoms, a pomade made with a bit of lime (from limestone) was recommended. In the nineteenth century, to prevent cracks and rashes on the baby's seat, burnt flour or vegetable sulfur in powder form were common remedies. In 1808, Saucerotte specifically mentioned "the powder that pharmacists use to dredge their pills and that is employed in the theater to imitate lightning." Fresh butter, diluted egg yolks, oil, wine, or alcohol were among the many products used in place of soap and, in fact, were still used in rural areas in the first half of the twentieth century. In 1943, a child-care manual noted, "Soap is scarce, but there are many good substitutes. In the country, you may make use of wood ashes." In the eighteenth century, Madame du Coudray wrote that "the infant's head should be washed with hot wine and fresh butter." In 1938, Jean Wall prescribed a mixture of alcohol and glycerine.

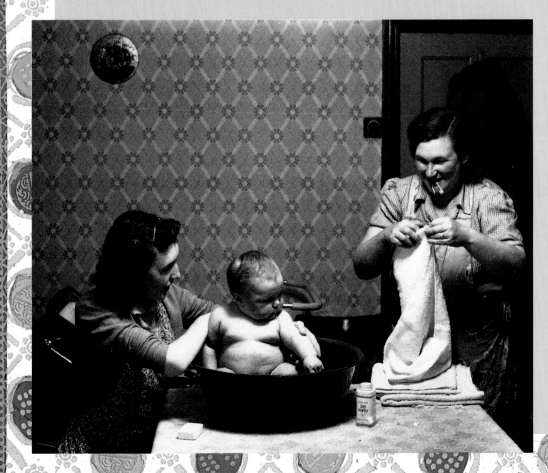

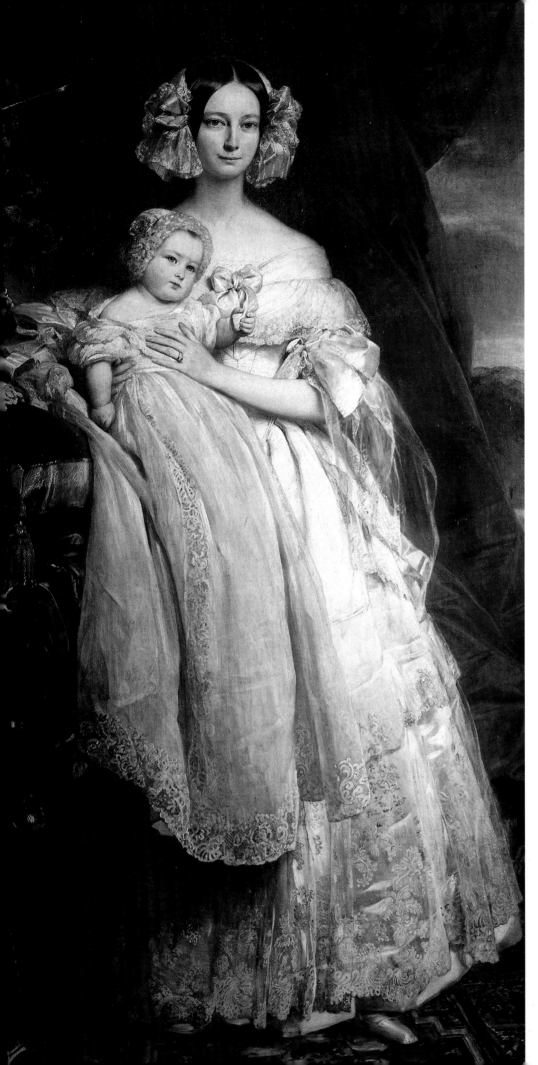

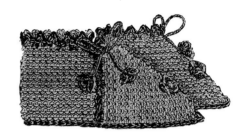

"*Every mother worthy of the name must herself know how to make her child's clothing; little girls should already practice cutting and sewing little jackets and little blouses.*"

Augusta Moll-Weiss,
Le foyer domestique, 1910

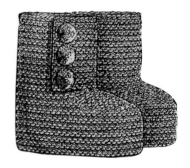

LEFT: Winterhalter (1805–1873).
The Duchesse d'Orléans with Her Son.
Château de Versailles

In the English Style or in the French Style

Clothed in short-sleeved shirts, underpants, and booties, English babies did not
have to wait for Rousseau before they could kick out at their pleasure. This style,
which crossed the English Channel, was increasingly taken up by the "modern"
European parents in the cities and the wealthy classes. Babies dressed in the English
style wore two or three small articles of clothing in layers: a short-sleeved blouse in
linen and one or two undershirts in flannel or cotton. The only remnant of the
swaddling clothes that remained was a band around the stomach, thought to support
the abdomen. The newborn wore a diaper, underpants, and woolen booties, topped
off by a long flannel dress that replaced the outer layer of swaddling clothes. It was
made longer than the baby and then was shortened when the infant began walking.
However, the majority of French urban parents continued to use swaddling clothes,
but "in the French style." The newborn was no longer tightly wrapped. Only the
bottom differed from the English style of dress: under the arms, over the undershirts
and blouse, a diaper and a swaddling cloth enveloped the lower part of the body.
These swaddling clothes were fastened with strings or safety pins, an improvement
over the bands.

Why did the baby stay swaddled in the cities and tightly wrapped in the country
for so long? Was the fragility of infants, their lack of resistance to the icy cold, the
main motive for the choice of clothing that enveloped the infant like a cocoon? Was
it an attempt to straighten at all costs the still-soft body, in response to the frequency
of rickets and congenital malformations? It was thought that the baby must also feel

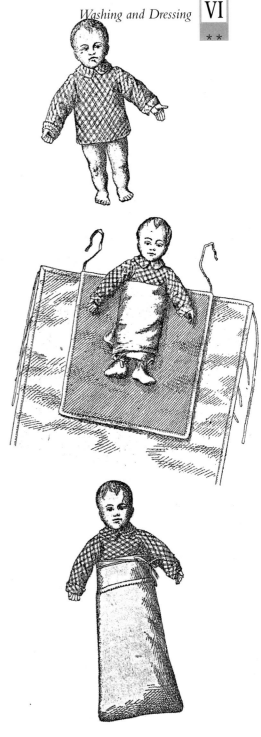

*The invention of the baby carriage
created the need for special outfits
reserved for the baby's walk.*

ABOVE: French swaddling clothes.
20th century. Prints

LEFT: Out for a walk. Photograph

OVERLEAF: Mothers and babies in
New York. 1946. Photograph

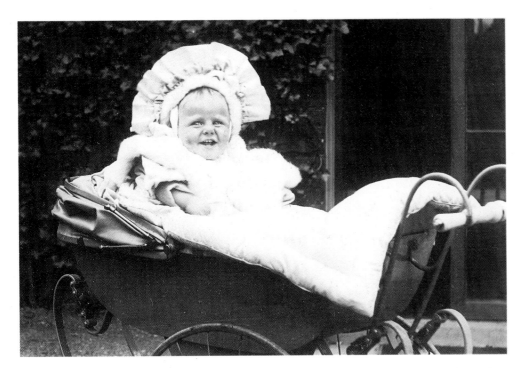

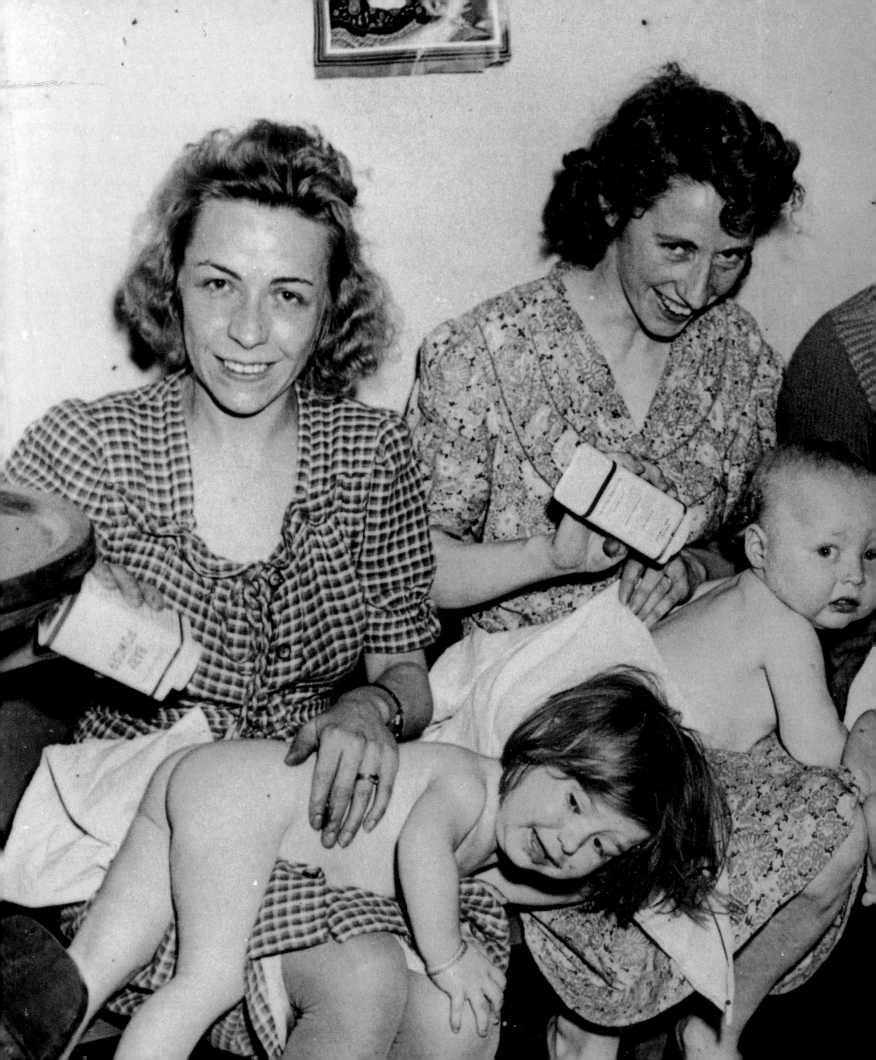

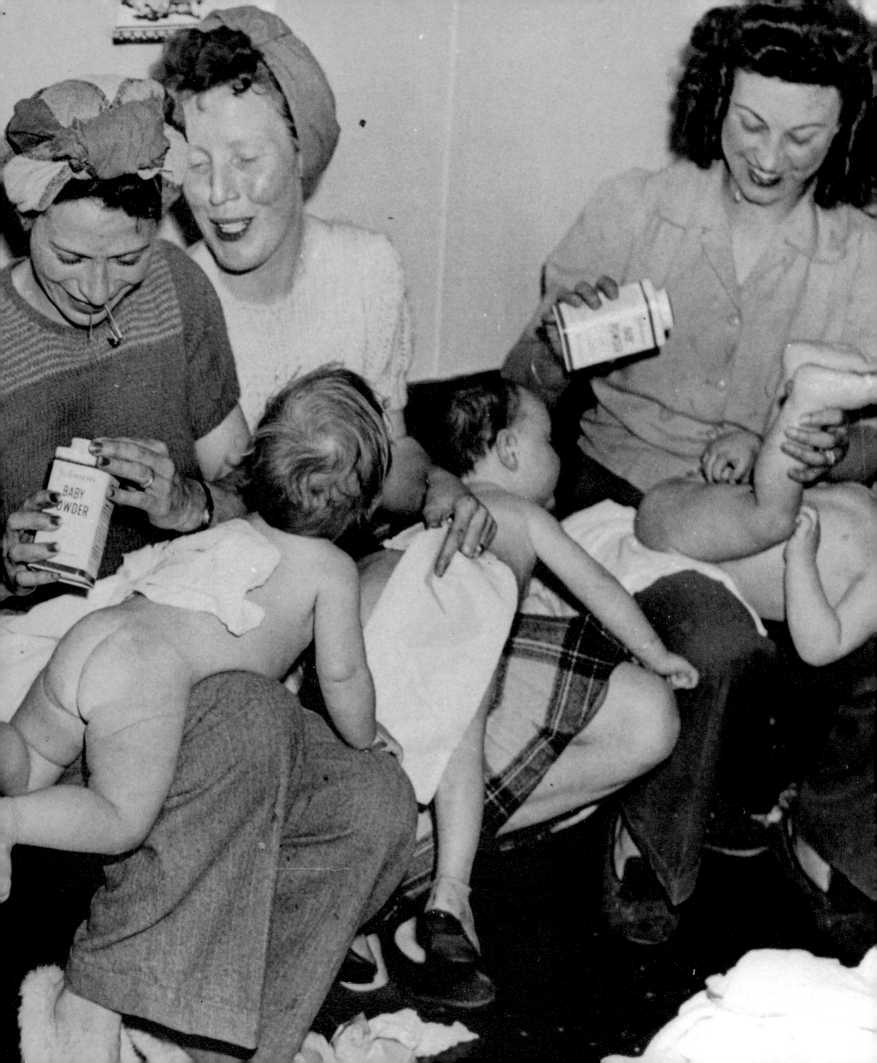

After the end of World War I, babies' long clothing, which impeded their movement, grew shorter and shorter. Countless baby-clothes manufacturers advertised in 1920s and 1930s periodicals. In the 1930s, styles changed. Pleats, flounces, embroidery, and lace were reserved exclusively for celebrations from then on, and the layers of clothing that had smothered generations of babies progressively evolved into a panty to cover the diaper, a body covering, and a small knitted vest or jacket.

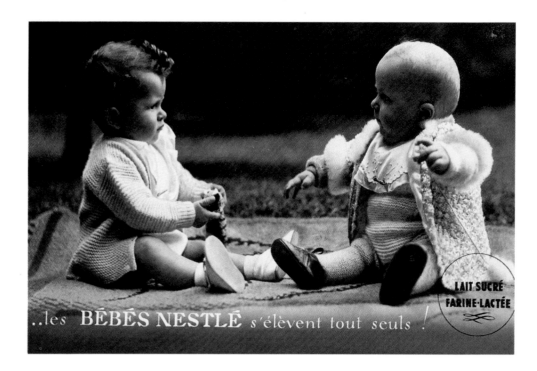

..les **BÉBÉS NESTLÉ** *s'élèvent tout seuls !*

LAIT SUCRÉ
FARINE·LACTÉE

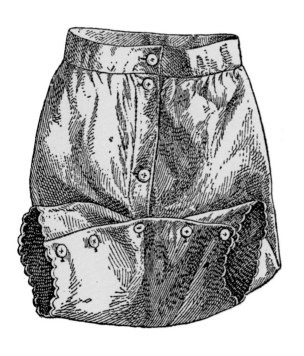

more secure nestled in his swaddling cloth, protected as he had been in its mother's belly. In a time when nurseries and child-care centers did not exist and it was necessary to work, mothers and wet nurses undoubtedly viewed swaddling clothes as a way of keeping babies safe. Wrapped up and sheltered from danger, they could be hung on a hook on a wall, carried in a basket, or placed immobile in their cradles. This form of dress was also highly economical: it could get longer as the baby got bigger. To clothe a baby in the first months of life, when he grows so quickly, it was unnecessary to have a large number of items, very expensive to buy and time-consuming to sew.

Underwear and Dresses

Undershirts, blouses, bonnets, headbands, and coats: in wealthy families, for many centuries a baby's layette had included close to a hundred different items. At the end of the nineteenth century in England, long dresses gradually disappeared, to be replaced, at the beginning of World War I, with shorter dresses and little woolen jackets. Many joined in the campaign against the multiple layers that continued to cocoon the baby. In English-speaking countries, baby clothes manufacturers heeded the advice of experts concerned with babies' health and well-being. Sterilization units, which controlled the cleanliness and purity of the clothing, were installed in some American factories. During World War II, knitting became a widespread pastime. Wool was considered an excellent material to use in terms of health, and knit layettes lasted until the 1960s, by which time synthetic fibers had proven their

In the twentieth century, doctors and child-care books agreed that a baby should have a daily bath. Books of advice, which began to proliferate at the end of the nine-teenth century, abounded in advice on how to hold the child in the bath, the proper temperature, and how long the bath should last.

miraculous qualities: they were easy to wash, quick to dry, wrinkle free, dazzlingly white. At the beginning of the century, guides for women told them not to buy baby clothes, as the healthiest pastime for the future mother was to sew and knit her baby's wardrobe. In addition, homemade clothes were considered more elegant and refined than those from stores, despite the progress made in their manufacturing. Until the 1920s, boys, like girls, wore dresses or, sometimes, one-piece undergar-ments. In this period, the convention that girls should wear pink and boys blue was established. The baby's wardrobe became simpler: embroidery, flounces, pleats, and lace gradually fell into disuse. At the end of the 1950s came the greatest revolution in the history of baby clothes since swaddling clothes were abandoned: the invention, in the United States, of the stretchy one-piece footed garment that closes with snaps, which is sold under a number of names.

On the Pot at Set Hours

It is never too soon to learn good habits. Rigorous discipline very quickly compels young children not to soil themselves; at the end of the seventeenth century, the philosopher John Locke recommended putting babies on a "pierced chair," a sort of potty-chair, every day after meals. They would not be allowed to play or eat again until they produced what was expected of them. From this time, small bottomless chairs existed for babies, some with a hole in the middle under which a chamber pot could be placed, others similar to small rocking chairs. Some might have a space in the back in which a hot brick could be put so that the occupant would not catch cold in the time— which could be sizable—spent waiting to satisfy the adults' demands. One hundred years later, doctors and teachers took inspiration from Locke's precepts. In the nineteenth century, energies turned to teaching cleanliness: going to the toilet had to be done from a very early age, at three or four months, at set hours—after all, this was a matter of education.

Some fifty years later, such strictness had not yet run its course: "It is stated that the newborn urinates almost every time he is undressed, some seconds after having felt contact with the air. Knowing that he will uri-nate, place him in a crouching position above a chamberpot, on which you support his buttocks: this posture will induce urination. After several days, the newborn will have made a strong

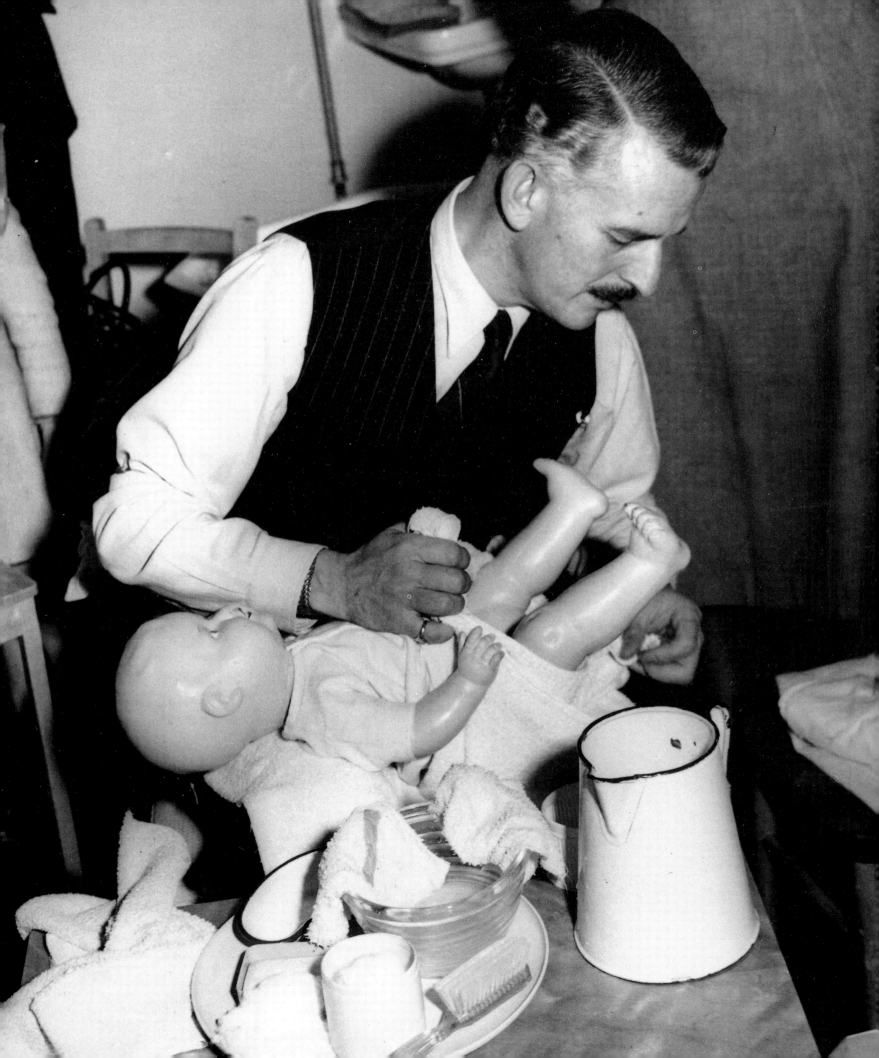

association between the two sensations: the flowing of urine and contact with the chamberpot; he will become accustomed to urinating only in his pot, that is, except during his sleep, and you will have made him clean from his earliest weeks," wrote Pouliot in 1921. If the poor baby was constipated, it was advised to insert a piece of soap sculpted to a point or a willow branch in her anus.

In the 1940s the potty-chair appeared, in the form of a small armchair in which a baby over four months of age could be strapped until he had completed his task. It was not until twenty years later that researchers demonstrated that mastery of the sphincter muscle could not be achieved before eighteen months, and that premature toilet training could result in psychological problems.

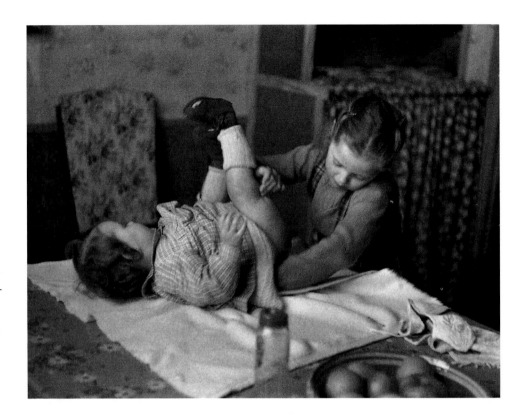

The Revolution of Disposable Diapers

The hemp or linen diapers—doubled at night with a swaddling cloth as thick as flannel—that were used for centuries to enclose babies' bottoms were hardly waterproof and proved very difficult to wash. In the eighteenth century some efforts were made to improve them: a swaddling cloth made of oiled silk, thought to prevent leaks, was added. At the beginning of the nineteenth century, a well-stocked layette included six dozen diapers, the minimum needed to change the baby regularly. Rubber pants stopped leaks, inevitable with cloth diapers, but they soon proved to be a source of irritation to the babies' tender skin. In the 1930s and '40s, a new wave of experiments brought out sponge-cloth diapers, the overlaying of diapers with squares of highly absorbent gauze or muslin, panties of oil-silk, and even, in Great Britain, underpants made of sterilized latex. During World War II, when soap was rationed, mothers were instructed to limit the washing of cloth diapers by using disposable cotton and wool diapers.

In 1959, the American company Procter & Gamble came out with the first real innovation, plastic underpants lined with a thick layer of cotton. Disposable diapers, such as those that are widespread today, began to be commonly used in the 1970s. This was the end of a long road from the time when a bundle of oats was placed in the cradle to absorb leaks from cloth swaddling clothes.

In the past, many people in rural areas did no more with babies' soiled swaddling cloths than dry them. Beginning in the twentieth century, they finally began to wash them with soap and water. In the 1930s, cloth diapers were washed and then boiled or sterilized with a very hot iron.

OPPOSITE: Baby-changing class for men, Westminster. 1952. Photograph

ABOVE: Robert Doisneau. Photograph

OVERLEAF: Babies in a center for maternal assistance. 1944. Photograph

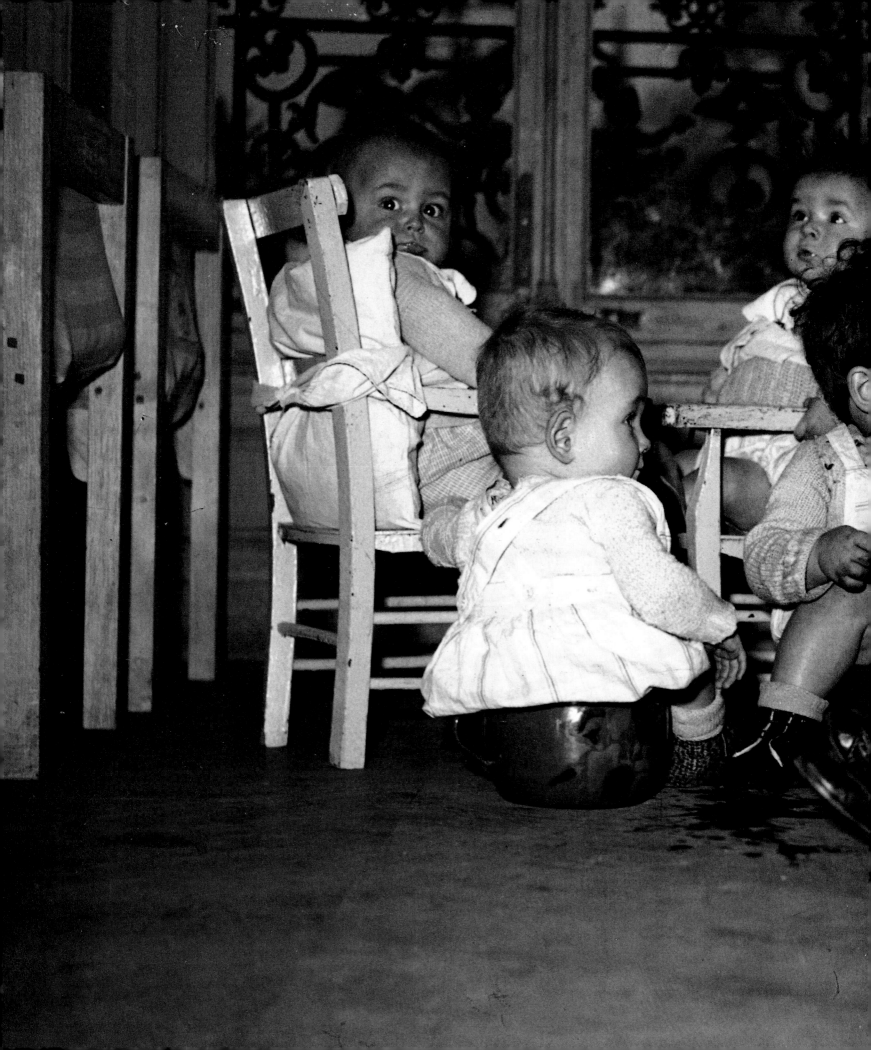

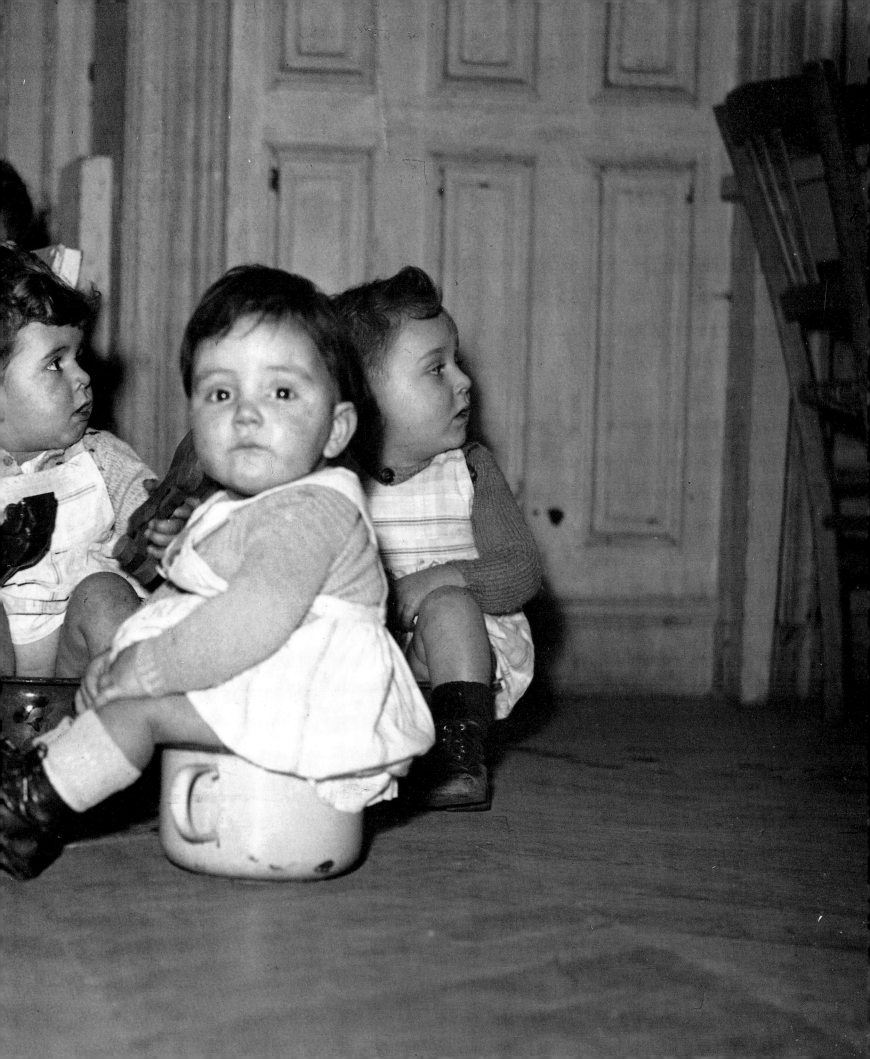

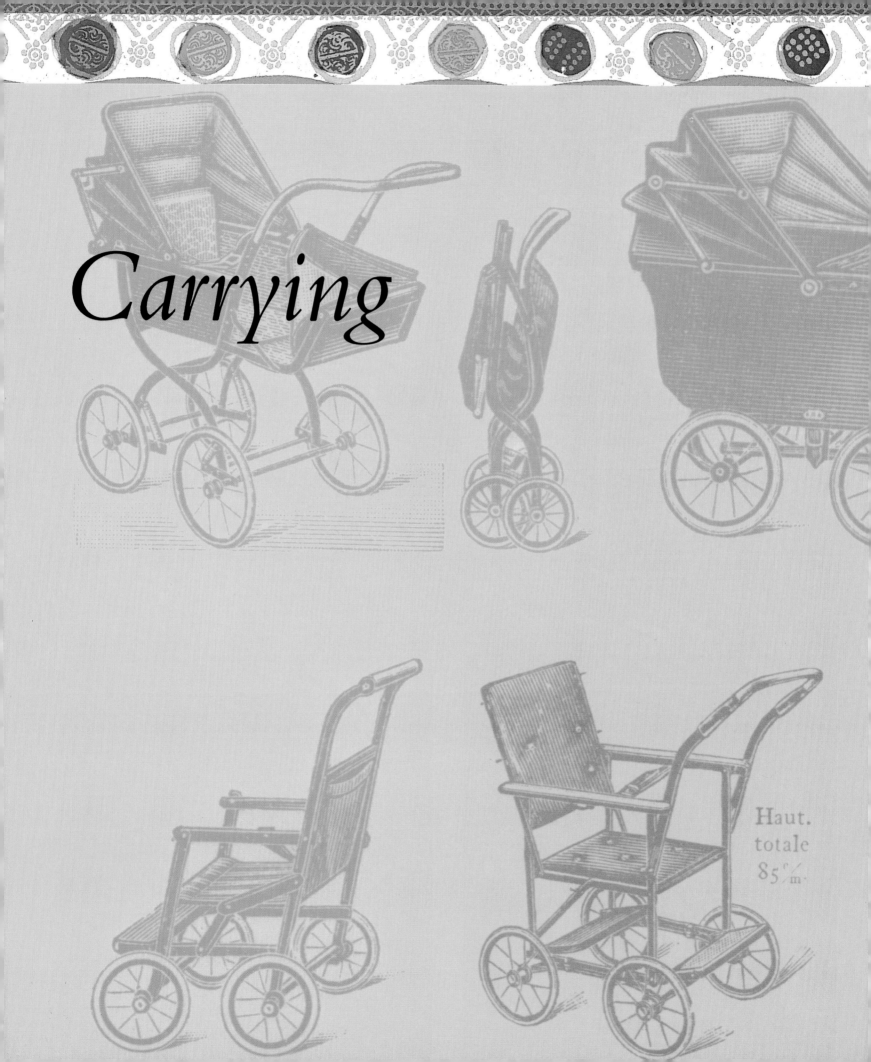

Carrying

Haut.
totale
85 c/m.

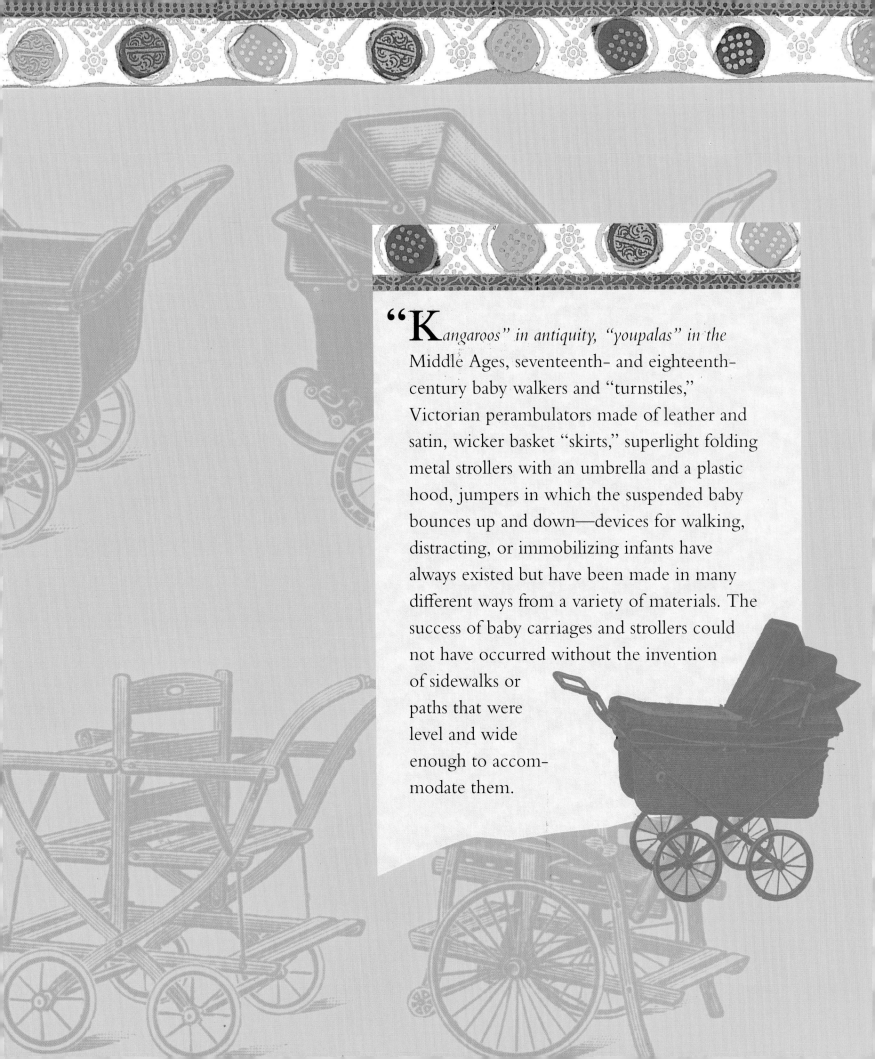

"Kangaroos" in antiquity, "youpalas" in the Middle Ages, seventeenth- and eighteenth-century baby walkers and "turnstiles," Victorian perambulators made of leather and satin, wicker basket "skirts," superlight folding metal strollers with an umbrella and a plastic hood, jumpers in which the suspended baby bounces up and down—devices for walking, distracting, or immobilizing infants have always existed but have been made in many different ways from a variety of materials. The success of baby carriages and strollers could not have occurred without the invention of sidewalks or paths that were level and wide enough to accommodate them.

Baby Sacks and Babies on Wheels

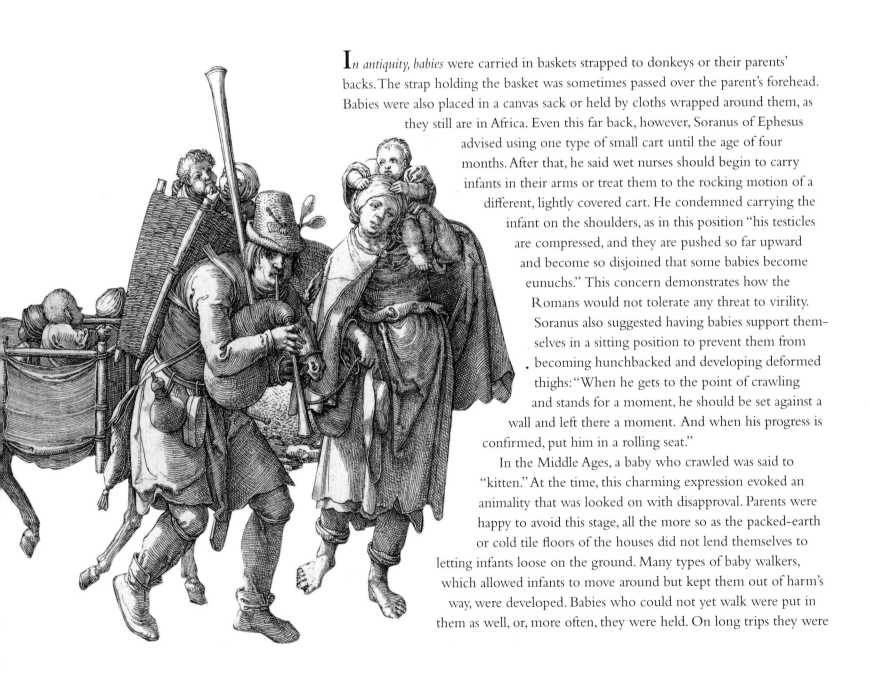

In *antiquity, babies* were carried in baskets strapped to donkeys or their parents' backs. The strap holding the basket was sometimes passed over the parent's forehead. Babies were also placed in a canvas sack or held by cloths wrapped around them, as they still are in Africa. Even this far back, however, Soranus of Ephesus advised using one type of small cart until the age of four months. After that, he said wet nurses should begin to carry infants in their arms or treat them to the rocking motion of a different, lightly covered cart. He condemned carrying the infant on the shoulders, as in this position "his testicles are compressed, and they are pushed so far upward and become so disjoined that some babies become eunuchs." This concern demonstrates how the Romans would not tolerate any threat to virility. Soranus also suggested having babies support themselves in a sitting position to prevent them from becoming hunchbacked and developing deformed thighs: "When he gets to the point of crawling and stands for a moment, he should be set against a wall and left there a moment. And when his progress is confirmed, put him in a rolling seat."

In the Middle Ages, a baby who crawled was said to "kitten." At the time, this charming expression evoked an animality that was looked on with disapproval. Parents were happy to avoid this stage, all the more so as the packed-earth or cold tile floors of the houses did not lend themselves to letting infants loose on the ground. Many types of baby walkers, which allowed infants to move around but kept them out of harm's way, were developed. Babies who could not yet walk were put in them as well, or, more often, they were held. On long trips they were

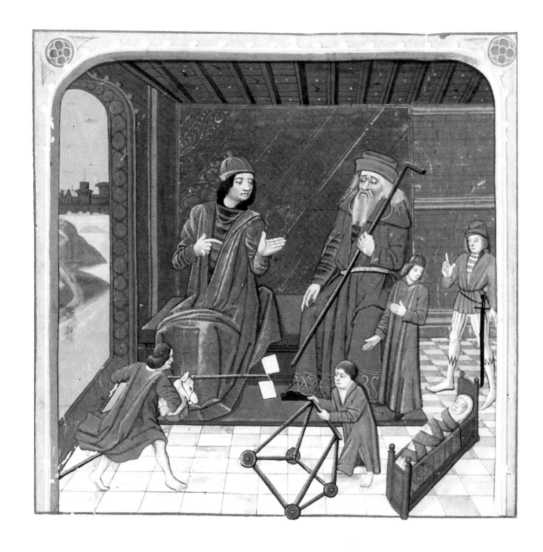

Medieval parents did not want their children to walk too soon. They feared it would deform their legs. Precocity was far from being considered an advantage; it signaled a shorter life.

OPPOSITE: Lucas de Leyde. *The Child Escort.* 16th century. Print. Bibliothèque Nationale, Paris

LEFT: Illumination from Bartholomaeus Anglicus, *De proprietatus rerum,* 15th century. Bibliothèque Nationale, Paris

slipped into a basket or a wooden chest tied vertically to the father's back. Cradles, small and portable, also served as carrying cases; this piece of furniture came into use mainly during the day, for at night, mothers often took their babies to bed with them. Men sometimes supported the cradle on their shoulders, while women carried them on their heads as they would a pot of milk. Other carrying devices varied according to the size and weight of the baby and the length of the trip—a bundle of canvas or leather strapped to the shoulders, a sling on the mother's hip, a small cask or a cradle in the shape of a wooden lobster pot fastened to the flanks of a donkey or mule.

At home, babies from most families were set on a rug or a cushion, free to divert themselves on the floor, or the children of the wealthy were shoehorned into walkers. For many, learning to walk was an adventure involving the patient help of a sister who held the baby, while the mother called and held out her arms from some feet away.

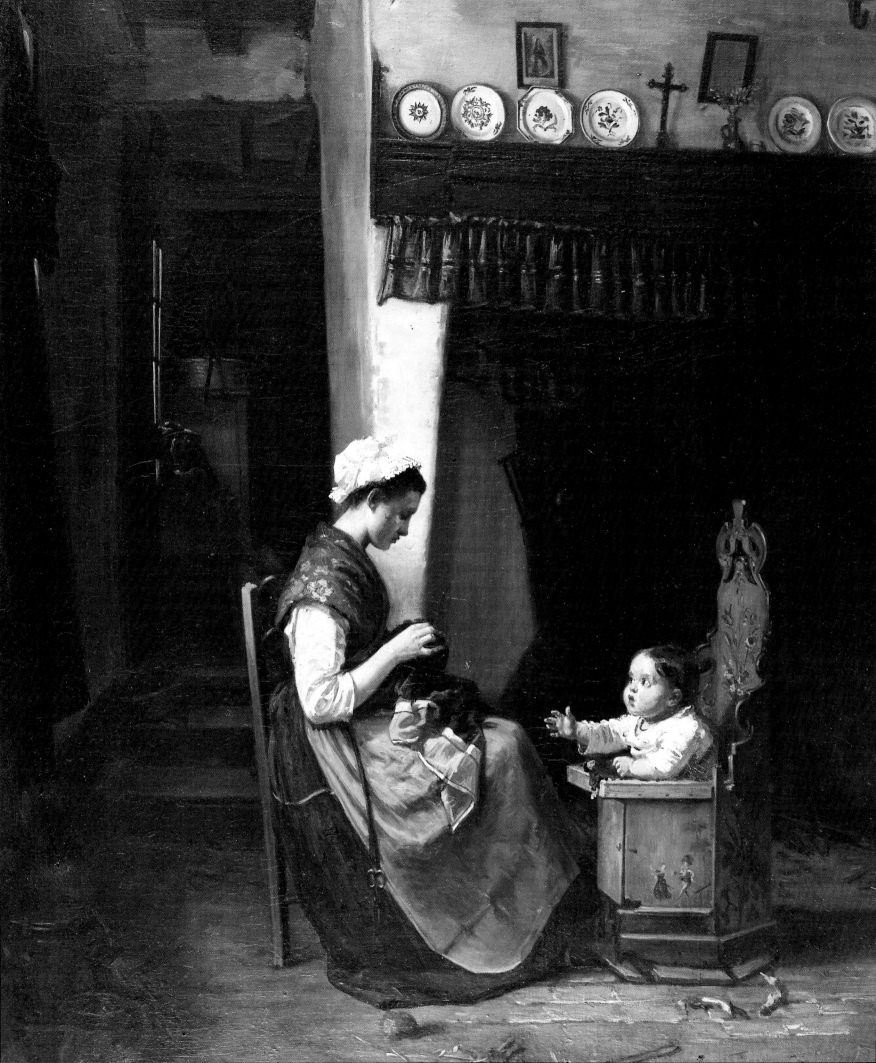

From the Handcart to the Pushcart

Well before the hygiene-minded doctors of the nineteenth century, some writers recommended taking babies on walks in their first months of life, not only for the benefits of fresh air but also, and especially, to entertain them and show them the world. "One should not always keep the baby in the bedroom," wrote Simon de Vallambert in 1565. "He should be brought outdoors in good weather to give him exercise and the opportunity to play. When he is two or three months old, he wants to be taken from a restricted space to one with more room, where the air is more open, as much to bring him relief from the heat while breathing fresh air as to provide him with diversion in looking at various things outdoors. If all he ever sees consists only of what is visible in his room, he will obtain no pleasure and he will find life boring."

In the sixteenth century, nurses and mothers pushed babies around the house in small carts when they tired of carrying them. Even after usable roads were built in the eighteenth century, taking babies out for a ride in these carts remained too jolting an experience. Not until the nineteenth century would the baby carriage be used exclusively outdoors.

When mothers had household chores to do, they placed older babies in small, low chairs, almost like opened-up boxes that were painted and furnished with a shelf on which the baby could play. In the country, even very young infants still in their swaddling clothes were slipped into a narrow basket, its bottom stuffed with straw that served as both insulation and support. Set vertically in this "baby caddy," infants could see the world better than when they lay in their cradles. In the seventeenth century, highchairs became common, which perhaps permitted the baby to join the family at table. The baby, however, could fall; for close to four centuries, falling from the highchair was among the most common childhood accidents. In the seventeenth century, at any rate, the baby's head would be protected by a bonnet with large pads.

In addition, many babies were tied to their chairs, which were usually made of solid oak and designed to be as stable as possible. Wealthy families had richly decorated highchairs that imitated adult furnishings, with elaborate carving and padding of leather, velvet, or other precious materials.

Children's chairs could be very rudimentary, little more than wooden boxes, or masterpieces of the cabinetmaker's art.

OPPOSITE: Louise Becq de Fouquières. *Picardy Mother.* 19th century

BELOW: Print. 17th century

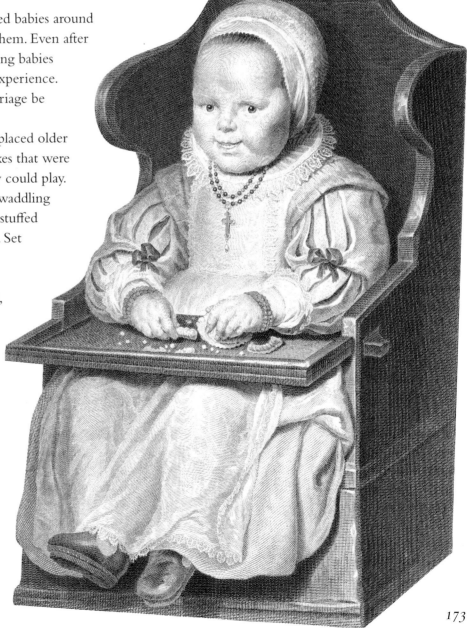

The Harnessed Baby

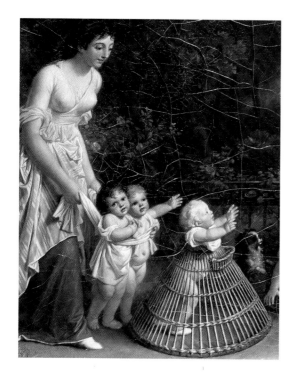

These wicker skirts were known as "baby carriers." Some had a small box that could hold a toy or a piece of bread.

ABOVE: Gérard Marguerite (1761–1837). *The First Steps.* Hermitage, St. Petersburg

BELOW: Walker. 19th century. Musée des Arts et Traditions Populaires, Paris

From the end of the eighteenth century up to World War II, doctors, teachers, and philosophers condemned all these baby-holding devices. Like swaddling clothes, they were seen to slow down the natural and harmonious development of the baby. "As soon as babies can move about by themselves," explained the doctor Nicolas Saucerotte at the end of the eighteenth century, "it is good to leave them for part of the day on the floor on a rug, a blanket, a straw or rush mat, or on the grass when it is dry, so they can have complete freedom of movement and do as they please. A small rolling cart in which they are seated also serves well to give them some exercise. The method of leaving them to themselves to stand up and begin to walk is infinitely preferable to that of placing them standing in rolling carts or holding them by the skirts or straps; these auxiliary aids compress their chests, make them raise their shoulders, strain their bottoms, and bring the blood rushing to their heads through the constraint that this compression entails. As soon as they try it themselves, it makes them become bolder, and as soon as they can remain standing, they should be encouraged to walk by enticing them or showing them an interesting object from several steps away, although never by promising them sweets." Opinions divided on the use of pads around the head; some claimed they reassured babies, but Saucerotte opposed them: "Myself, I think that if these young beings are left to test their strength early on, they will soon acquire enough confidence to take risks for themselves, declining to confine their heads in an impediment that heats and compresses them."

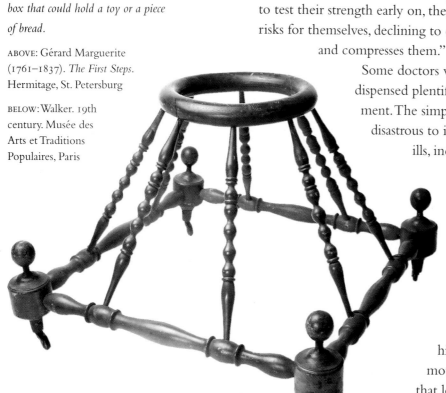

Some doctors who were too careful, too fearful, or too busy dispensed plentiful advice on the baby's psychomotor development. The simple act of carrying a baby in one's arms could be disastrous to its health; it could result in an infinite number of ills, including dislocation or detachment of the epiphysis. "These imprudent games in which wet nurses throw the infant from one arm to the other bring about numerous deformities," one authority wrote. Another warned, "Stand the infant up too early, and he will end up limping: this lameness often results when the baby is enclosed in a kind of basket made of wicker or wood, commonly called the baby carrier, and in which he is forced to remain on his feet for six or seven hours in a day." But what mother would leave a baby in one of these objects for that long? It was certainly simpler just to put a sleepy baby to bed.

Harness, Pads, and Forced Walking

Another doctor recommended, "When carrying infants in one's arms, one must be careful to change arms occasionally, so that they will not form the habit of leaning to one side rather than another, as this can result in a structural deformity in the vertebrae and in the entire side that is thus squeezed." Some doctors pronounced themselves in favor of putting the baby in pads, which they advised should be quite large. These protective bags stuffed with rags and straw were meant to protect the nose if the baby fell forward.

In the eighteenth century, one boaster claimed that using this method, his baby had learned to walk alone very early: "Forty days after birth, he made his mother, after she got out of bed, let him roll in the still-warm bed at his ease. She could entice him by offering him her breast from a distance; he tottered at first, he fretted, but soon he advanced, so much more easily that she often repeated these innocent games. When holding him securely in her arms, she would lift him slightly above the bed and make him concentrate all his energy as he became aware of a kind of danger. I love to see her induce her tender infant to stop in his tracks and hold onto her dress, trying to reach her breast. Nothing is more admirable than seeing the skill with which the little devils climb their way up clothing."

In 1760, the sympathetic observer Des Essarts chose a very different method, which he recounted in his *Traité de l'éducation corporelle des enfants ou réflexions pratiques sur les moyens de procurer une meilleure constitution aux citoyens* (Treatise on the Physical Education of Children or Practical Reflections on the Means of Obtaining a Better Constitution for Our Citizens): "As soon as the infant reaches the age of three or four months, an intelligent wet nurse will not let a single day pass without giving him practice in holding himself upright on his little feet. The willingness and care that some of them display deserve great praise. When the infant is freed of his

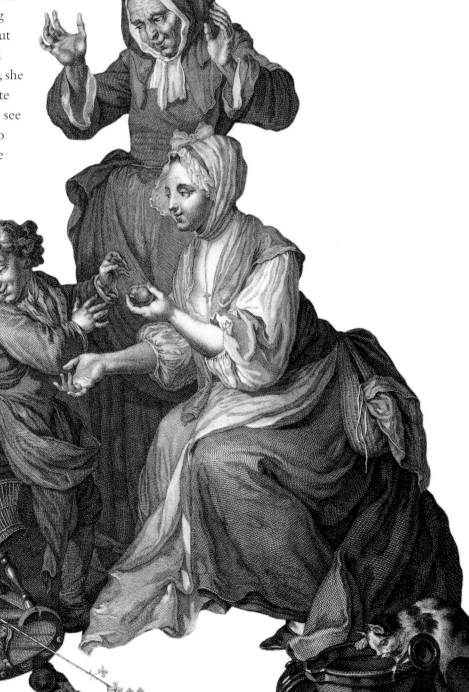

His bottom exposed to the air, this baby wears a helmet in his youpala. Clearly, child-care paraphernalia in the eighteenth century was no less impressive than that available today.

BELOW: *The First Steps of Childhood.* 18th century. Print. Bibliothèque Nationale, Paris

swaddling clothes, they set him upright on their knees and, supporting him gently between their hands, they make him move forward until he reaches their face. Each little walk usually ends in a kiss."

Baby on the Wall

In the half-darkness of a farmhouse where hens and pigs come and go, it is hard to make out a sack hanging from a nail on one of the walls. But the sack moves, and a small nodding head emerges from it. The peasant woman has slipped her tightly swaddled baby there so she can do her chores. Perched on the wall, her baby is safe from the animals and the dampness of the floor. A simple sack, a wooden or straw basket, or, instead, straps fastened to the baby's waist band and hung on a nail—these rudimentary methods were employed in rural areas for centuries, up to World War I, to keep babies out of harm's way. However, the little ones were not inevitably hung on a perch. As soon as they could hold themselves up, they could be set in a variety of different objects from simple tree trunk shapes woven of straw, to small, rudimentary chairs made of four pieces of wood, to high and narrow cylindrical braided baskets. When babies had no problem holding themselves upright, their swaddling clothes were removed and they were clothed in short dresses that allowed them freedom of movement. They then needed to move about, exercise their small legs, and learn to walk, so the various objects or baskets that kept them immobile no longer suited them. Other systems, differing from region to region, allowed babies to move while keeping them safe from the dangers they would encounter if left to themselves.

Tethers and Turnstiles

Alone in her room, a ten-month-old baby moves in a circle like a bird in a cage. She is imprisoned in a strange contraption. From a tall wooden post rising in the middle of the room and wedged against the main beam of the ceiling a plank extends horizontally; there is a hole in it into which the child has been slipped. Supported under her arms, she moves this "turnstile" by pushing with her feet. In 1911, the author of a book entitled *Les appareils populaires destinés à apprendre à marcher* (Common Devices Used to Learn How to Walk) still promoted the merits of this device, whose use was then on the decline, even in the most secluded rural areas: "And often the baby turns and tacks as if possessed, almost as fast as the arms of the neighboring windmill! One who has never witnessed this sight would believe himself at the circus, where a small monkey in disguise, attached to the center pole, circled the ring.... Be that as it may, in comparison with other, more modern devices, this one makes the process of teaching babies to walk very convenient, effective, and dependable. Its only drawback is that it is stationary and cannot be taken outside in good weather. But does not the child have its entire life ahead in which to breathe the fragrant and salutary bosky breeze?"

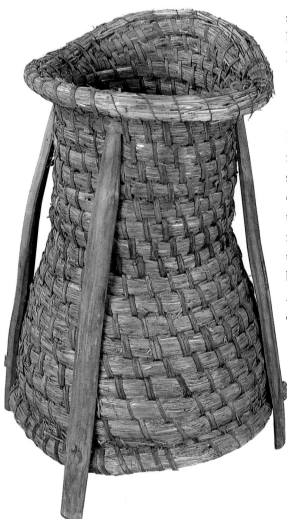

To keep the infant from adopting an "animal posture" and to protect her from the cold floor and danger from animals and fire, she was held upright by stays in her small dress and various other devices of varying sophistication.

ABOVE: Baby carrier made of straw. 19th century. Musée des Arts et Traditions Populaires, Paris

OPPOSITE: *The Baby Caretaker.* 19th century. Print

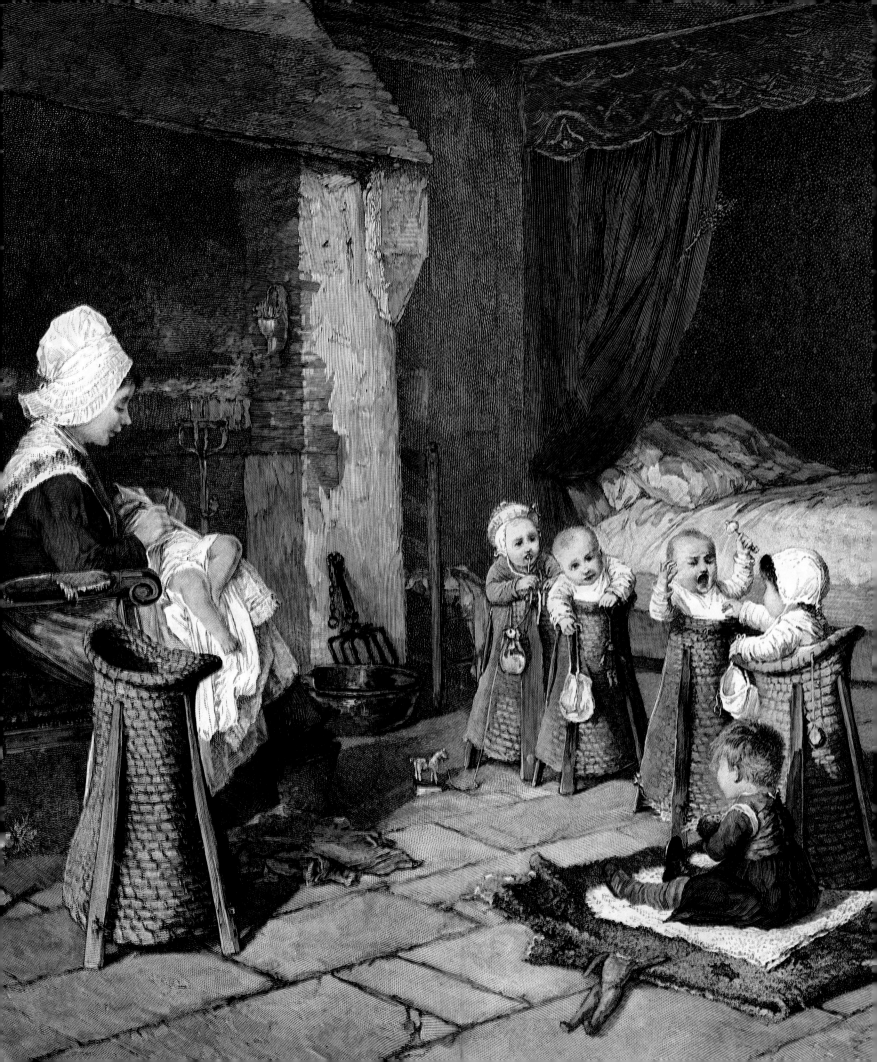

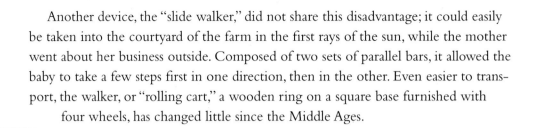

Another device, the "slide walker," did not share this disadvantage; it could easily be taken into the courtyard of the farm in the first rays of the sun, while the mother went about her business outside. Composed of two sets of parallel bars, it allowed the baby to take a few steps first in one direction, then in the other. Even easier to transport, the walker, or "rolling cart," a wooden ring on a square base furnished with four wheels, has changed little since the Middle Ages.

The Victory of the First Step

All these contraptions were intended to keep the baby in one place while promoting the standing position and walking. Babies on all fours made their parents worry. What if they never gave up that position? Until the twentieth century, serious nutritional deficiencies and inbreeding, common in rural areas, made a good number of children suffer from rickets or deformities. The baby's first step signaled a victory over these potential defects; it meant that a malevolent force did not make the baby "rickety" and prevent him from standing up. His mother had of course done all she could to improve the situation: she had carefully avoided cutting his nails and passing him over a table. If her child was slow to begin walking, she would have energetically massaged his legs with butter, bear fat, or urine to strengthen them. If no progress was made, she took her baby on a pilgrimage to a place where contact with the water of a spring or a stone devoted to a particular saint—Saint Fessé, Saint Marche, or Saint Lié, depending on the locale—would make the infant stand on his legs.

Parents who pushed their children to walk at an early age—who can still be found in all social classes—met with the disapproval of experts in every realm. In most late-nineteenth-century and early-twentieth-century books, all the devices and methods of teaching babies to walk too young elicited vehement criticism: "The young infant has no need to learn to walk, and any premature training of his muscles brings disadvantages. This precocity in which mothers glory has its dangers, and the defective incurvature of the legs, as yet unfit to support the weight of the structure, is the least consequence of a too great haste to make babies walk."

Fathers in the past often fashioned devices—such as turnstiles, slide walkers, and walkers—to hold their children upright before they learned to walk on their own.

LEFT, TOP TO BOTTOM: Turnstile, easel, and slide walker. 19th century. Prints

OPPOSITE: Colin Libour. *The Turnstile.* 1892. Musée des Arts et Traditions Populaires, Paris

OVERLEAF: Gaetano Chierici (1838–1920). *The First Steps.* Gallery of Modern Art, Genoa

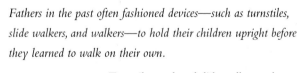

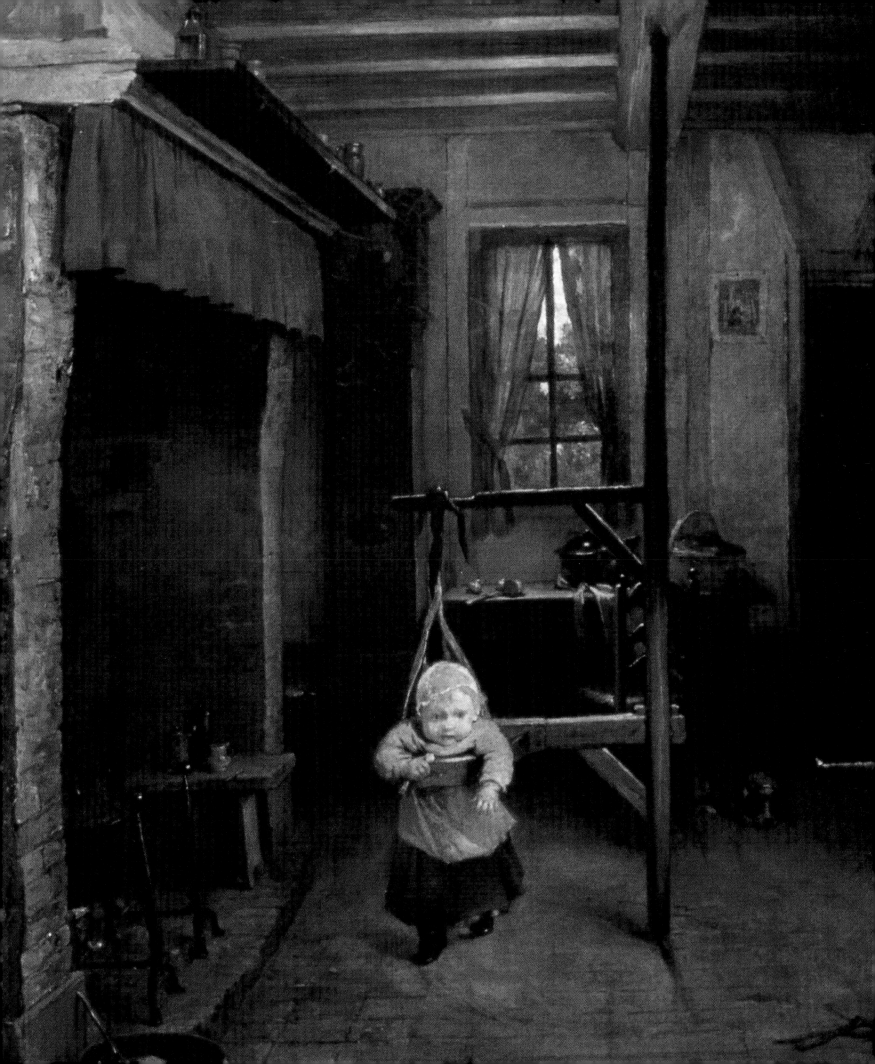

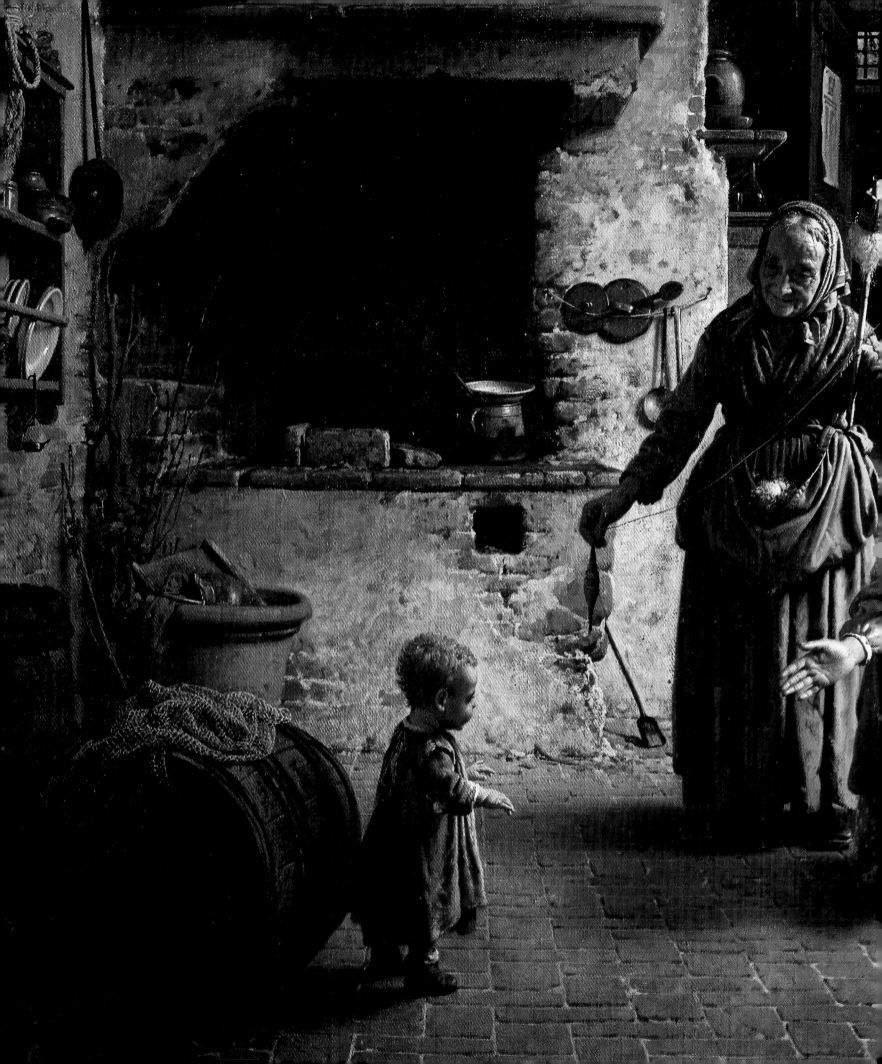

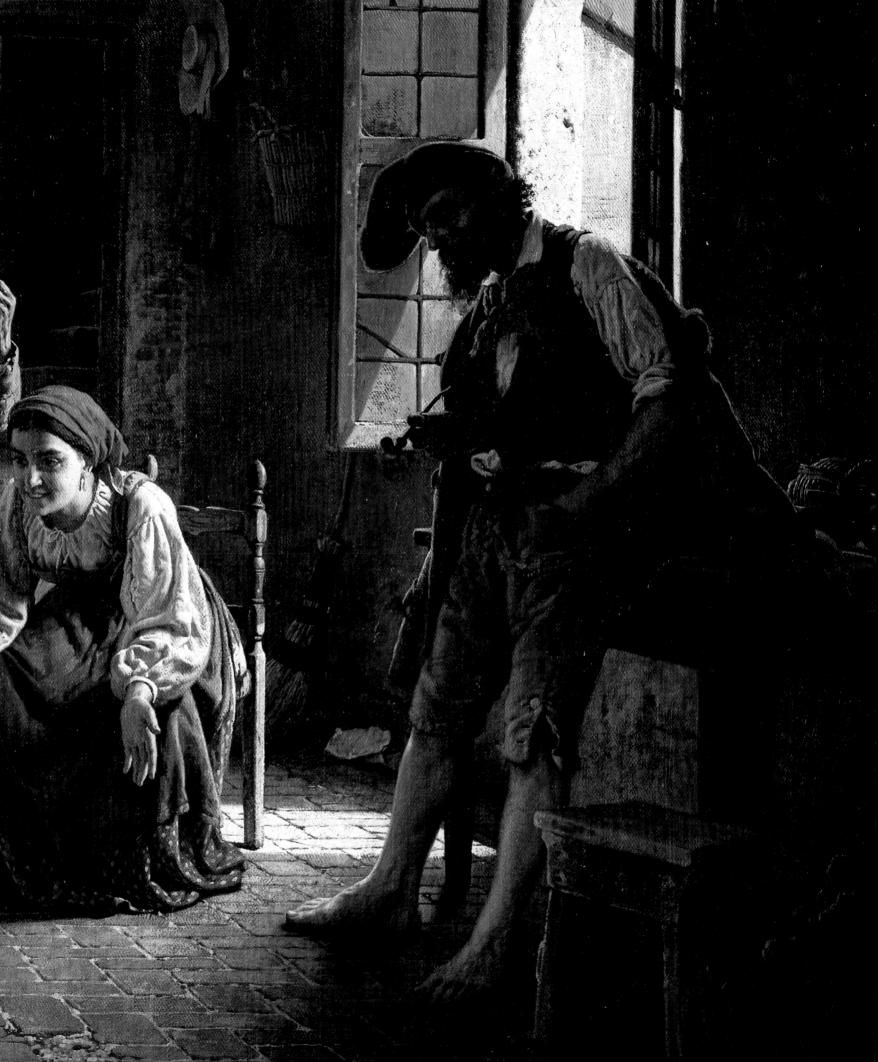

The Passion for the Open Air

"Where the sun never visits, the doctor visits often" goes the proverb. Child-care experts enthusiastically recommended giving babies the benefit of fresh air. This new passion took off at the beginning of the nineteenth century. In England, babies could sample the oxygen so necessary to their good health not only when they went out on walks but also in their rooms. Nursery windows were usually left wide open, and the babies played and walked in front of them and even slept in small baskets hung from the window sills. In France as well, doctors prescribed taking babies outside: "Except on days of heavy rain, excessive cold, and storms, the extended walk, in summer as well as winter, is very good for them; it promotes their development and gives their skin tone and color," claimed one. "You must make taking the baby out every day as much as possible a fixed rule," directed another.

Doctors set specific parameters for these walks: they were to begin only after the newborn was ten or fifteen days old in the summer and twenty or thirty days in the winter. Babies had to be covered warmly and wear a veil, a kind of gauze to protect them from the wind, dust, and insects. They were to be taken out once a day up to the age of three months, and thereafter twice a day. Until the age of six months, they would rest their heads against a small pillow and be carried in the nurse's arms to be warmed by her body heat. When they were bigger and could sit up properly, they were put in a small baby carriage, with their feet resting on a hot-water bottle.

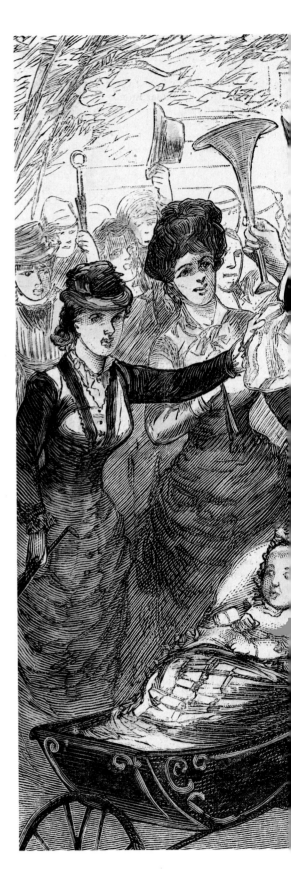

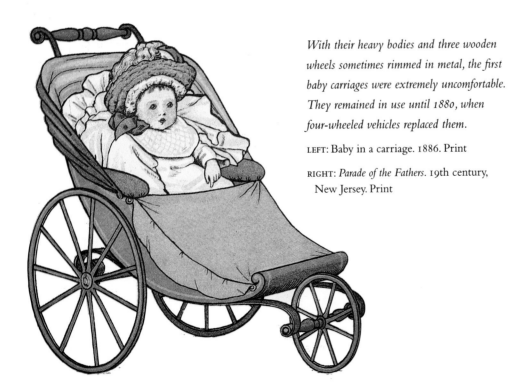

With their heavy bodies and three wooden wheels sometimes rimmed in metal, the first baby carriages were extremely uncomfortable. They remained in use until 1880, when four-wheeled vehicles replaced them.

LEFT: Baby in a carriage. 1886. Print

RIGHT: *Parade of the Fathers.* 19th century, New Jersey. Print

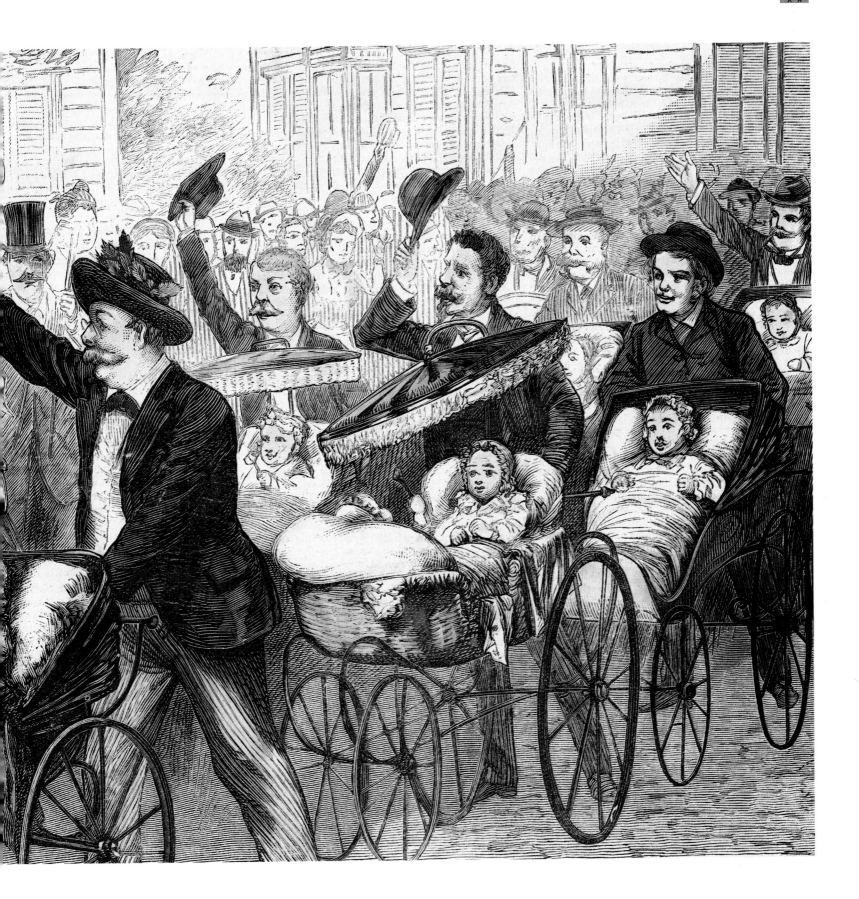

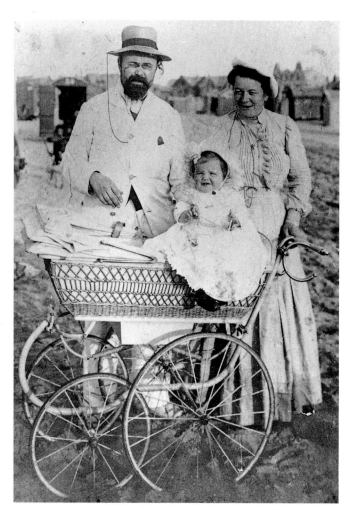

At the end of the nineteenth century and the beginning of the twentieth, the first four-wheeled baby carriages, perched on their large wheels like giant insects, appeared in the photographs of wealthy families.

ABOVE: Family on the beach at Berck, France. 1910. Photograph

RIGHT: Baby carriage. 1900. Photograph

The Baby Carriage

Since the beginning of the nineteenth century in the big cities, walking the baby was a ritual. This salutary exercise, indispensable to her health, presented challenges when the baby got too heavy to be carried but could not yet walk on her own. A new means of transport had to be invented, one more suitable than a peasant's small wooden cart or the opulent miniature carriages pulled by a large dog or a pony owned by wealthy families. Invented in England, the baby carriage—a three-wheeled vehicle designed to be pushed from behind, not pulled—caused a sensation. The first baby carriage factory opened its doors in England in 1840. Some years later, Queen Victoria endorsed this new mode of transportation by buying three of them to wheel her children about.

In 1855 a Reverend Armstrong noted in his journal that the streets of London were full of nurses pushing perambulators, or baby carriages; he had never seen these devices before. The perambulator became all the rage, a new status symbol, taking its place alongside the nurse in the parks of London. The baby had to sit up in these first three-wheeled baby carriages, so they could not easily be used before the baby was six months old.

In 1876, a carriage manufacturer designed a baby carriage with four wheels for smaller infants, but this vehicle was banned from the sidewalks by the police, who initially classed it as a wagon meant to ride in the street. This problem was not restricted to England; nineteenth-century Germany required a pushcart license. A new vehicle that eluded this rule was developed about 1880. It permitted babies to be transported lying down; a wicker cradle, imported from France, sat atop a chassis and wheels. Delicate and hard to clean, these rolling baskets were replaced at the end of the nineteenth century by ones made of other materials, including wood, papier-mâché, and thick leather.

The citizens of England's big cities participated in unofficial contests to display the most beautiful perambulator. Their various models of baby carriages, selected from catalogues, bore such grandiloquent or bucolic names as the Ascot, the Albany, the Parisian, the Dover, the Coronation,

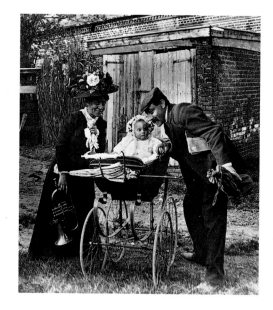

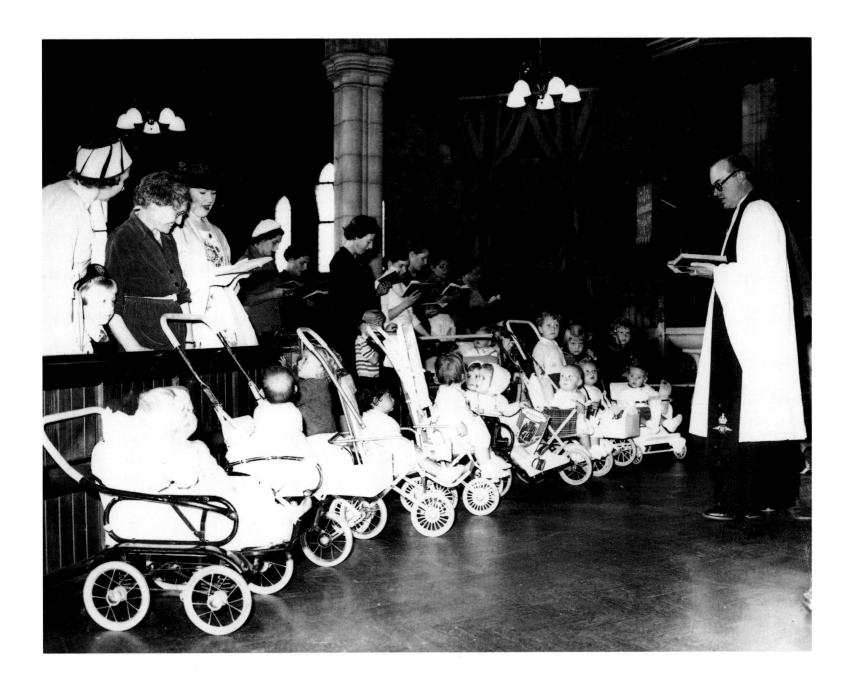

the Windsor, the Canoe, the Park, the Nest. Like the horse-drawn carriages that inspired them, perambulators could be ordered with coats of arms painted on their sides.

At the beginning of the twentieth century, they grew more and more sophisticated as manufacturers vied to be more ingenious than each other. All sorts of novelties—both useful and frivolous—abounded: baby carriages that could be converted to cradles, to carts, to sleds, and even to seesaws; baby carriages with built-in folding seats for the nurses; and so on.

In this London church, the priest seems to be celebrating mass for a group of babies in their strollers, which were not as willingly tolerated in other public spaces.

ABOVE: Photograph

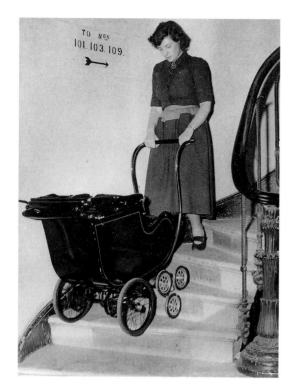

Wooden Strollers and Steel Baby Carriages

In the 1920s, elegance and luxury gave way to safety and comfort. The baby carriage was no longer an object of display. It became very deep to prevent babies from falling out, its wheels grew smaller, and its suspension and padding improved. Stronger as well, it utilized steel instead of wood, leather, or wicker. While the first baby carriages had been based on full-size carriages, in the era of the automobile the design of baby carriages took its inspiration from cars. The use of steel made it possible for the first time to mass-produce good-quality vehicles at reasonable prices. As mothers gradually replaced nannies in the parks, they pounced on every feature that could make their lives easier, such as folding baby carriages, which were produced in the United States at the beginning of the century, along with wooden strollers that also folded. Manuals urged certain precautions in the use of these vehicles: after a "short apprenticeship to practice going up and down the sidewalks of cities without making the baby bounce around…it is important to avoid stops and starts as much as possible, as the shaking they cause throughout the little body could have harmful consequences. You must always walk very slowly and evenly. Finally, the last recommendation to give to the nurses: never leave the carriage, even for a moment, while it is in motion; the least negligence can lead to the most awful accidents."

Today, parents living in industrialized countries can choose from a great number of models of carriages and strollers. Baby transportation—only recently involving wheels—has come a long way since the days when there were few alternatives to arms.

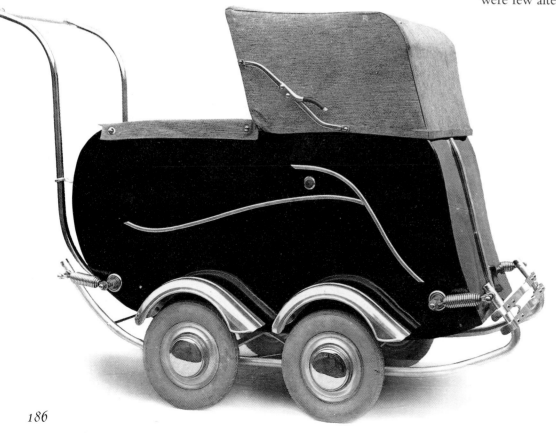

Leather upholstery, umbrella stands, waterproof hoods, fenders, brakes—the steel baby carriages manufactured after World War I appeared to be veritable nurseries on wheels. The more sophisticated they were, the more practical they became.

ABOVE AND LEFT: The massive, big-bodied forms of prewar baby carriages

OPPOSITE: Wayne Miller/Magnum. Photograph. 1950

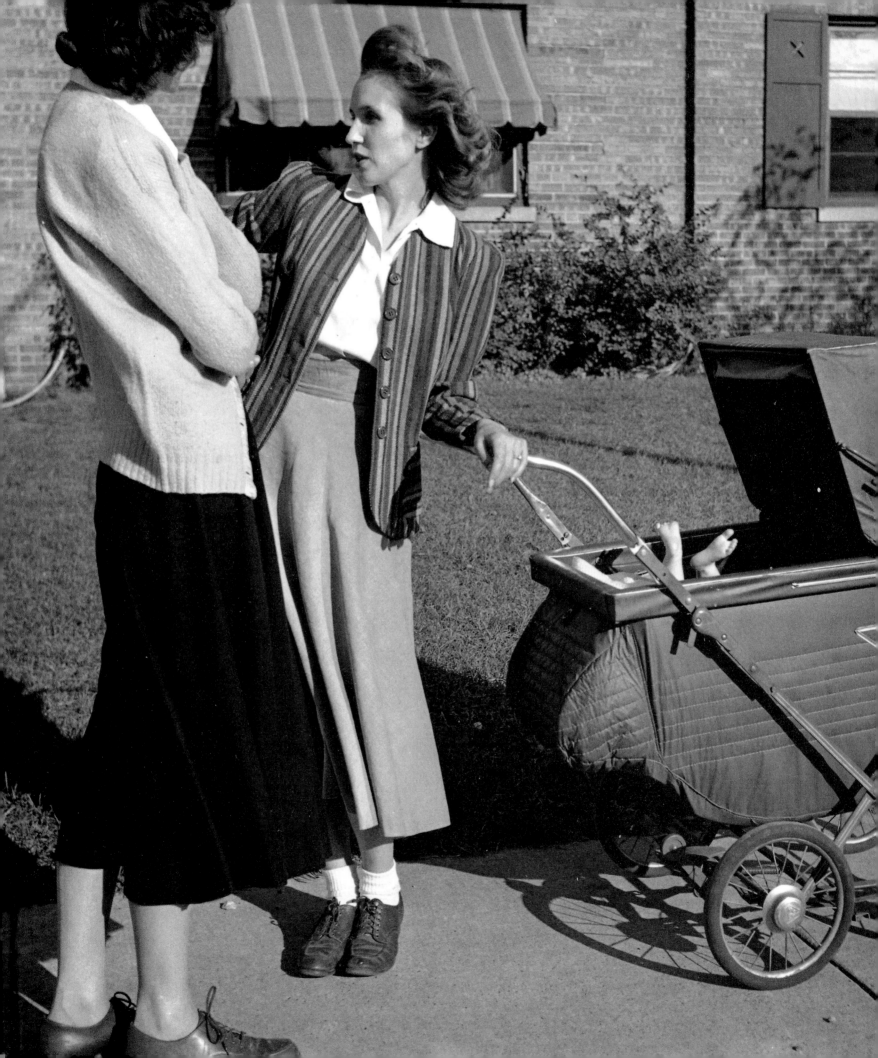

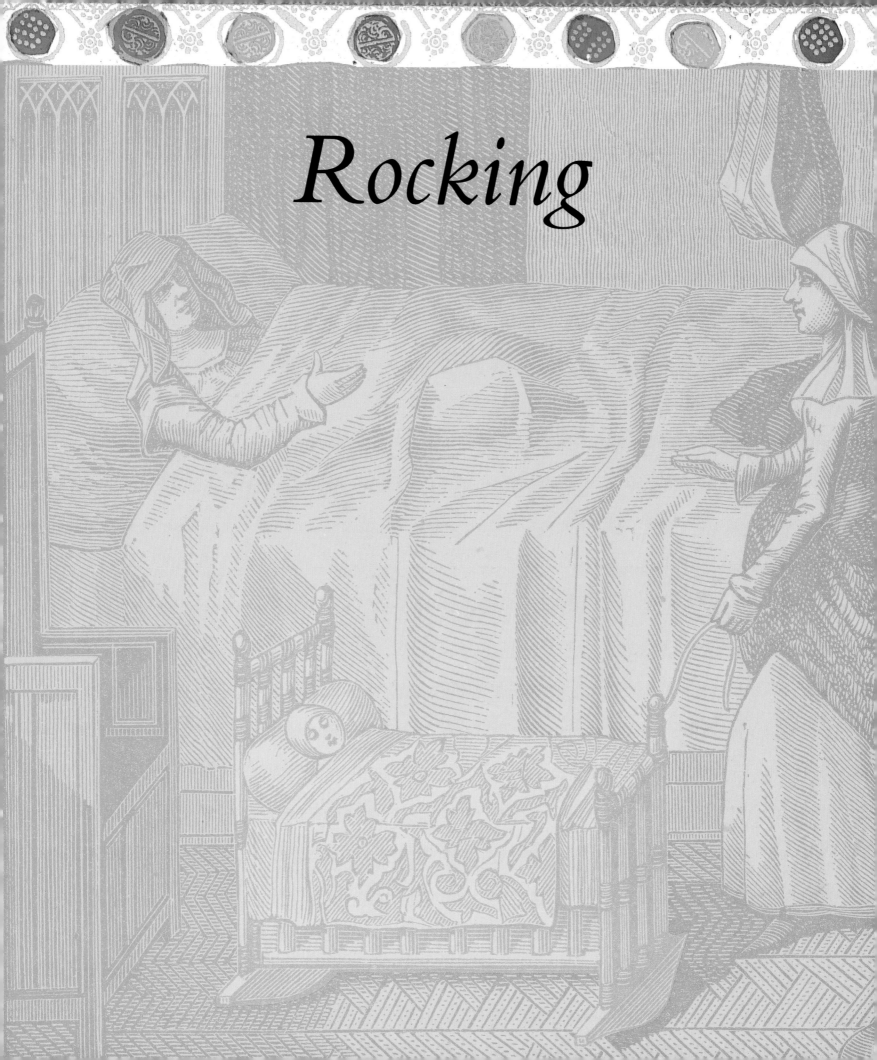

Rocking

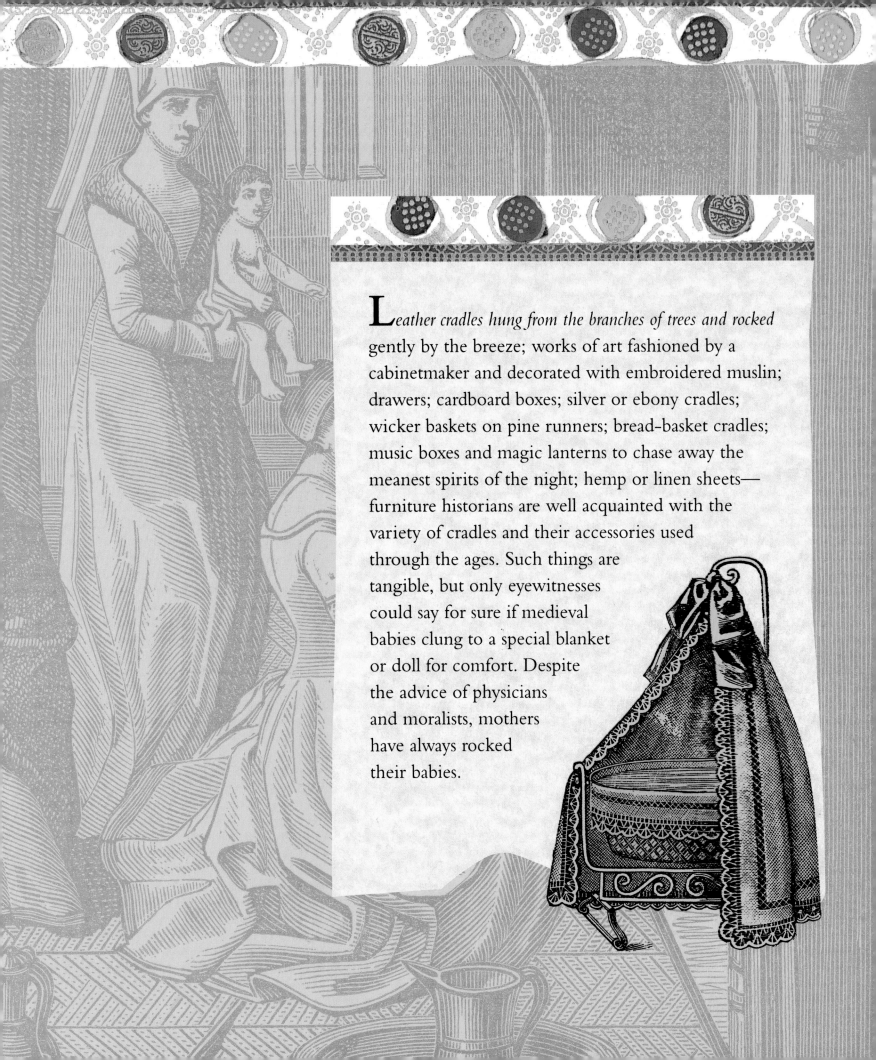

Leather cradles hung from the branches of trees and rocked gently by the breeze; works of art fashioned by a cabinetmaker and decorated with embroidered muslin; drawers; cardboard boxes; silver or ebony cradles; wicker baskets on pine runners; bread-basket cradles; music boxes and magic lanterns to chase away the meanest spirits of the night; hemp or linen sheets—furniture historians are well acquainted with the variety of cradles and their accessories used through the ages. Such things are tangible, but only eyewitnesses could say for sure if medieval babies clung to a special blanket or doll for comfort. Despite the advice of physicians and moralists, mothers have always rocked their babies.

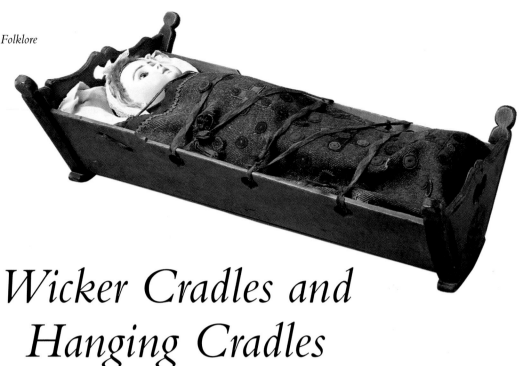

Wicker Cradles and Hanging Cradles

ABOVE: Cradle. 19th century. Musée des Arts et Traditions Populaires, Paris

BELOW: Miniature. 15th century. Bibliothèque de l'Arsenal, Paris

"**F**or the bodies as well as the souls of very young infants, it is beneficial for all, but especially for the youngest, to experience as much as possible during the night, as during the day, in addition to nourishment, a sort of swinging; in short, it would do them good to live, if possible, as if they had never stopped floating in the sea," wrote the philosopher Plato. In antiquity, babies were rocked all the time. The Romans made rocking into an actual profession, taken up by both men and women; so parents could choose between a *cunarius* or a *cunaria*—terms taken from the goddess Cunina, who presided over rocking and was responsible for driving away all the evil spirits prowling around the baby. The cradles of patrician families were decorated with mosaics and paintings, lined with precious fabrics, and sprinkled with flower petals. A sheepskin placed at the bottom collected the baby's excrement. Soranus of Ephesus once again surprises us with the modernity of his views. He advised against placing babies on a hard surface, which was common among the Thracians and Macedonians, who either strapped their infants to flat planks to flatten the area around the neck or placed them on a surface that was too soft. He directed that diapers under babies be changed regularly to prevent their catching cold or becoming imbued with bad odors.

A layer of bay leaves or myrtle placed under babies gave off a pleasant scent.

In the Middle Ages, parents rarely let their babies cry. They thought that tears could be dangerous to the baby's health and led to the risk of convulsions, which, resembling possession, would attract the devil. In a society without electric lights, where the nights became completely black, perhaps adults felt themselves more bound up with their babies and their nocturnal frights, which they undoubtedly shared. So women rocked their babies night and day, sometimes even when they were not crying. The image of the mother spinning wool while rocking a cradle at her feet has been endlessly repeated in popular iconography. When the mother finished one task, she got up, took the cradle under her arm, and went to another, even to working in the field. Easily managed and not very heavy, the cradle was employed mostly during the day, for at night mothers preferred to take their unweaned young to bed with them, where they fed them, warmed them, and calmed them. However, under the pretext of preventing infants from being accidentally suffocated, the Church opposed this practice. The mothers therefore, with regret, left their babies in cradles, but pulled them against or hung them over their beds. Then, if the infant suffered harm, the fault could be laid to the cradle. However, this small piece of furniture was designed as a sort of protective shell. In its narrowness, it echoed the form of the swaddled infant, like a mummy in its sarcophagus. It completed the work of shaping the baby's body. It had holes cut or cleats set into its sides, which allowed a lace, often red, to zigzag over the top like a shoelace to keep the infant from falling out if the cradle capsized.

The cradle, in which the baby was securely tied, did not have a fixed position in the house, except at the feet of the adult who kept an eye on the baby and kept him company.

RIGHT: Michael Pacher (1434–1498). *Saint Ambroise*. Alte Pinakothek, Munich

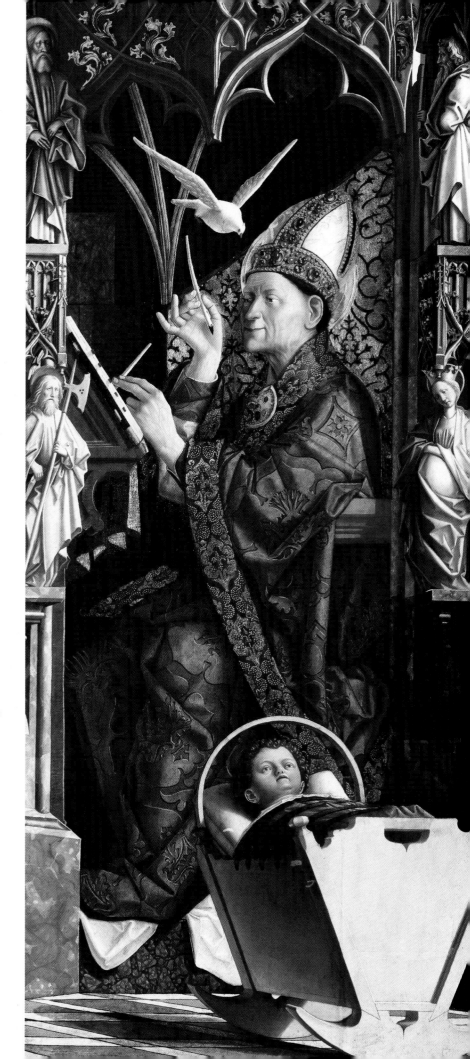

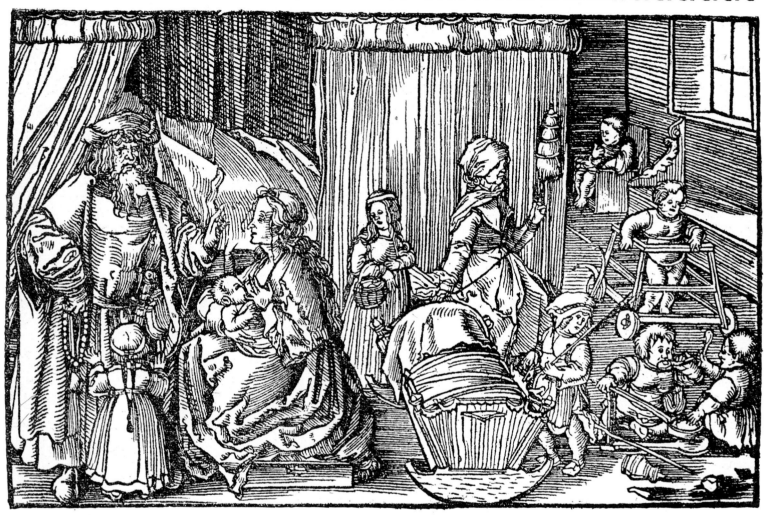

The cradle hood was invented in the mid-fifteenth century. A cloth draped over an arch above the baby's head served to protect her from harsh light, drafts, and insects.

ABOVE: Wood engraving. 15th century

Boxes, Baskets, and Barrels

In the Middle Ages, a great variety of cradles existed, different from setting to setting and region to region: the trough cradle, hollowed from a half trunk of a tree; the box cradle, which was made from a few planks of wood the father had pinned together and was painted red and decorated with simple motifs that had protective powers; the wicker hamper cradle; the half-barrel cradle (in the Middle Ages barrels had many uses in addition to those involving wine-making); the basketwork hod cradle with leather thongs for long trips; the court cradle for royal families, on which artisans and artists labored for months. The peasant baby lying in an apple basket and the royal baby sleeping under the canopy of a golden, beribboned cradle were both rocked to their heart's content. Several cradles were made of fragrant and rot-resistant pine, larch, and cypress wood. Widely available and easy to work with, these woods stood up to babies' urine, and their resinous aroma opened up the respiratory tract. Young princes rested in cradles made of ebony, extremely rare during this period. Considered a protective material, ebony's dark color was thought to help babies overcome their fear of the dark. Families of lesser means attached a small piece of ebony to the cradle for the same reason.

Mattresses of Straw and Sheets of Gold

The bedding also varied according to setting. Even if a cradle had a perforated bottom, the bedding—wheat straw, rye straw, chaff, or thistledown—had to be changed often. A hempen or woolen sheet covered the mattress. Blankets were expensive, another reason poor parents took their babies to bed with them. Aristocratic families could cover their offspring with sumptuous sheets of gold lined with ermine. These young princes also enjoyed the services of a "rocker," a woman employed exclusively for that task. Some infants dozed off to the sound of veritable orchestras comprised of harps, oboes, and flutes. All babies listened to lullabies, and the French peasant sang sweetly to her baby, "Little Saint Margaret, put my child to sleep, until she is fifteen; when fifteen years have gone by, married she must be, with a boy who is good, they will make a good household, in a little room, full of pecans, with a hammer to crack them, and white bread to eat." Why did Saint Margaret have to put the child to sleep until the age of fifteen? Did childhood hold too many dangers to overcome, and did parents have too many woes, and were they too exhausted to take care of a child?

In any case, even if the father made the cradle, he had no place in the history of rocking; that occupation remained the exclusive province of the woman. Nonetheless, some texts, recounted by Danièle Alexandre-Bidon and Monique Closson in *L'enfant à l'ombre des cathédrales* (The Child in the Shadow of the Cathedrals), reveal that although the father did not do the rocking, he might end up bent over the cradle, half secretly, during the night. A tale describes a father who gets up to urinate in the night and on his way checks the baby to see if all is well: "He got into the habit at night, when the urge to urinate possessed him, to touch the cradle first off."

In the fifteenth and sixteenth centuries, rich and poor continued to be rocked, although some critics, in order to stigmatize rustic wet nurses, attacked this practice, which they claimed could sour the milk in the baby's stomach and shake her brain. Sensible authorities, however, such as Simon de Vallambert, advised mothers to

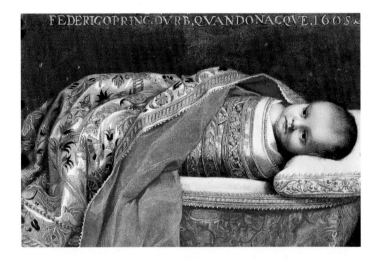

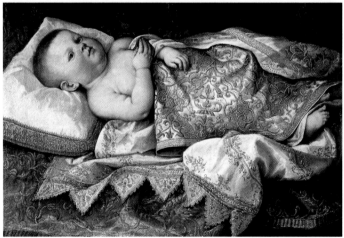

TOP: Federico Barocci (1526–1612). *Prince Federico d'Urbino.* Galleria Palatina, Florence

ABOVE: Tiberio Titi (1573–1627). *Prince Leopold de' Medicis.* Galleria Palatina, Florence

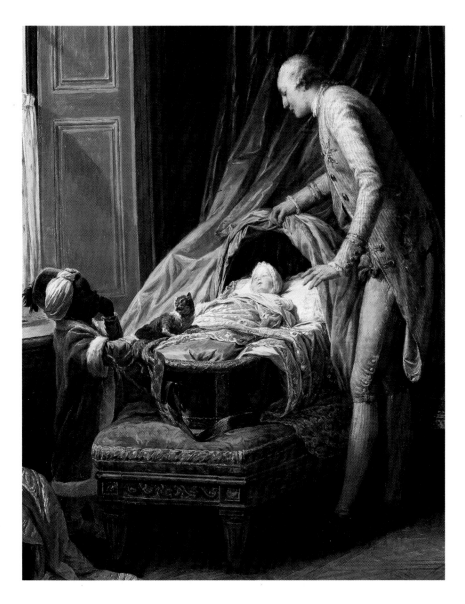

"send their babies to sleep by rocking them, singing to them softly, placing them near running water, if possible, by making water fall drop by drop into a basin, avoiding all noise, giving them fresh scents to smell." He added, "To bring on sleep, place some oil of violet or rose in his nose with lettuce juice, adding a drop of oil of anise, and put on top of the head oil of poppy or waterlily, sometimes adding a grain of opium." He insisted that the child not be covered too heavily nor the room overheated, "Being that the infant in his mother's belly, suffering from too much heat, desires coolness and wants to emerge into the open air. Having thus emerged, it is a big mistake to keep him shut in, as if the idea were to make him go back inside." Elsewhere, to those who held that rocking was bad for digestion, he responded that, to the contrary, a gentle and rhythmic rocking "prepares and stimulates the heat of the digestion of milk, makes it go down into the stomach, and as a result it puts the child to sleep, just as gentle massages and songs do, for through these means the soul draws back to itself gently, and inside the spirits of animals all other actions cease and sleep comes."

"Gentle Shakes"

In the Renaissance, the large hangings that enclosed the parents' bed and undoubtedly enveloped the small cradles as well disappeared. The concept of cradles took a new turn; the hood was invented, and later, small curtains were adapted to protect the baby. In the eighteenth century, enlightened doctors explained how beneficial rocking could be, since the movement brought babies back to their life in the womb. "As the fetus in the heart of his mother, suspended on the umbilical cord, moves easily in every direction while his mother is active, it was thought, not without reason, that a similar movement must give newborns pleasure. Daily experience tells us that the most miserable babies calm down and fall into a sweet slumber when they are gently rocked," recalled the physician Van Swieten. His colleague Johan Peter Frank pushed the arguments in favor of rocking even further: "This movement in truth has its benefits in what its gentle shakes produce: the infant's body gains strength; then, due to the stirring of the air it creates, her lungs are more effectively dilated. I might add that with this movement inspiring the

In the eighteenth century, rocking babies began to be seen as a bad habit. Jean-Jacques Rousseau asserted that it could corrupt the child.

ABOVE: Nicolas Lépicié (1735–1784). *Louis-Philippe at the Cradle.* Collection of Monseigneur le Comte de Paris

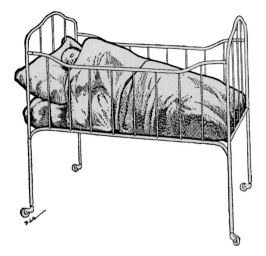

infant to breathe more strongly and more deeply, the very tips of the arteries find themselves shaken, gain in activity, and react on the humors." On the other hand, he criticized those "perverse artifices used by some maids who to calm a baby titillated his genital parts and in this way paved the way from the tenderest youth for an inclination toward sensuality, or who to make babies sleep give them opium or other similar narcotics."

While some authorities found rocking good for the health, others thought it a dangerous habit: "The baby's sleep, after this violent agitation, is less a true sleep than stupefaction, similar to the effect produced by turning a hen after it has put its head under its wing. The blood and liquids stop in the head, compress the brain, and create, by this pressure, a mild apoplexy rather than a true sleep," explained Des Essarts. That is, rocking the baby produced a forced sleep.

Des Essarts went on to point out an even more pernicious danger than rocking: the cohabitation of two individuals of different ages and constitutions. "In every period doctors have tried to revive exhausted bodies dying of weakness by having them sleep with others who are young and in good health. We noticed that of many young children used to sleeping in the same bed as their grandfathers and grandmothers or with their governess that the area of their bodies in the closest contact with those with whom they sleep were weaker, thinner, and had less color."

For or against curtains and lace? Doctors and bourgeois families carried on a lively debate at the end of the nineteenth century.

ABOVE: Print. 20th century

BELOW: Postcard. 1914

OVERLEAF: Eugène le Roux (1833–1905). *The Newborn.* Musée des Beaux-Arts, Rennes

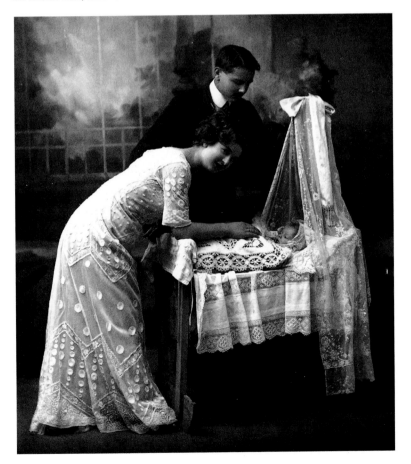

Iron Bedsteads and Lace

For thousands of years, mothers rocked their children in complete peace. In the nineteenth century, these small, gentle actions, these murmured little songs would become altogether prohibited. The baby had become, it seemed, a calculating and capricious personality who had to be disciplined at a very early age. Child-care experts championed the parents' cause and undertook to abolish what was seen as intolerable slavery to which they had fallen victim. "The best cradle is one that cannot be rocked," declared Professor Pinard, who nevertheless displayed great solicitude toward babies. "Whatever fortune it may be your happiness to possess, nothing will make a cradle that rocks a good cradle," another doctor lectured.

And a third went further: "Rocking is very much in favor with nurses, who by this means more easily calm their charges. This habit is best given up, as the baby used to being rocked can no longer do without it; she

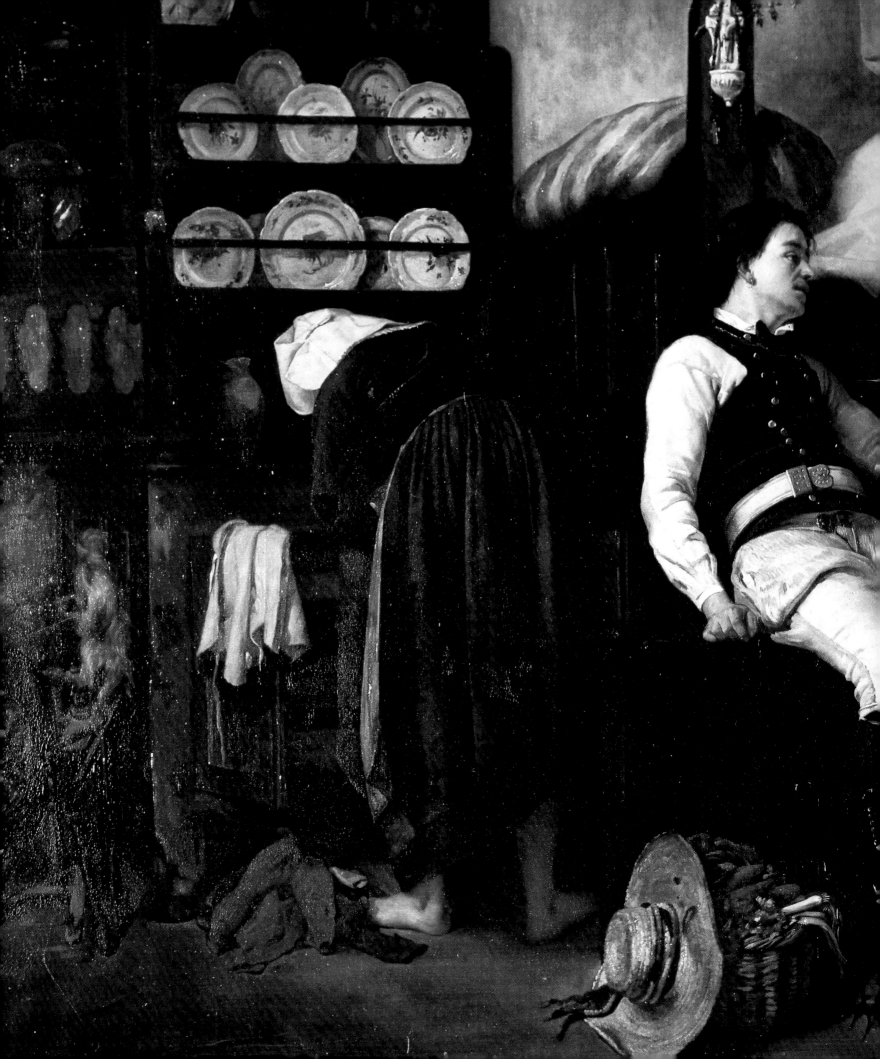

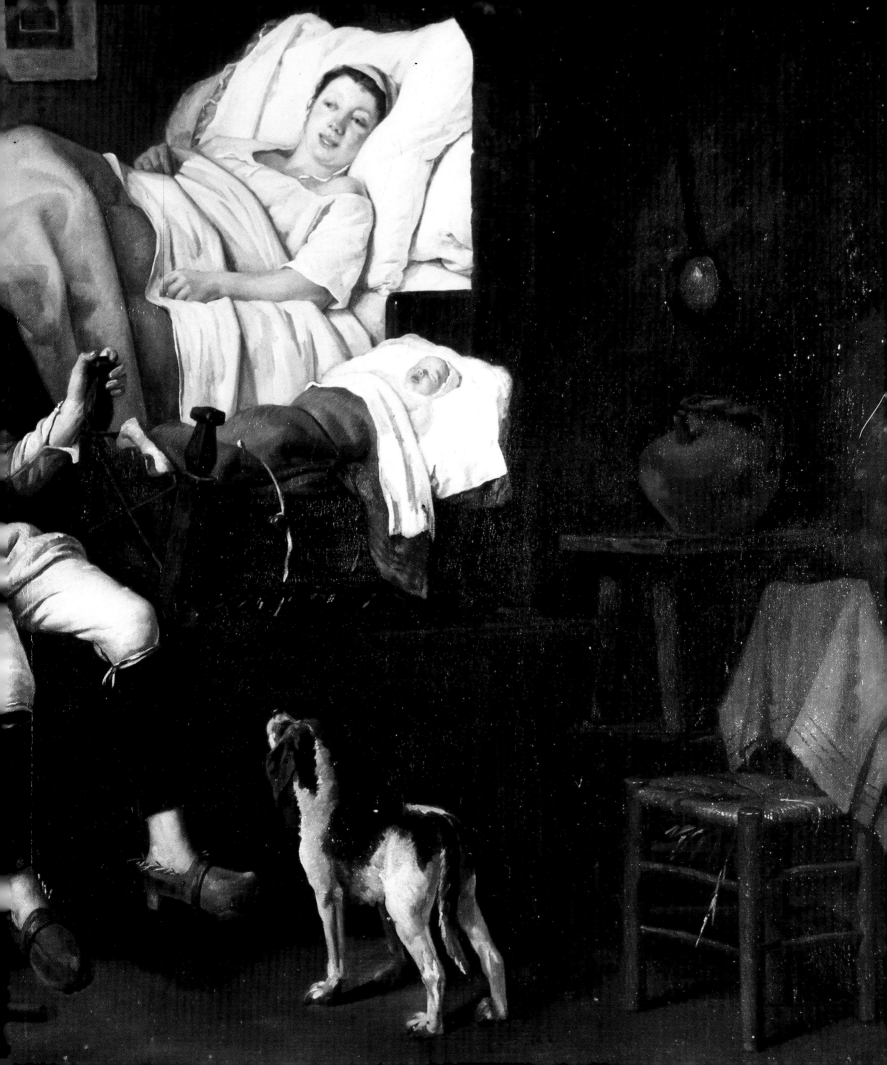

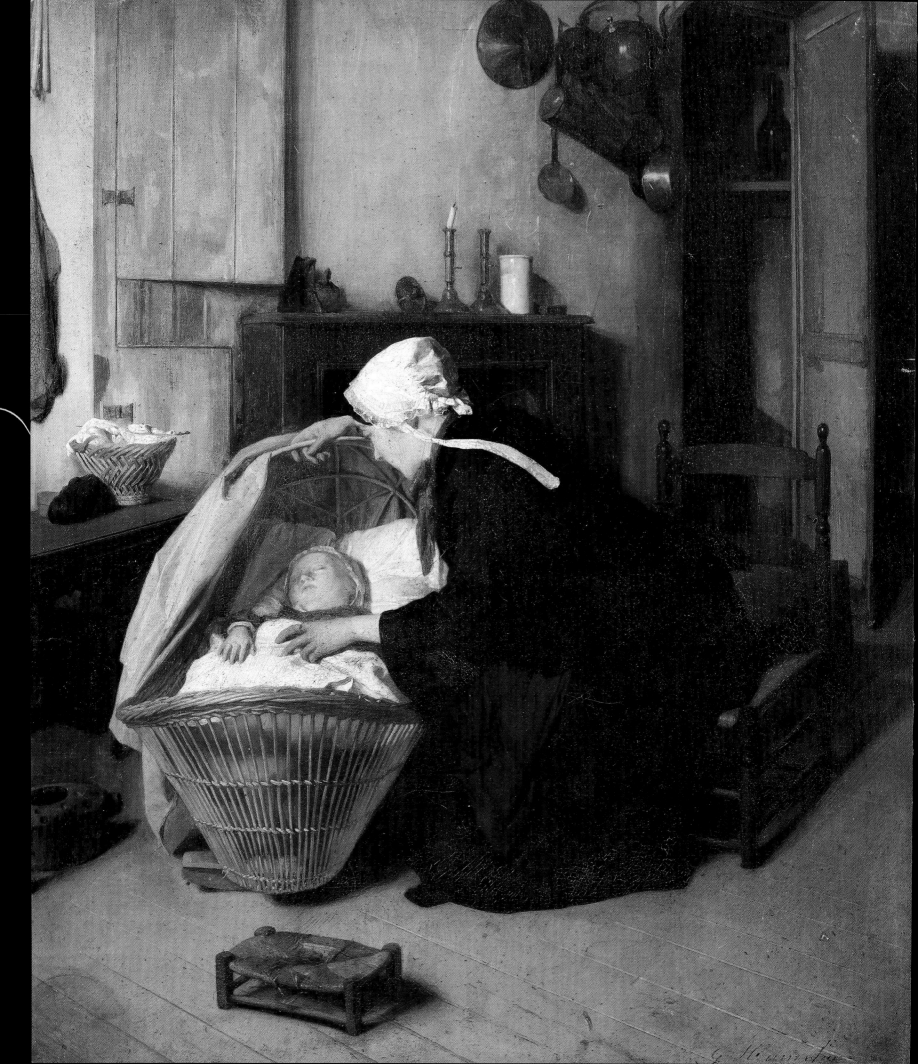

acquires a mania for rocking, and there is no proof that this oscillating movement, frequently repeated, is not harmful to the nervous system, so delicate at that age."

Although it produced such strict principles, the nineteenth century was also the century of hygiene, from which babies greatly benefited. Doctors repeatedly enjoined mothers to air out often the room where their babies slept, for it should not be "an alcove, a receptacle for miasmas"; not to shroud them under several layers of blankets; and to choose an iron bedstead rather than a wooden cradle, which could easily be infested with fleas and other bugs. Small iron beds could be washed and even disinfected. Nineteenth-century books on child care gave numerous details on bedding, then composed of several kinds of mattresses: canvas sacks stuffed with horsehair, seaweed, chaff, or the largest stems of fern leaves, which gave the baby's bed a pleasant smell. These mattresses, however, had to be changed frequently, for most doctors still advised against waterproof fabrics—taffetas treated with gum or waxed canvas—which they considered unhealthy.

Curtains became the object of a lengthy controversy. One doctor of the period sanctioned them if it were certain "that these curtains were of a flexible and thin fabric that permitted the passage of a filtered air. But too often they give the cradle the air of a catafalque; they are many and thick, and to uncover the baby they hide it is necessary to throw aside a multitude of muslins and other, heavier fabrics." A woman doctor of the time praised a blanket in knit wool, velvety and very soft. In winter, stoneware hot-water bottles wrapped in a cloth could be placed in the cradle to warm the baby.

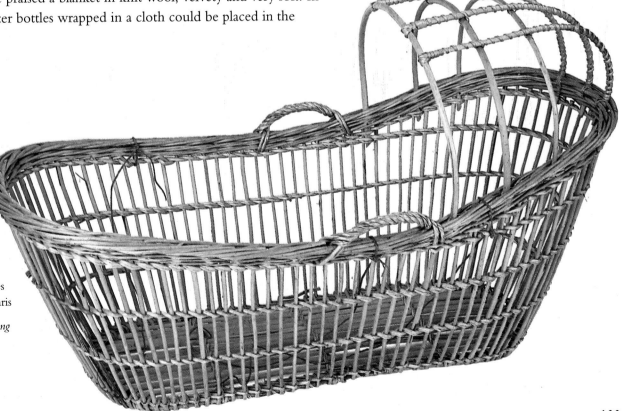

Before the invention of rubberized cloth, it was necessary to wash cradles in the sea or a river.

ABOVE: Print. 19th century

RIGHT: Wicker cradle. Musée des Arts et Traditions Populaires, Paris

OPPOSITE: Jacques Hamelin. *Young Mother*. Musée des Beaux-Arts, Le Havre

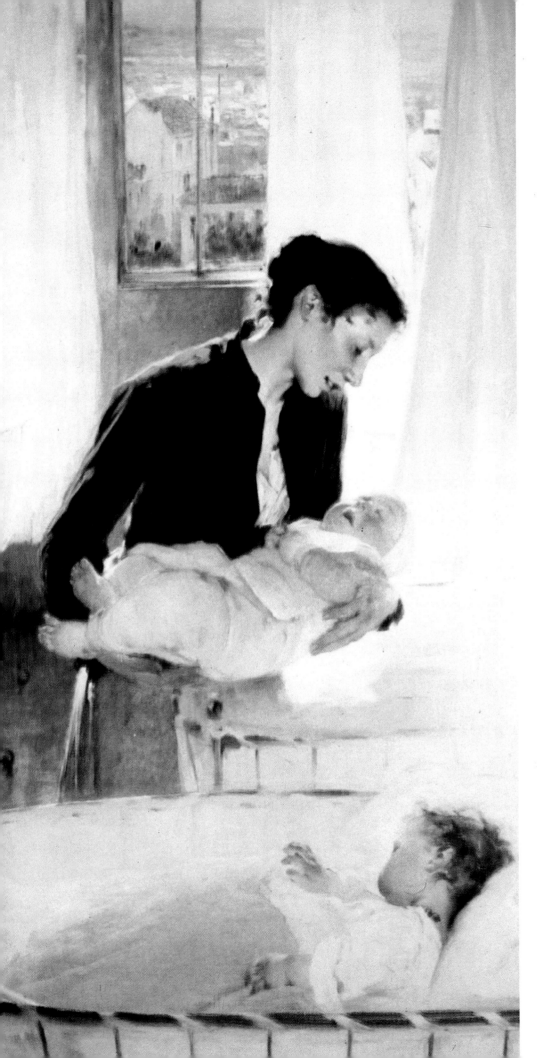

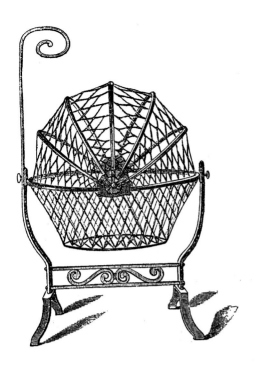

"My child is an angel
God gave him to me,
I am not worthy
They tell me to sell him
Angel of heaven,
He is beyond price for me."

Portuguese lullaby

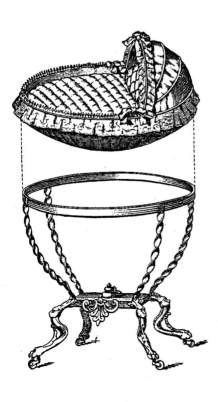

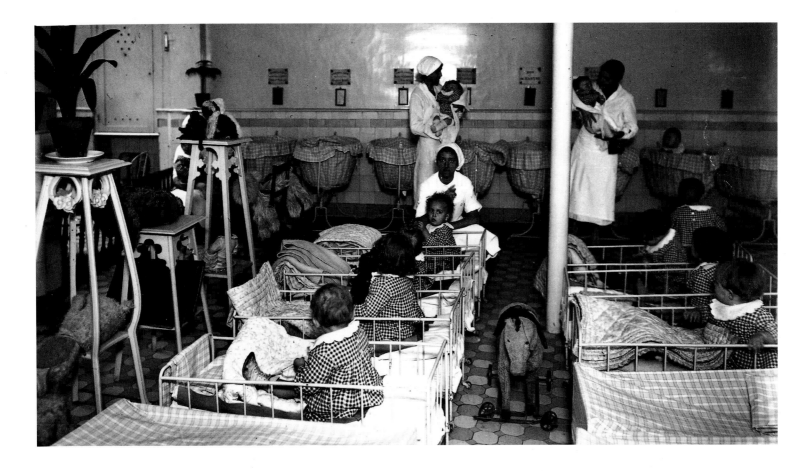

Cradle Litter

Some authors mention an original idea for handling babies' waste—filling the bottom of the cradle with bran. "Most cradles do not call for more than thirty to forty liters," one specified. Heating the bran in a baker's oven sterilized it. Each day, the nurse removed and replaced the soiled bran; both liquids and solids clumped it into balls that could easily be gathered and picked out. The baby was unclothed below the navel; she wore only a short-sleeved blouse, a jersey, and an undershirt, so her legs had complete freedom of movement. She could not sink in the bran and certainly could not be buried in it, as some people feared. However, this method carried some drawbacks: it was impossible to keep the bran from overflowing onto the surrounding area when picking up the baby, and some bran dust inevitably stuck to the baby's skin. Beyond these problems, it worked only for part of the first year; after that, babies began to play with the bran, picking it up by the fistful and throwing it as well as putting it in their mouths. "This highly economical child-rearing method practiced in Normandy could be suitable for poor households little concerned about the risk of the child wallowing in dirty swaddling clothes," one doctor scornfully concluded. In reality, its use remained the exception, not the rule.

ABOVE: Day nursery. 20th century. Photograph

OPPOSITE: Jean Geoffroy. *At the Day Nursery*. Musée de l'Assistance Publique, Paris; above: iron cradle; below: removable wicker cradle. 20th century. Prints

BELOW: Small mattress used to carry infants. 20th century. Print

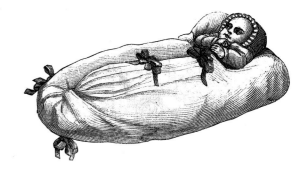

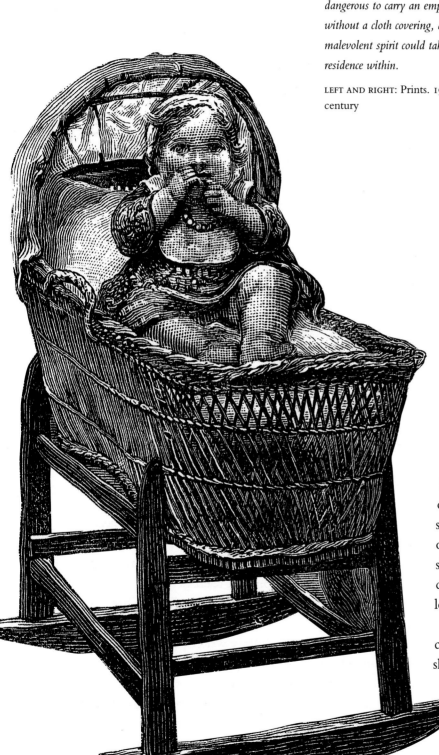

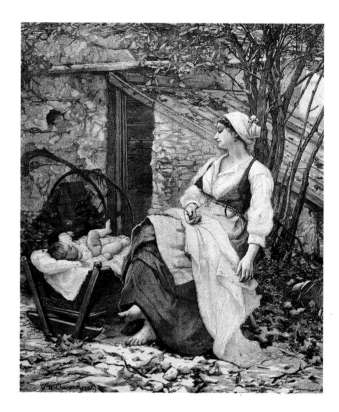

Pediatricians have only recently begun to recommend putting babies to sleep on their backs; throughout the nineteenth century, parents were advised never to put the baby in this position. Instead, they were stretched out on alternate sides, first one, then the other. Pinard warned, "Their little heads are soft, and having them always sleep on the same side would flatten it. Many adults have lopsided heads because in their infancy they were always put to bed or carried on the same side." It may be the baby himself who insists on staying in the same position. One woman doctor advised, "Put on him a small bonnet or band that has a large button on the side that the baby does not want to move from, or move his cradle sideways so he will be forced to turn over if he wants to look out at the room."

Some doctors favored wicker cradles, in which the baby could be carried without being removed from her bed. Many shared the opinion that "in this way the baby is spared a bad position in the arms." For reasons of hygiene as well as the delicate nature of the baby's skeleton, it was thought best to touch the baby as little as possible. Other doctors rebelled against this strange advice: "Babies

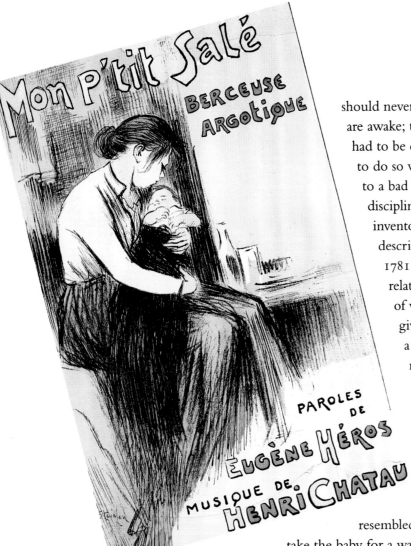

Mon P'tit Salé
BERCEUSE ARGOTIQUE

PAROLES DE EUGÈNE HÉROS
MUSIQUE DE HENRI CHATAU

ABOVE: Sheet music of a lullaby. Early 20th century

OVERLEAF: Auguste Pinchart. *The Cradle.* 1887. Musée des Beaux-Arts, Fécamp

should never be left lying on their backs in their cradles when they are awake; they should be picked up and held vertically." But parents had to be careful: "Take the baby out of the cradle, but be sure not to do so when the infant demands it while crying, as this can lead to a bad habit." While doctors considered child care a form of discipline, in the frenzy of patents that characterizes this century, inventors developed mechanical cradles. Accounts of cradles past describe some that were fastened to cows' tails to be rocked. In 1781, an Englishman developed a cradle with a mechanism related to the slow turning of a spit. Others worked by means of waterwheels or clockworks. An English dictionary of 1830 gives the first technical description of a cradle that provided a regular and gentle rocking automatically for forty-five minutes. "Too regular!" objected a doctor who himself preferred manual rocking.

Rolling, Pitching, and Vibrations

German author Friedrich von Zglinicki, in his book *The Cradle,* explained how the sixteenth-century baby cart would make the cradle obsolete. At first, it resembled a small cart and did not go outdoors. It could be used to take the baby for a walk indoors or put the baby to sleep, with a to-and-fro movement preferable, according to some doctors, to the pitching of the cradle, which was thought to induce seasickness. When baby carriages left the house in the mid-nineteenth century, they produced a new type of rolling that seemed to be as effective at putting infants to sleep as the cradle's rocking.

Mothers also sang lullabies to quiet their babies. In traditional France, these songs often evoked the dangers of infancy and the death of the baby. "Chabri chabra, my little heart is sick, Chabri chabra, perhaps it will die, Chabri chabra, my little heart is sick, Chabri chabra, perhaps it will revive" goes one of them. These sometimes sad and resigned songs not only expressed the mother's distress in the face of the dangers that threatened her baby, but they also revealed ambivalent feelings toward a child who was not always wanted. The lullaby soothed the mother as well as the baby by reconciling one to the other.

Peasant women who, according to nineteenth-century writers, did not know how to talk to their babies undoubtedly found other ways to be close to them. Lullabies gave them a means to express reproach, praise, and tenderness, as in the following lullaby from Picardy: "Go 'way grandma dust that goes by shaking its skirt, while I keep an eye on your sleep, take a nap, my little gnat, take a nap, take a nap. How these children today give such trouble. There's no longer a way to get

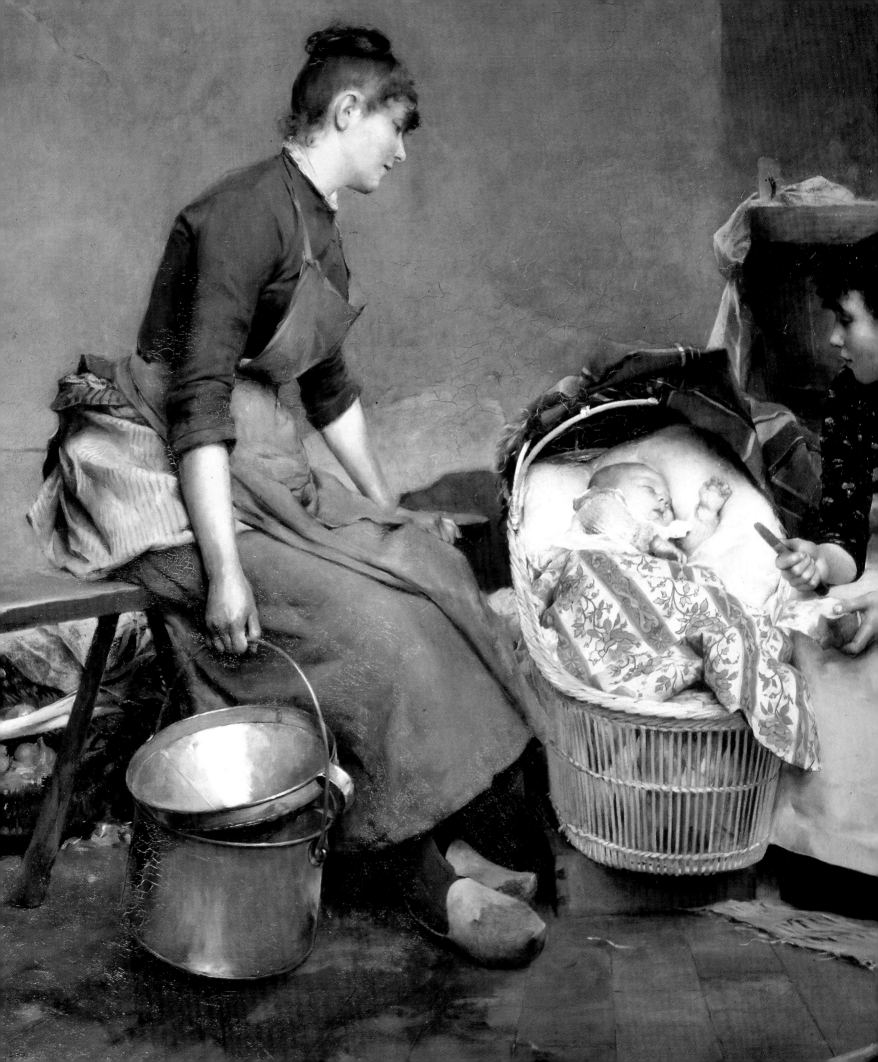

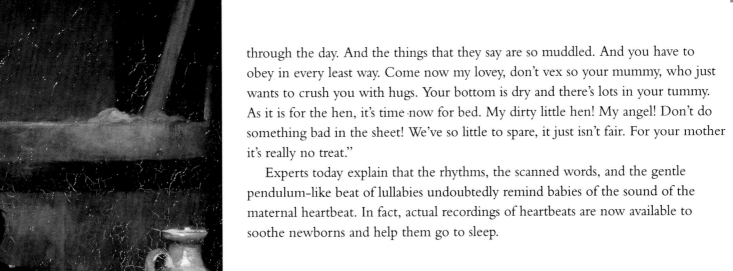

through the day. And the things that they say are so muddled. And you have to obey in every least way. Come now my lovey, don't vex so your mummy, who just wants to crush you with hugs. Your bottom is dry and there's lots in your tummy. As it is for the hen, it's time now for bed. My dirty little hen! My angel! Don't do something bad in the sheet! We've so little to spare, it just isn't fair. For your mother it's really no treat."

Experts today explain that the rhythms, the scanned words, and the gentle pendulum-like beat of lullabies undoubtedly remind babies of the sound of the maternal heartbeat. In fact, actual recordings of heartbeats are now available to soothe newborns and help them go to sleep.

The Baby in Exile

First babies were driven from their parents' beds, then from their parents' rooms, and finally from their own little rocking cradle, that instrument of sleep. A piece of tied cloth, often dipped in wine or poppy juice, was forbidden, as well as the innocent pacifier and the thumb, until recently. Mothers forgot the words and tunes to old lullabies. Babies had to learn to go to sleep all alone, in their own rooms.

How did all these misfortunes come to visit these small beings, who in other ways have become more and more spoiled? Their rooms are filled with colorful mobiles, toys, and an entire collection of gadgets meant to prevent them from knocking against anything or having their fingers caught. To begin with—and this is unquestionably one of the major causes of their eviction from their mothers' bed—their lives are no longer in danger. When they had a lesser chance of survival, their physical closeness to their parents served as protection (today, premature babies are still placed on their mothers, among other methods, to help them survive). The passion for hygiene, parents' desire for intimacy with each other, higher standards of living, the involvement of psychologists and psychoanalysts, the constraints of modern life, and the fact that many mothers now work outside the home have done the rest. Babies often must get through the night on their own before the age of three months. This demand may contribute to the ever-increasing numbers of children who have sleep disorders.

Still, after apparently expending their stores of patience to get their children to bed, how many parents return on tiptoe to contemplate their sleeping offspring proudly? And what parent, no matter how sleep deprived, is not gratified to see the baby open her eyes in the morning and smile?

Des Essarts, in 1760, advised mothers how to wake up their babies: "First they should gently shake their bed, then rub and caress their small hands in order to arouse a tickling sensation, a mild titillation that prepares them for merriment; and if their mothers show them a smiling face when they open their eyes, they will not lack for a smile themselves."

Understanding

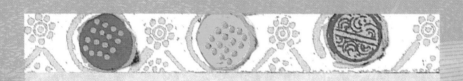

The *twentieth century is the century of the baby;*
observed, analyzed, and psychoanalyzed,
babies are a focus of doctors, psychologists,
and scientists; of manufacturers and advertisers; and, finally, of their parents, who
have structured their material and emotional
world around their cherished offspring.
Nonetheless, neither this century nor the
last has an exclusive claim to affection for
the little ones.

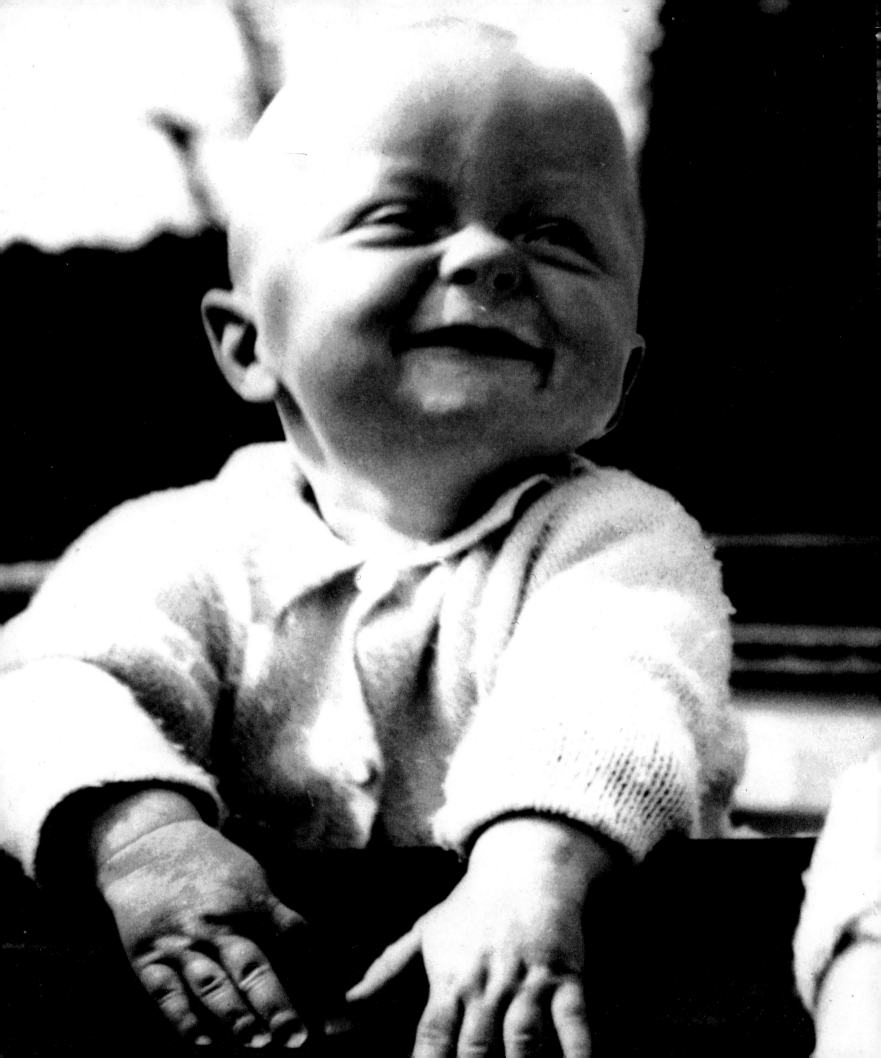

intended for all, the importance of this communication between baby and parents from the moment of birth.

Paralleling the psychoanalytic work, a field of research has developed around the study of child behavior. The use of tape recorders, cameras, and then computers has brought researchers a giant step forward in the observation of babies. The American Arnold Gesell, a pioneer in the study of child psychology, has investigated the neuropsychological maturation of the infant. To carry out his research, he adopted completely new experimental techniques, employing one-way mirrors and reworking tests of motor function, language, adaptation, and reactions to make them applicable to the very young. He uses the camera to refine the precision of his observations. The American professor T. Berry Brazelton, pediatrician and neonatologist, has earned a worldwide reputation. He examined babies' behavior by using a rattle, a box of rice, and a red ball. Spurred on by a real passion for infants, he was the first to bring to light a baby's extraordinary abilities.

"For years, early childhood had been like the hidden face of the moon. We had few means at our disposal with which to discover what was going on in the minds of babies. While extremely charming, they are not particularly inclined to collaborate with psychologists," wrote one expert. In order to study infants and gain an understanding of what was happening inside their small, preverbal heads, scientists have gone in unexpected directions, such as connecting an artificial nipple to a computer and measuring the frequency of babies' sucking in response to various stimuli. The rate of sucking is analyzed and interpreted carefully in order to learn more about these little guinea pigs.

For some decades now, babies have been at the heart of a bidding war; psychologists, educators, and advertisers are fighting over these small beings who, it turns out, are so gifted. In the face of this recognition of infants' consciousness and their developmental needs, parents feel ever more challenged to actively engage all the senses of their tiniest babies. In fact, they now shoulder the responsibility of rising to the level of these uncommon infants in a world filled with new stresses and challenges. A pinch of common sense and lots of love are no longer enough. Will exhausted mothers and fathers now turn increasingly to books of advice that, with a sense of humor, tell them how *not* to be perfect parents?

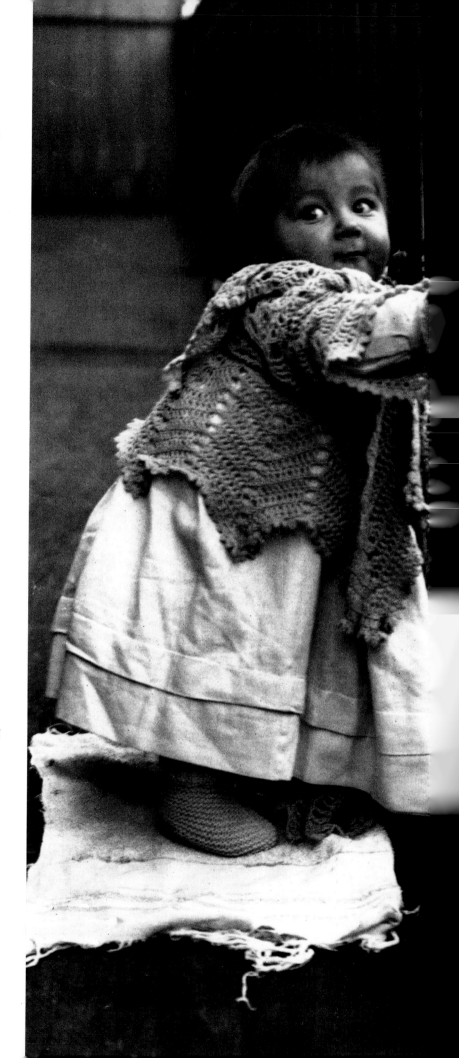

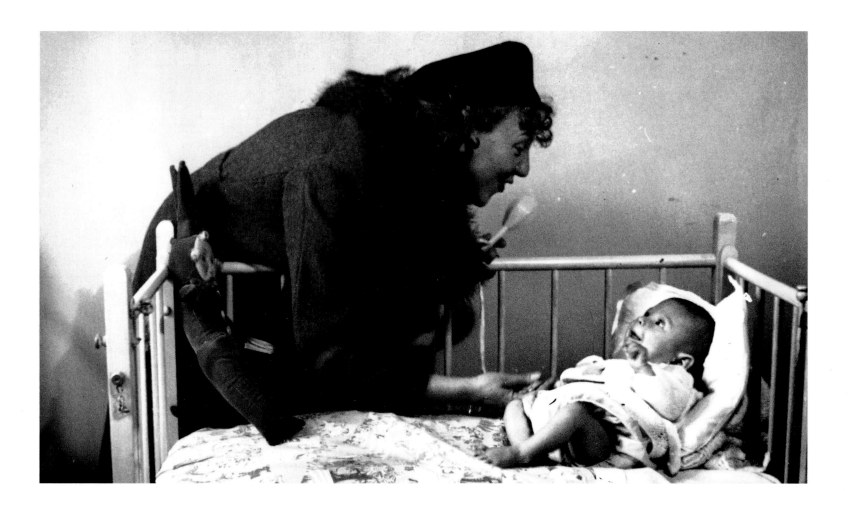

In 1972 Donald Winnicott wrote that a baby pays close attention to her mother in her first days, focusing on her style of care as well as the shape of her breast, the curve of her ear, the nature of her smile, and the smell of her breath.

ABOVE: Photograph

OPPOSITE: Photograph

OVERLEAF: Photograph

"The history of civilization has a gap. At the first stage of life, there is a blank page on which no one has yet written, because no one has investigated the first needs of humans," wrote an educator in 1936. While psychologists had begun to be interested in children, they did not lean over the infant's cradle for a very long time. Sigmund Freud, the father of psychoanalysis, analyzed the first stages of the child's development: during her first months, the baby primarily experiences oral gratification—she enters into contact with the world through the mouth. In 1947, René Spitz, an American doctor and psychoanalyst, reported that babies in orphanages who lacked nothing materially but everything emotionally became physically ill and listless—an unprecedented discovery. Melanie Klein, a British psychoanalyst and pioneer in the field of child psychology, hypothesized the existence of fantasies from birth; the baby is immediately capable of feeling anguish, of being subject to a life or death drive. English pediatrician and psychoanalyst Donald Winnicott placed supreme importance on the quality of the baby's physical contact and the regularity of the mother's care, which must be, according to his felicitous expression, good enough. French psychoanalyst Françoise Dolto emphasized, in clear language

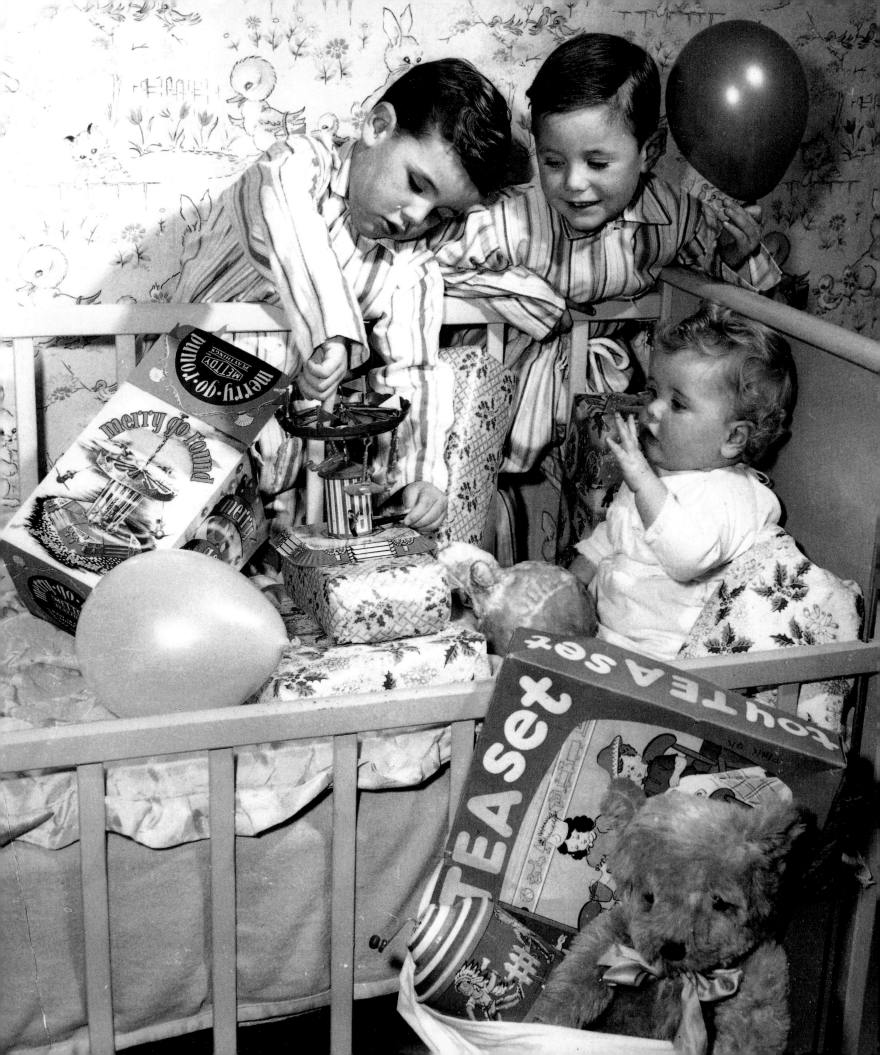

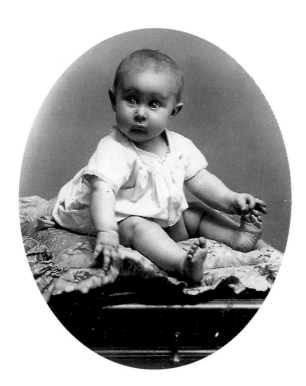

At home with their own children, researchers can often devote themselves to the kind of observation of infants that leads to new knowledge. In the nineteenth century, Charles Darwin studied his son's behavior day after day. At the end of the same century, French psychologist Alfred Binet created a new method of intelligence testing after observing his daughters.

ABOVE: Photograph. 20th century

OPPOSITE: Photograph. 1937

The Trial of the Pacifier

"The pacifier is the despair of the children's doctor. So often she sees the baby suck on it for hours without a break, ruining the shape of her jaw by this constant sucking, so often she sees the pacifier rolling on the floor or going into the mouth of an adult before it finds its way back to the child. If the mother who is responsible for this frightful dirtiness knew how filthy the floor was, how many particles of food, of germs, of unhealthy secretions from cavities, etc., her mouth harbored, she would be horrified," wrote the woman doctor Champendal in 1928. This small, inoffensive-appearing object has inspired controversies not only among authors of books on child care and doctors but also among politicians. In 1910, the French Assembly even passed a law forbidding the manufacture and sale of rubber pacifiers. Yet this item had already—and beneficially—replaced the makeshift pacifiers that wet nurses had always made for their charges from a bit of stale bread wrapped in a rag. The pacifier has ceased to be considered a harmful accessory used exclusively by the lower classes and has become instead a "transitional object," recognized as useful by many psychologists, that satisfies a natural need to suck. The same is true of the thumb; for a long time, parents tried to dissuade babies from forming the bad habit of sucking their thumbs by painting them with a bitter substance, such as aloe or mustard. Other methods consisted of placing small gloves on their hands, sliding their arms in cardboard tubes so they could not bend them, or even tying their arms to the cradle.

Hidden Talents

Discoveries about the workings of babies' minds and bodies have abounded in the twentieth century, especially since the 1960s. They make clear the early capacities of babies in the realms of all the different senses: sight, hearing, touch, taste, smell— a long way from the perception of the deaf, blind, and unconscious newborn. For years, it was believed that babies could not see at birth. It has since been established that, while their visual field is less extensive and their visual acuity is less than those of the adult, babies see from birth and after a few weeks can distinguish colors. Their sense of touch is highly developed; babies touch with their mouths, their hands, in fact, their entire bodies. Far from being deaf, newborn babies already are accustomed to hearing numerous sounds, which they have heard in muffled form in their mothers' womb, and they already display a preference for certain ones. Like adults, they can distinguish among flavors that are bitter and acidic, salty, and sweet, and they show a predilection for the last. They smell odors perfectly well and prefer those that are sugary, fruity, and milky; above all, they respond to the odor of their mothers. In the nineteenth century, Charles Darwin observed that his one-month-old son could recognize his mother's breast by its smell.

Laws for Babies

In the nineteenth century, Western society gave a new worth to the baby. The creation of day nurseries, the "Drops of Milk," and the associations for the protection of childhood made it possible for infants to take full advantage of the advances in medicine (especially vaccines) and hygiene (especially sterilization). At the end of the nineteenth century, these advances had effected a significant decline in the infant mortality rate. The beginning of legal protection was also established internationally. In 1875, New York became the first state to institute child protection laws, with other states soon following. The French Roussel Act (1874) stated: "Every child under two years of age who is placed with a salaried wet nurse, to be weaned, or to be watched outside the home of his parents, by this act becomes subject to the care of the public authority with the goal of protecting his life and health."

In England, the word *baby* began to be used exclusively to refer to infants in the nineteenth century; before this, only the word *nursling* had designated the child in his first year, and *baby* referred to children of all ages, especially schoolchildren.

Books offering parenting advice flourished throughout the nineteenth and twentieth centuries. Until then, such books were written for doctors, midwives, or the elite of society. Now they are intended for all parents, even though many cannot afford to buy them or are unwilling or unable to read them. Previously, these books of advice could be extremely rigid: "The cry is an indispensable pulmonary exercise after birth. Let [the baby] calm herself all alone and in the following days, and do not let the baby's cries keep you from setting the hours for her meals to suit you! Let her cry. You must refrain from rocking her, talking to her, taking her in your arms, and, above all, feeding her." And again: "One cannot begin teaching good habits to children too early. Therefore, from the earliest days of your children's existence, be firm, for their happiness, rest assured, as well as yours." At times, this rigidity gave way to affectionate care: "In order to develop as she should, a child needs to be lively and, especially, loved" and "Every day the child seeks to become familiar with everything that surrounds him, giving him a store of accumulated impressions. Study, young mothers, this countenance coming to awareness, guess the thoughts it contains, search closely what is hidden deeply within his nascent soul. Whether a natural cry or a spontaneous cry, do not disregard this language of infancy; the cry of the infant, however fleeting and varied, reveals real and deep feelings beneath his different states of suffering or contentment."

For three or four decades, first-time parents have had at their disposal a great number of more practical, less moralizing books, including those by the famous Dr. Spock.

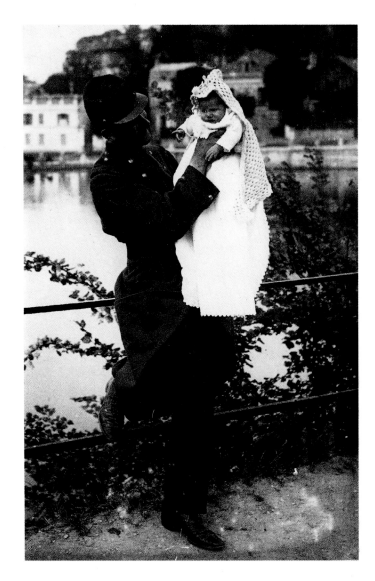

After devastating wars, population decline always concerned the authorities, who would then launch extensive campaigns against infant mortality.

ABOVE: Photograph. 1901

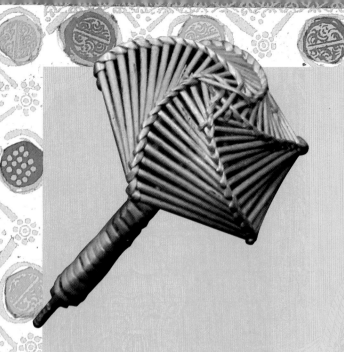

"The Little King and His Scepter with Bells"

Since antiquity, the making of toys, especially rattles, intended to divert the infant testifies to the attention given babies from their first months. The crepitaculum *(from the verb* crepare, *to make noise)*, or rattle, most often made of terra-cotta, was also a protective object, thought to drive away evil spirits. The only medieval rattles that have come down to us are made of gold or silver, from aristocratic circles. It is not known whether the babies of poor peasants had any diversions other than a hunk of bread, a stick of licorice, or their mother's breast, given on demand. In the seventeenth and eighteenth centuries, silver rattles, which encased pieces of coral, were often decorated with a row of small hand bells—making them simultaneously musical toys, protective amulets, and teething accessories. These rattles were often given to the baby at baptism.

In every period, authors have dreamed of toys that stimulate and educate, and there were supporters of early childhood education centuries ago. In antiquity, Quintilian wished that wet nurses who were able to learn the alphabet by means of ivory letters would begin teaching their charges from the cradle. In the eighteenth century, an author recommended that "in place of the toys called rattles, infants be given the different letters of the alphabet made of ivory or another material, and gradually they would become familiar with and get to know the shapes; these would be joined successively with several more to form syllables and words; I believe that by this method they would learn to read as soon as they learned to talk." In the twentieth century, babies' toys have become very varied. Germans and Americans share the responsibility for the plush bear: the famous teddy bear was being manufactured in Germany by Steiff at the beginning of the century. In the 1950s, rubber toys for babies abounded; easy to clean, they could be placed in the mouth without risk. Since then, plastics have made it easy to vary the design of rattles.

"Bells made of silver, gold, coral, faceted crystals, rattles of every price and every variety: what useless and pernicious affectations! Nothing of the kind. No more bells, no more rattles; small branches of trees with their fruits and leaves, a poppy head in which the seeds can be heard, a stick of licorice that they can suck on and chew will amuse them more than these magnificent trinkets."

Jean-Jacques Rousseau

ABOVE LEFT: Wicker rattle. 19th century. Musée des Arts et Traditions Populaires, Paris

ABOVE RIGHT: Rattle belonging to the king of Rome. 19th century. Musée Carnavalet, Paris

The Feelings of Infants

What was known of infants' perceptions, of their needs for contact and communication in centuries past? In the sixteenth century, Simon de Vallambert took into account the psychological and emotional needs of the infant as well as the stimulation of her senses. "In all things the important point is to start well. This means that over the course of our life it must follow that, if our early age went well, all the other ages will go well to the very end. It thus becomes a matter of great consequence to know how to take care of a newly born child, by smiling, singing him songs, taking him on your lap, taking hold of him under the arms, supporting him in your arms, making him dance and leap, and cuddling him. The wet nurse would do well to offer a lovely bouquet of flowers, hold it to her nose and then to the baby's nose. The infant should be stimulated and learn to tell hot from cold, bitter from sweet, things that are good for him, and things that are bad. The nurse should make it possible for him to see many things, and when the time comes, and the weather is good, he should be taken outside and entertained by looking at the sun, the sunlight, the flowers of the lush meadows, the trees with their leaves, and the colors, and he should be diverted by hearing sweet voices, temperate sounds such as that of a lyre, a spinet, a violin."

Vandermonde, a doctor of the eighteenth century, considered the newborn a "vegetating substance," although he conceded that a few months after birth all children are susceptible to love and hate, joy and sadness: "One cannot take enough pains to make them joyful and remove from them all the causes of unhappiness. Joy opens the blood vessels, sets the mind in motion, enhances nutrition. Unhappiness, on the other hand, produces a constriction throughout the body, the blood vessels contract in diameter, the liquids circulate more slowly." During the same period, Rousseau asserted in *L'Emile*, "We are born with the capacity to learn.... Human education begins at birth; before she speaks, before she understands, she is already teaching herself.... She wants to touch everything, hold everything: in no way should you try to counter this restlessness; it indicates in her a very necessary period of learning. It is only through movement that we learn that there are things that are not us.... We have long sought to ascertain if there is a natural universal language for all humans; undoubtedly, it exists, and it is that language that infants speak before they learn how to talk. This language is not articulated, but it is stressed, voiced, intelligible."

"I rarely left him and I strove to leave the mark of my soul in his."

Honoré de Balzac, Les mémoires de deux jeunes mariées *(The Memoirs of Two Young Wives), 1840*

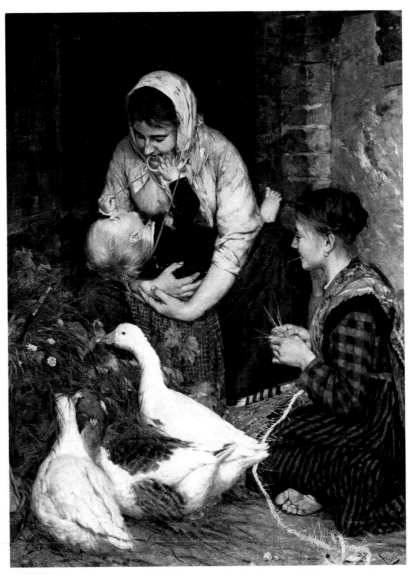

ABOVE: Giannicci Niccolo (1846–1906). *Maternal Joy.* Gallery of Modern Art, Florence

these books. When the Dutch poet Vondel lost his one-year-old son, he wrote a poem in which, speaking in the voice of the dead child, he betrayed his emotional response as well as the immense distress of his wife:

Mother, why this flood of tears
Why do you grieve so on my bier
I live on high, I fly in the air
Little angel above the skies.

In the seventeenth century, theologians and moralists highly disapproved of parents when they were indifferent to their children, but they also criticized them for being lax, easy-going, and far too indulgent. They denounced "dotingness," a tender and amused attitude toward babies, as harmful, approaching that of the animals. They also found too-frequent kissing and hugging revolting. At the end of the sixteenth century, Montaigne exclaimed, "I cannot harbor that passion that makes others kiss barely born children, having neither movement nor soul, nor even a recognizable shape of the body that could make them lovable, and I have not willingly suffered having them near me."

In the eighteenth century, one baby in four died before his first birthday. Some historians see the high infant mortality rate as an explanation for the apparent indifference of parents toward their babies—they did not want to become attached to a child who was at such high risk of dying, and they did not begin to love her until she had passed the danger point of the first or first few years. According to historians, parental love arose in different periods. Philippe Ariès believed the feeling made a hesitant appearance at the end of the sixteenth century and in the seventeenth century. American historian Edward Shorter thought that "among the ordinary people" maternal love did not fully develop until the nineteenth century: "Good mothering is an invention of modernization. In traditional society, mothers viewed the development and happiness of infants younger than two .with indifference. In modern society,

"As soon as you're hungry,
as soon as you cry
I was always ready to come
to your aid.
Summer as winter,
these seasons so bad,
Though icy with cold
or covered with sweat
I bent my breast toward
your ravenous mouth;
To go back to bed,
I'd wait till you slept.
Even when you were stuck
in your muck
Or were covered
with blisters and crust,
I never gave in to disgust
and always my tenderness
Carried me high
above and beyond my delicacy."
Napian, 1781

they place the welfare of their small children above all else." Shorter claims that seventeenth- and eighteenth-century mothers did not pass "the 'sacrifice' test": the life and happiness of their infant did not come first.

While the practices and attitudes of parents have changed since then, there is no justification for challenging the genuineness of their affection in any given period. No document, revealing as it may be, can fathom the feelings of an entire population. Few people had the education to know how to formulate their feelings toward their babies, and their behavior was guided by the culture of their society of the time. Is it possible to write a history of feelings, especially feelings as subtle and intimate as those experienced by parents toward their babies? Jacques Gélis, a historian of birth, rightly concludes, "Do not confuse maternal love, a constant sentiment, and its expression, variable through the course of centuries."

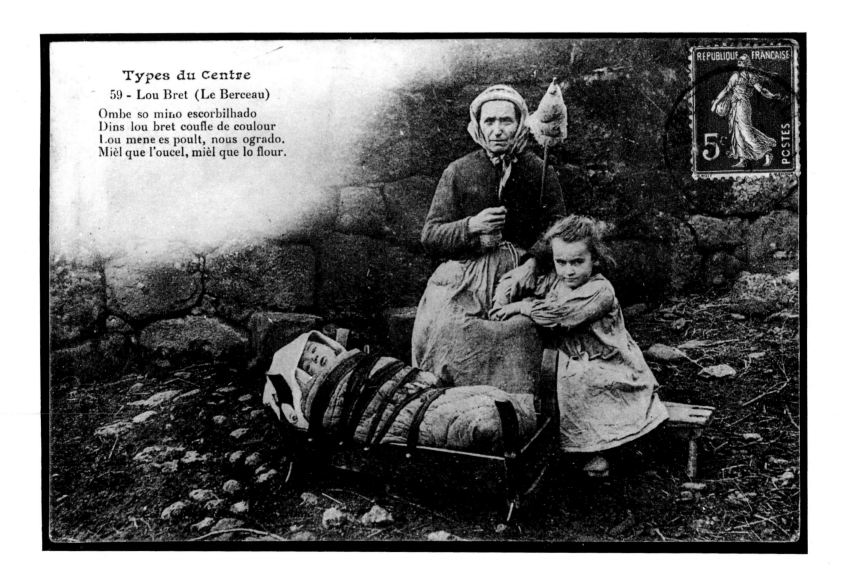

"If mothers tied their children head to feet so that they couldn't respond to tickling, clucking, and cajoling, it must mean the mothers had little interest in such things in the first place."
Edward Shorter, The Making of the Modern Family, *1975*

ABOVE: Rubber nipple. Musée de l'Assistance Publique, Paris

BELOW: Postcard. 20th century

Types du Centre

59 - Lou Bret (Le Berceau)

Ombe so mino escorbilhado
Dins lou bret coufle de coulour
Lou mene es poult, nous ogrado.
Mièl que l'oucel, mièl que lo flour.

gesture of protection—for the adult as well as for the infant—when paired with caresses it also indicated the mother's tenderness. Medieval miniatures and literary texts conveyed the image of loving and attentive mothers.

But what of the fathers? They, apparently, were often put out by infants' bawling and dirty swaddling clothes. In the twelfth century, the abbess Heloise asked the teacher and philosopher Abelard, who stubbornly persisted in wanting to marry her, "Is there a man who, given to meditations on Letters and Philosophy, can bear the wails of the newborn, the songs of the wet nurse who consoles her, the unending dirtiness of very young children?" "Infants consist only of cries, dirtiness, boredom, and anxiety," we read in Eustache Deschamps's *Le miroir du mariage* (The Mirror of Marriage). Yet, while the mother occupied herself with seeing to all the baby's needs, the father could play tenderly with him, entertain him with a rattle, or even feed him his pap.

"In medieval society, which we are taking as our point of departure, a feeling for childhood did not exist…. This does not mean that children were neglected, abandoned, or mistreated. A feeling for childhood was not the same as affection for children; it corresponds to an awareness of the particularity of childhood, that particularity that distinguishes the child from the adult…. The baby's games must have always seemed engaging to mothers, wet nurses, and 'rockers,' but this belongs to the vast domain of unexpressed feelings." Many historians have followed the same train of thought as Philippe Ariès, a twentieth-century pioneer researcher in the history of children. Some have gone so far as to assert, sometimes rather gruffly, that there was a total indifference to children during this period.

In *L'enfant à l'ombre des cathédrales* (The Child in the Shadow of the Cathedrals), Danièle Alexandre-Bidon and Monique Closson came to the opposite conclusion. They feel that a tender affection linked parents to their young ones. Childhood in the Middle Ages was brief, as the child quickly moved on to adulthood. The "miniature adult" did not enjoy the same role or place in society as she does today, but certain accounts, like one reported by Emmanuel Le Roy Ladurie in *Montaillou, village occitan* (Montaillou, Village of Occitania), testify to genuine feeling for the baby. The wife of a lord in the fourteenth century, before leaving to join the heretics, wanted to see and embrace her baby one last time: "Then the baby started to laugh; as she had begun to leave the room where the baby had been sleeping, she went back toward him; the baby began to laugh again; and this went on repeatedly, until finally she could not bring herself to leave the baby. Seeing this, she told the servant, Take him outside."

Some early artists captured the poses characteristic of very young children.

RIGHT: Prints. 15th century, Germany

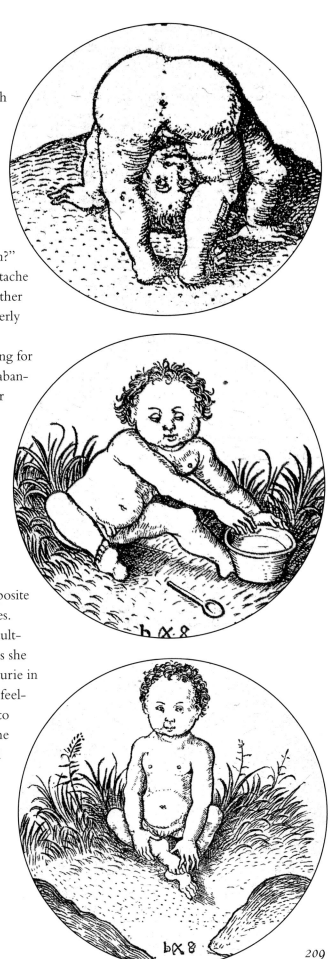

209

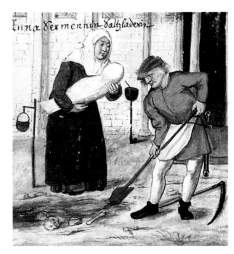

ABOVE: Miniature. 16th century, Germany. Bibliothèque Nationale, Paris

OPPOSITE: Print. 18th century. Bibliothèque Nationale, Paris

BELOW: J. G. Meyer (1813–1886). *The Three Sisters.* Joseph Mensing Hamm Gallery

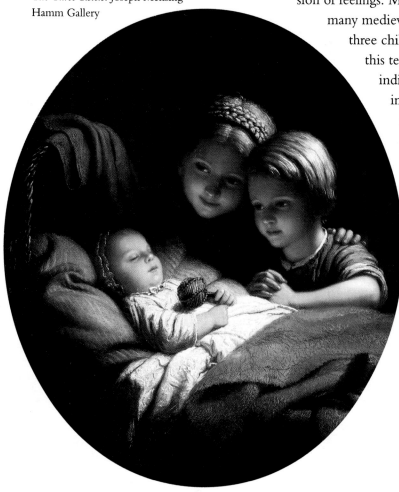

"Angels for Paradise"

"Corrupted at my mother's breast, I was conceived in sin," wrote Saint Augustine in the fourth century. Not all medieval authors shared this idea, and many in fact glorified the baby's purity and innocence, in which form the infant Jesus was incarnated. Religion during the Middle Ages reflected this double aspect of the baby, at once sinful and innocent. Profoundly pious, medieval society placed enormous weight on baptism, which saved those who died very young from wandering eternally in the mysterious world of limbo and assured them a place in paradise. The concern to save babies' souls reached its peak in the seventeenth century. The Calvinists among the Protestants and the Jansenists among the Catholics stressed babies' impurity from birth, while other authors saw the child as a precious creation of God that should be respected as such. Among men of the Church, the most outrageous assertions can surely be laid to the cardinal of Bérulle, who qualified childhood as "the vilest and most abject [state] in human nature after that of death."

The comfort of knowing their baptized baby would go to heaven undoubtedly eased the pain of parents in mourning, especially when all they had to offer their offspring on earth was a miserable existence. Religious faith influenced the expression of feelings. Mothers of today, however, find it hard to understand how so many medieval parents failed to attend their babies' funerals. "I lost two or three children to the wet nurse, not without regret but without anger": this testimony of Montaigne has often been interpreted as a proof of indifference. However, numerous *livres de raisons*, a kind of diary in which a family's material existence and major events were recorded, took a more intimate tone starting in the seventeenth century, and the child played the most important role in them. Some described dead children in the most minute detail. Although it remained constrained by their submission to the dictates of providence, parents' grief showed itself fully in

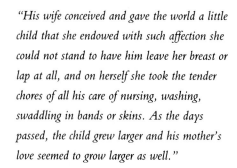

"His wife conceived and gave the world a little child that she endowed with such affection she could not stand to have him leave her breast or lap at all, and on herself she took the tender chores of all his care of nursing, washing, swaddling in bands or skins. As the days passed, the child grew larger and his mother's love seemed to grow larger as well."

Geoffroy d'Auxerre,
twelfth century

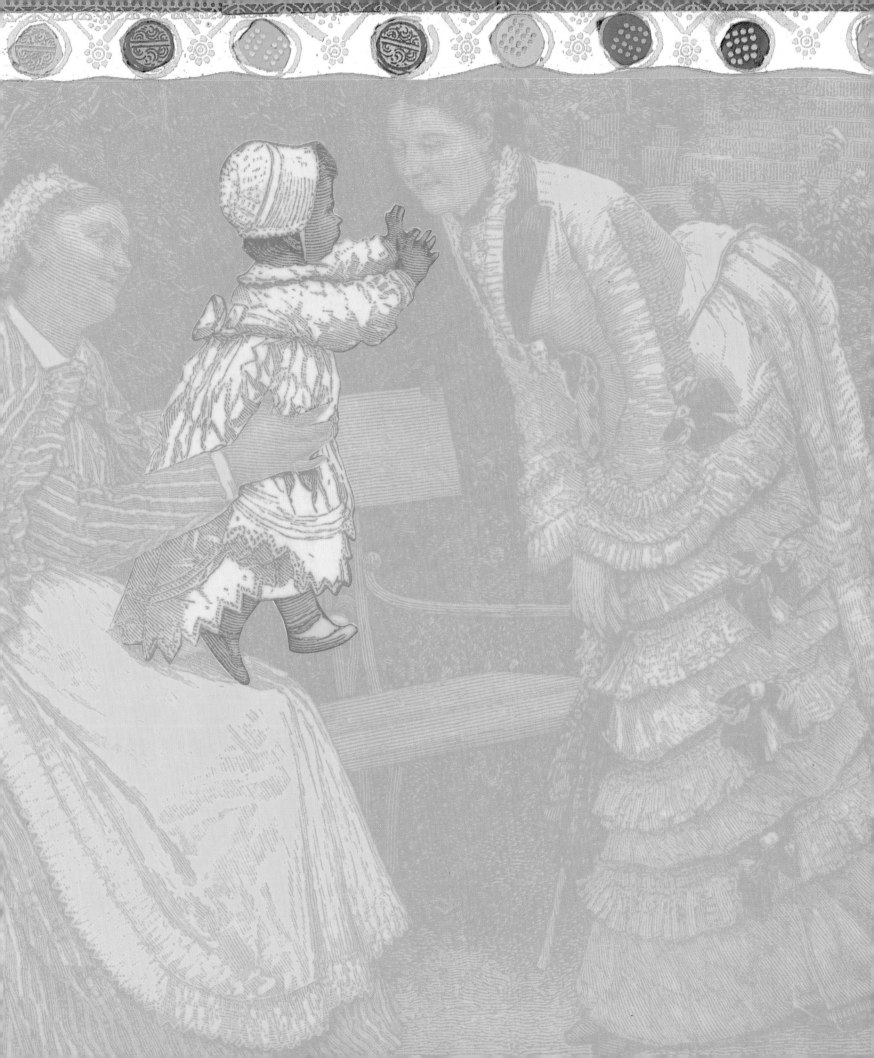

"The Baby Is a Person"

BELOW: Family tree. 15th century.
Illumination. Bibliothèque
Nationale, Paris

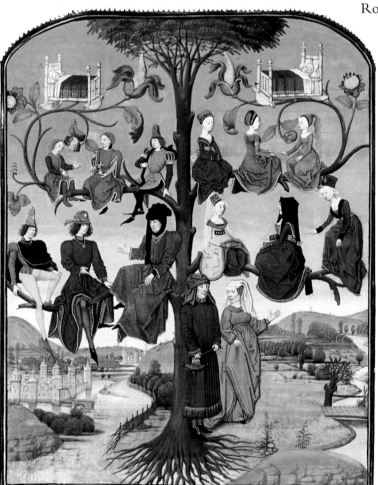

In *classical Rome,* until the end of the fourth century, fathers had the right to choose life or death for their babies. Killing and abandoning babies were ordinary and perfectly legal actions. Roman mothers who could afford to do so eagerly handed their babies over to wet nurses for nursing. The numerous ways in which parents and Roman society carried out their responsibilities seem to indicate a certain lack of feeling toward babies. Yet how do we account for the wrenching epitaphs engraved on the tombstones of very young children that bitterly lament their demise and describe their age and traits in minute detail? The interest aroused by newborns also appears through the pens of authors in antiquity. Soranus of Ephesus provided extremely detailed instructions on how to care for infants, emphasizing that it was important to be gentle in one's gestures toward them, to communicate with them, and to quiet their tears "with a few twittering noises, babbling, and gentle words."

Medieval Coaxing

> For they must be swaddled up
> And tenderly enveloped
> Rocked and cleaned and offered joys,
> Carried, sung to, given toys
> And sent flying white streamers
> And covered with soft furs,

declaimed the poet Eustache Deschamps in the fourteenth century. These daily acts and the numerous rituals meant to protect and care for babies bear witness to a true solicitude for them. Mothers placed their crying infants on their bosoms to comfort and console them, night and day. They took them in their arms and hugged and kissed them. While the medieval kiss was a ritual

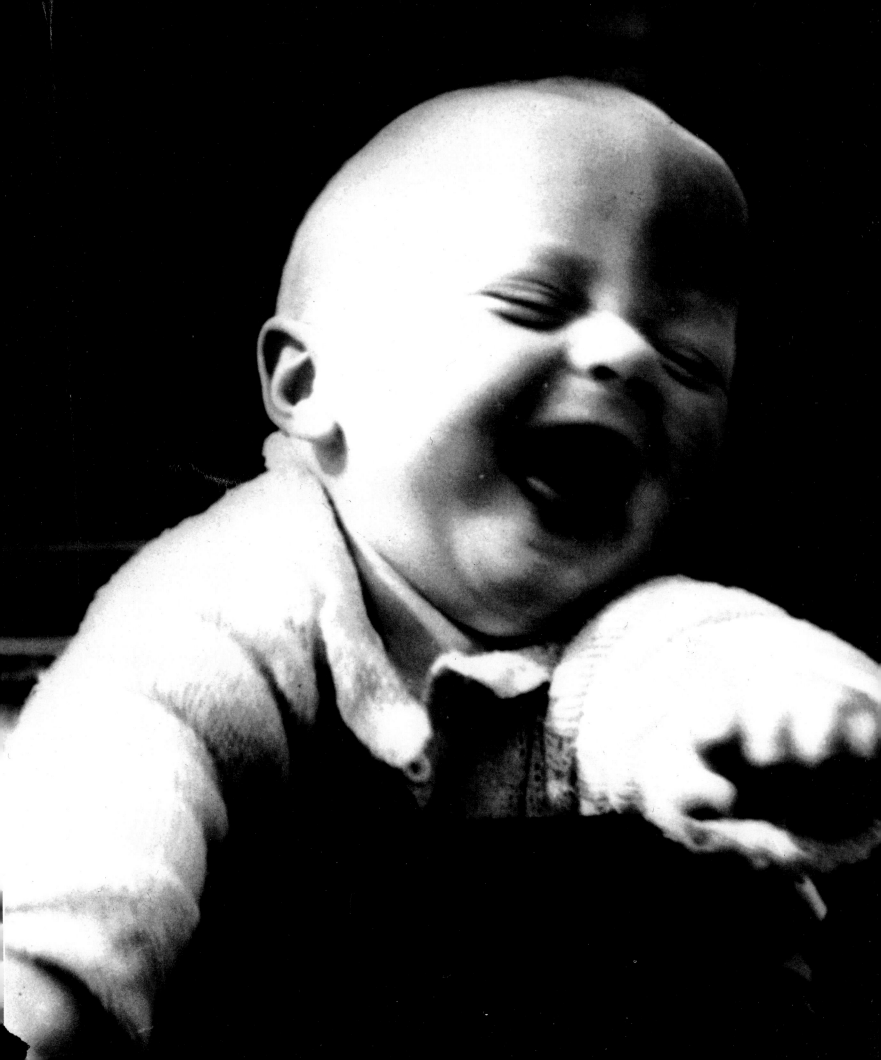

Bibliography

Abt, Arthur. *Abt-Garrison History of Pediatrics.* Philadelphia and London: W. B. Saunders, 1965.

Alexandre-Bidon, Danièle, and Monique Closson. *L'enfant à l'ombre des cathédrales.* Lyons: Editions du CNRS, Presses Universitaires de Lyon, 1985.

Ansley Worrell, Estelle. *Children's Costume in America, 1607–1910.* New York: Scribner, 1980.

Ariès, Philippe. *L'enfant et la vie familiale sous l'Ancien Régime.* Paris: Seuil, 1973; *Centuries of Childhood.* New York: Alfred A. Knopf, 1962.

Ariès, Philippe, and Georges Duby, eds. *Histoire de la vie privée.* Paris: Seuil, 1985; *A History of Private Life.* 5 vols. Cambridge, Mass.: Belknap Press of Harvard University, 1987–91.

Auvard, A. *Le Nouveau-Né.* Paris: A. Delahaye, 1888.

Auvard, A., and Pingat. *Hygiène infantile, ancienne et moderne.* Paris: Rongier, 1889.

Badinter, Elisabeth. *L'amour en plus.* Paris: Champs Flammarion, 1980; *Mother Love: Myth and Reality.* New York: Macmillan, 1981.

Ballexserd, Jacques. *Dissertation sur l'éducation physique des enfants.* Paris: Chez Vallat-La-Chapelle, 1762.

Barbaut, J. *Histoires de la naissance.* Paris: Calmann-Lévy, 1990.

Bartholomaeus Anglicus. *De proprietatus rerum.* Paris, 1480; *Le propriétaire de toutes choses.* Paris: A. Verard, 1878; *On the Property of Things.* 3 vols. Oxford: Clarendon Press, 1975–88.

Baudelocque, J.-B. *L'art des accouchements.* Paris: Méquignon l'aîné, 1815; *An Abridgement of Mr. Heath's Translation of Baudelocque's Midwifery.* Philadelphia: Desilver, 1823.

Baudoin, M. *Les appareils populaires destinés à apprendre à marcher.* Paris, 1911.

Billard, C. *Traité des maladies des enfants.* Paris: Ballière, 1828; *A Treatise on the Diseases of Infants.* New York: Langley, 1840.

Bouchut, Eugène. *Hygiène de la première enfance.* Paris: Ballière, 1885.

Bourgeois, Louise. *Observations diverses sur la stérilité, perte du fruits, fécondité et accouchements,* followed by *Instructions à sa fille.* 1609.

Brochard, André-Théodore. *Almanach illustré de la jeune mère.* 1875.

Budin, Pierre. *Le nourrisson, alimentation et hygiène.* Paris: Doin, 1900; *The Nursling; the Feed and Hygiene of Premature and Full-Term Infants.* New York: Imperial, 1906.

———. *De la puériculture après la naissance.* Paris: Doin, 1900.

Burguière, André, et al., eds. *Histoire de la famille.* Paris: Armand Colin, 1986; *A History of the Family.* Cambridge: Polity Press, 1996.

Cabanes, Dr. Augustin. *Moeurs intimes du passé.* Vols. 6 and 7. Paris: Albin Michel, 1908–9.

Cadogan, William. *An Essay upon Nursing, and the Management of Children.* London, 1749.

Caron, A.-C. *Le code des jeunes mères, traité théoretique et pratique pour l'éducation physique des nouveau-nés.* Paris, 1859.

———. *La puériculture.* Rouen: Orville, 1866.

Champendal, Dr. *Le petit manuel des mères.* Paris, 1928.

Coudray, Angélique du. *Abrégé de l'art des accouchements.* Châlons-sur-Marne: Bouchard, 1773.

Coulon, Gérard. *L'enfant en Gaule romaine.* Paris: Errance, 1994.

Coulon-Arpin, M. *La maternité et les sages-femmes, de la préhistoire au XXe siècle.* Vols. 1 and 2. Paris: Roger Dacosta, 1981.

Cunnington, Phillis, and Anne Bloch. *Children's Costume in England.* New York: Barnes and Noble, 1965.

Darmon, Pierre. *Le mythe de la procréation à l'âge baroque.* Paris: Seuil, 1981.

Debré, Robert. *L'honneur de vivre.* Paris: Stock Hermann, 1974.

Delahaye, M.-C. *Tétons et tétines: Histoire de l'allaitement.* Paris: Trame Way, 1990.

Delaisi de Parseval, Geneviève, and Suzanne Lallemand. *L'art d'accommoder les bébés: cent ans de puériculture française.* Paris: Seuil, 1980.

de Mause, Lloyd, ed. *The History of Childhood: The Untold Story of Child Abuse.* New York: The Psychohistory Press, 1974; New York: Peter Bedrick Books, 1988.

Demirleau, Dr. *Manuel de catéchisme de puériculture pratique et moderne.* 1920.

Desclais Berkvam, Doris. *Enfance et maternité dans la littérature française.* Paris: Honoré Champion, 1981.

des Essarts, J.-C. *Traité de l'éducation corporelle des enfants en bas âge.* Paris: Hérissant, 1760.

Devraigne, Louis. *La puériculture: son histoire, son domaine.* Paris: Les Publications Sociales Agricoles, 1943.

Fay-Sallois, Fanny. *Les nourrices à Paris au XIXe siècle.* Paris: Payot, 1980.

Fildes, Valerie. *Breasts, Bottles, and Babies: A History of Infant Feeding.* Edinburgh: Edinburgh University Press, 1986.

———. *Wet Nursing: A History from Antiquity to the Present.* Oxford: B. Blackwell, 1988.

Firmin-Marbeau, Jean-Baptiste. *Des crèches pour les petits enfants des ouvrières.* Paris: Amyot, Guillaumin et Le Clère, 1863.

———. *Manuel de la crèche.* Paris: J. Tardieu, 1867.

Flandrin, Jean-Louis. *Familles.* Paris: Seuil, 1984; *Families in Former Times.* Cambridge: Cambridge University Press, 1979.

———. *Le sexe et l'Occident.* Paris: Point Histoire Seuil, 1986.

Foisil, Madeleine. *L'enfance de Louis XIII.* Paris: Perrin, 1996.

Fonssagrives, Jean Baptiste. *Le rôle des mères dans les maladies des enfants.* Paris, 1870.

Frank, J. P. *Traité sur la manière d'élever sainement les enfants.* Paris, 1799.

Franklin, A. *La vie privée d'autrefois: L'enfant, la layette, la nourrice, la vie de famille.* Vols. 17 and 19. Paris, 1896.

Galtier-Boissière, Dr. Emile. *Pour élever les nourrissons.* Paris: Larousse, 1907.

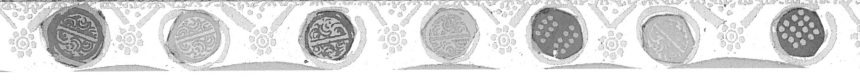

Gélis, Jacques. *L'arbre et le fruit: La naissance dans l'Occident moderne.* Paris: Fayard, 1984; *History of Childbirth.* Cambridge: Polity Press, 1991.

———. *La sage-femme ou le médecin: Une nouvelle conception de la vie.* Paris: Fayard, 1988.

Gélis, Jacques, Mireille Laget, and Marie-France Morel. *Entrer dans la vie: Naissances et enfances dans la France traditionnelle.* Paris: Coll. "Archives" Gallimard/Julliard, 1978.

Golden, Mark. *Children and Childhood in Classical Athens.* Baltimore: Johns Hopkins University Press, 1990.

Guillemeau, Jacques. *De la nourriture et du gouvernement des enfants.* Paris: Buon, 1585; *The Nursing of Children.* London, 1612.

Hanawalt, Barbara A. *Growing Up in Medieval London: The Experience of Childhood in History.* New York: Oxford University Press, 1993.

Hecquet, Philippe. *De l'indécence aux hommes d'accoucher les femmes.* Paris: Etienne, 1707; Paris: Cote-femmes, 1990.

Héroard, Jean. *Journal sur l'enfance de Louis XIII.* Paris: Soulié et Barthélemy, 1868; Paris: Fayard, 1989.

Hiner, N. Ray, and Joseph M. Hawes, eds. *Growing Up in America: Children in Historical Perspective.* Urbana: University of Illinois Press, 1985.

Icard, S. *L'alimentation du nouveau-né.* Paris: Alcan, 1894.

Joubert, Laurent. *Des erreurs populaires et propos vulgaires touchant la médecine.* Paris, 1587; *Popular errors.* Tuscaloosa: University of Alabama Press, 1989.

Kevill-Davies, Sally. *Yesterday's Children: The Antiques and History of Childcare.* Woodbridge, Suffolk, Eng.: Antique Collectors' Club, 1991.

Knibiehler, Yvonne, and Catherine Fouquet. *Histoire des mères du moyen age à nos jours.* Paris: Montalba, 1980.

Konner, Melvin. *Childhood.* Boston: Little, Brown, 1991.

Lacasse, Robert. *Hygiène de la grossesse, conseils pratiques aux jeunes mères.* Paris: Fourier, 1913.

Laget, Mireille. *Naissances: L'accouchement avant l'âge de la clinique.* Paris: Seuil, 1982.

Laurent, Sylvie. *Naître au moyen age.* Paris: Léopard d'or, 1989.

Le Conte Boudeville, Dr. A. *Auprès du berceau.* Paris: Delagrave, 1922.

Leroy, Alphonse. *Médecine maternelle ou l'art d'élever et de conserver les enfants.* Paris: Méquignon l'aîné, 1803.

Le Roy Ladurie, Emmanuel. *Montaillou, village occitan.* Paris: Gallimard, 1975; *Montaillou: The Promised Land of Error.* New York: Braziller, 1978.

Locke, John. *Some Thoughts Concerning Education.* London: Churchill, 1693; Oxford: Clarendon Press, 1989.

Loux, Françoise. *Le jeune enfant et son corps dans la médecine traditionnelle.* Paris: Flammarion, 1978.

Mauquest de La Motte, Guillaume. *Accoucheur de campagne sous le Roi-Soleil; Le traité des accouchements de G. Mauquest de La Motte,* edited by J. Gélis. Paris: Imago, 1989; *A General Treatise of Midwifery.* New York: Garland, 1985.

Mauriceau, François. *Traité des maladies des femmes grosses et de celles qui sont accouchées.* Paris, 1668; *The Diseases of Women with Child, and in Child-Bed.* New York: Garland, 1985.

Mercier, Louis-Sébastien. *Tableaux de Paris.* Paris, 1781; Paris: Laffont, 1990; *The Waiting City* (abridged). Philadelphia: Lippincott, 1933.

Millet-Robinet, Cora Elisabeth, and Dr. Emile Allix. *Le Livre des jeunes mères.* Paris: Librairie Agricole de la Maison Rustique, 1887.

Mitford, Jessica. *The American Way of Birth.* New York: Dutton, 1992.

Moll-Weiss, Augusta. *La femme, la mère, l'enfant.* Paris: Maloine, 1917.

Mozere, Liane. *Le printemps des crèches.* Paris: L'Harmattan, 1992.

Néraudau, Jean-Pierre. *Etre enfant à Rome.* Paris: Les Belles-Lettres, 1984.

Paré, Ambroise. *De la génération de l'homme et manière d'extraire les enfants du ventre de leur mère.* Paris, 1573; *Collected Works.* Pound Ridge, N.Y.: Milford House, 1968.

Pinard, A. *La puériculture du premier âge.* Paris: Armand Colin, 1931.

Pouliot, L. *Hygiène de maman et de bébé.* Paris: Nouvelle Librairie Nationale, 1921.

Prost de Royer, Antoine. *Mémoire sur la conservation des enfants.* Lyons, 1778.

Saucerotte, Nicolas. *Instructions concernant les femmes enceintes, celles qui sont accouchées et de la manière d'élever les petits enfants.* Strasbourg: Gay Libraires, 1777.

———. *De la conservation des enfants et de leur éducation depuis la naissance jusqu'à l'âge de six ans.* Paris: Guillaume, 1796.

Schorsch, Anita. *Childhood: An Illustrated Social History.* New York: Mayflower Books, 1979.

Shorter, Edward. *The Making of the Modern Family.* New York: Basic Books, 1975.

———. *A History of Women's Bodies.* New York: Basic Books, 1982.

Soranus of Ephesus. *Maladie des femmes.* Book 2. Paris: Les Belles-Lettres, 1990; *Soranus' Gynecology.* Baltimore: Johns Hopkins University Press, 1991.

Stork, Hélène. *Les rituels du coucher de l'enfant.* Paris: E.S.F., 1993.

Svévole de Sainte Marthe. *Paedotrophia ou la manière de nourrir les enfants à la mamelle.* Paris, 1698; *Paedotrophia; or the Art of Nursing and Rearing Children.* London, 1797.

Underwood, Michael. *A Treatise on the Diseases of Children.* Philadelphia, 1793.

Vallambert, Simon de. *Cinq livres sur la manière de nourrir et de gouverner les enfants dès leur naissance.* Lyons, 1541.

Vandermonde, Charles Augustin. *Essai sur la manière de perfectionner l'espèce humaine.* Paris, 1756.

Van Swieten, Gerard. *Traité des maladies des enfants.* Paris, 1759.

Variot, Gaston. *La puériculture pratique.* Paris: Doin, 1920.

Witkowski, Gustave Joseph. *Histoire des accouchements chez tous les peuples.* Paris: Steinheil, 1890.

———. *Accoucheurs et sages-femmes célèbres.* Paris: Steinheil, 1902.

Zglinicki, Friedrich von. *Die Wiege.* Regensburg: Pustet, 1979.

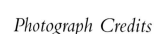

Photograph Credits

A.K.G.: 11b, 53a, 111, 124–25, 133, 145, 152a, 153, 155. Archive Photos: 7, 56. Assistance publique: 76, 78–79c, 97b, 108–09, 119, 130, 200, 210, 212a. Bibliothèque Nationale, Paris: 13, 27, 48–49, 66, 68, 71, 92, 93, 95, 97 (background), 100, 170, 171, 175, 190b, 199a, 206–07 (background), 208, 210a, 211. Bulloz: 39, 150, 194. J.-L. Charmet: 17, 18–19, 20b, 30, 38b, 44–45, 64, 69, 72–73, 77a, 82, 84, 87, 91, 102, 103b, 117, 153, 154, 156, 172. Dagli-Orti: 11a, 14b, 15, 26, 28, 29, 31, 91, 94, 103a, 146, 148, 149r, 151. Mary Evans: 37, 43, 57, 118b, 119, 154, 159, 182, 202l, 206, 214. Giraudon: 14a, 35, 42 (Bridgeman), 51, 106, 114–15, 136, 152 (Bridgeman), 78l, 79r, 198, 210b (Bridgeman), 214r. Hulton Deutsch: 157, 218. H. Josse: 101, 142, 157, 196–97, 204–05. Keystone: 23, 58–59, 86, 127, 160–61, 163, 164, 184a, 185, 186a, 217, 220–21. Kharbine Tapabor: 75, 121, 122, 148–49, 162a, 192, 202r, 203, 209, 212. Magnum: 40, 65, 85, 187. Rapho: 140, 143, 165. R.M.N.: 34, 36b, 38a, 47l, 57, 132, 152b, 174b, 176, 179, 190a, 199b, 214. Roger-Viollet: 10, 54 (Harlingue-Viollet), 60, 61, 69b, 81 (Boyer-Viollet), 83, 90, 116 (Harlingue-Viollet), 137 (Boyer-Viollet), 144–45 (background), 160, 178, 184b, 186b, 195, 201, 215, 219, 220. Scala: 32–33, 41, 70, 96, 98, 104–05, 107, 131, 134–35, 147, 166–67, 174a, 180–81, 191, 193, 213. Tallandier: 14 (background), 60. Endpapers: © Michel Tcherevkoff/The Image Bank.

Acknowledgments

Jacqueline de Bourgoing, Didier Busson, Luc Jacob-Duvernet, Laure Paoli, Dominique du Peloux, Antoine Sabbagh, Patrick Sergant, Jacques de Taisne, Philippe Tristan, Chantal Waltisperger, Daniel Wolfromm

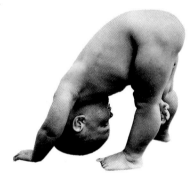

Project Coordinator, English-language edition: Ellen Cohen
Editor, English-language edition: Sharon AvRutick
Design Coordination, English-language edition: Dirk Luykx and Tina Thompson

Library of Congress Cataloging-in-Publication Data
Fontanel, Béatrice.
[Epopee des bébés, une histoire des petits d'hommes. English]
Babies: history, art, and folklore / Béatrice Fontanel and Claire d'Harcourt;
translated from the French by Lory Frankel.
p. cm.
Includes bibliographical references.
ISBN 0–8109–1244–9 (cloth)
1. Infants—Folklore. 2. Childbirth—Folklore. 3. Birth customs—History.
4. Infants—Care—History. I. D'Harcourt, Claire, 1960– . II. Title.
GR475.F65   1997
398'.354—dc20   96–43560

Printed and bound in Italy by Vincenzo Bona, Turin

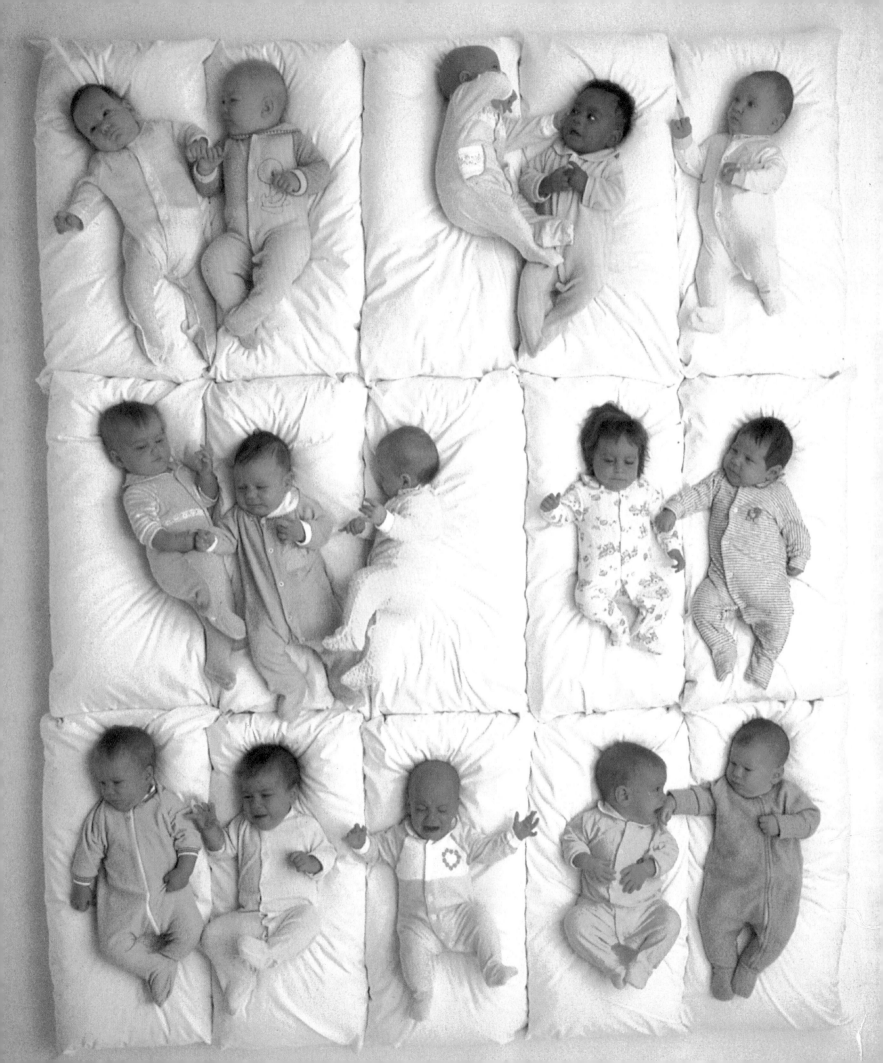